Learning Disabilities Sourcebook, 3rd Edition
Leukemia Sourcebook
Liver Disorders Sourcebook
Lung Disorders Sourcebook
Medical Tests Sourcebook, 3rd Edition
Men's Health Concerns Sourcebook, 2nd Edition
Mental Health Disorders Sourcebook, 4th Edition
Mental Retardation Sourcebook
Movement Disorders Sourcebook, 2nd Edition
Multiple Sclerosis Sourcebook
Muscular Dystrophy Sourcebook
Obesity Sourcebook
Osteoporosis Sourcebook
Pain Sourcebook, 3rd Edition
Pediatric Cancer Sourcebook
Physical & Mental Issues in Aging Sourcebook
Podiatry Sourcebook, 2nd Edition
Pregnancy & Birth Sourcebook, 2nd Edition
Prostate & Urological Disorders Sourcebook
Prostate Cancer Sourcebook
Reconstructive & Cosmetic Surgery Sourcebook
Rehabilitation Sourcebook
Respiratory Disorders Sourcebook, 2nd Edition
Sexually Transmitted Diseases Sourcebook, 3rd Edition
Sleep Disorders Sourcebook, 3rd Edition
Smoking Concerns Sourcebook
Sports Injuries Sourcebook, 3rd Edition
Stress-Related Disorders Sourcebook, 2nd Edition
Stroke Sourcebook, 2nd Edition
Surgery Sourcebook, 2nd Edition
Thyroid Disorders Sourcebook
Transplantation Sourcebook
Traveler's Health Sourcebook
Urinary Tract & Kidney Diseases & Disorders Sourcebook, 2nd Edition
Vegetarian Sourcebook
Women's Health Concerns Sourcebook, 3rd Edition
Workplace Health & Safety Sourcebook
Worldwide Health Sourcebook

Teen Health Series

Abuse & Violence Information for Teens
Accident & Safety Information for Teens
Alcohol Information for Teens, 2nd Edition
Allergy Information for Teens
Asthma Information for Teens, 2nd Edition
Body Information for Teens
Cancer Information for Teens
Complementary & Alternative Medicine Information for Teens
Diabetes Information for Teens
Diet Information for Teens, 2nd Edition
Drug Information for Teens, 3rd Edition
Eating Disorders Information for Teens, 2nd Edition
Fitness Information for Teens, 2nd Edition
Learning Disabilities Information for Teens
Mental Health Information for Teens, 3rd Edition
Pregnancy Information for Teens
Sexual Health Information for Teens, 2nd Edition
Skin Health Information for Teens, 2nd Edition
Sleep Information for Teens
Sports Injuries Information for Teens, 2nd Edition
Stress Information for Teens
Suicide Information for Teens, 2nd Edition
Tobacco Information for Teens, 2nd Edition

Environmental Health SOURCEBOOK

Third Edition

Health Reference Series

Third Edition

Environmental Health SOURCEBOOK

Basic Consumer Health Information about the Environment and Its Effects on Human Health, Including Facts about Air, Water, and Soil Contamination, Hazardous Chemicals, Foodborne Hazards and Illnesses, Household Hazards Such as Radon, Mold, and Carbon Monoxide, Consumer Hazards from Toxic Products and Imported Goods, and Disorders Linked to Environmental Causes, Including Chemical Sensitivity, Cancer, Allergies, and Asthma

Along with Information about the Impact of Environmental Hazards on Specific Populations, a Glossary of Related Terms, and Resources for Additional Help and Information

Edited by
Laura Larsen

Omnigraphics

P.O. Box 31-1640, Detroit, MI 48231

Bibliographic Note

Because this page cannot legibly accommodate all the copyright notices, the Bibliographic Note portion of the Preface constitutes an extension of the copyright notice.

Edited by Laura Larsen

Health Reference Series

Karen Bellenir, *Managing Editor*
David A. Cooke, MD, FACP, *Medical Consultant*
Elizabeth Collins, *Research and Permissions Coordinator*
Cherry Edwards, *Permissions Assistant*
EdIndex, Services for Publishers, *Indexers*

* * *

Omnigraphics, Inc.
Matthew P. Barbour, *Senior Vice President*
Kevin M. Hayes, *Operations Manager*

* * *

Peter E. Ruffner, *Publisher*

ISBN 978-0-7808-1078-5

Library of Congress Cataloging-in-Publication Data

Environmental health sourcebook : basic consumer health information about the environment and its effects on human health ... -- 3rd ed. / edited by Laura Larsen.
p. cm. -- (Health reference series)
Summary: "Provides basic consumer health information about the health effects of environmental hazards and diseases linked to environmental causes, with facts about the impact on specific populations. Includes index, glossary of related terms, and other resources"--Provided by publisher.
Includes bibliographical references and index.
ISBN 978-0-7808-1078-5 (hardcover : alk. paper) 1. Environmental health. 2. Environmentally induced diseases. 3. Environmental toxicology. I. Larsen, Laura.
RA565.E484 2010
616.9'8--dc22

2009044771

∞

This book is printed on acid-free paper meeting the ANSI Z39.48 Standard. The infinity symbol that appears above indicates that the paper in this book meets that standard.

Printed in the United States

Table of Contents

Visit www.healthreferenceseries.com to view *A Contents Guide to the Health Reference Series*, a listing of more than 15,000 topics and the volumes in which they are covered.

Part III: Outdoor Environmental Hazards: Air, Water, and Soil

Part IV: Household and Indoor Hazards

Part V: Foodborne Hazards

Part VI—Consumer Products and Medical Hazards

Part VII: Additional Help and Information

Preface

About This Book

The environment has always contained hazards to health, but modern and man-made factors compound the risks. Humans are now exposed to pollution in the air, water, and the soil. Contaminants are increasingly found throughout the food chain, in homes and schools, and in manufactured goods. Furthermore, in today's global economy, health hazards can even come from far away through tainted fish, imported toys, and technologically altered foods. Although some environmental hazards lead to immediate illness, often the risks are not identified until medical researchers link long-term exposures to chronic disease.

Environmental Health Sourcebook, Third Edition, offers updated information about the effects of the environment on human health. It discusses specific populations—including pregnant women and their fetuses, children, the elderly, and minorities—in which the effects of environmental exposures are especially harmful and, in some cases, can have a lasting impact that extends to future generations. Airborne, waterborne, foodborne, and chemical hazards are discussed, and facts about cancer, respiratory problems, infertility, autism, and other diseases with suspected environmental triggers are presented. A section on consumer products and medical hazards examines health risks associated with some common household items. The book concludes with a glossary and a directory of resources for additional information.

How to Use This Book

This book is divided into parts and chapters. Parts focus on broad areas of interest. Chapters are devoted to single topics within a part.

Part I: Understanding the Health Effects of Environmental Hazards provides information and risk assessment tools to help readers determine what health threats may be present in the world around them. It offers suggestions for reducing possible exposure to dangers, and it discusses issues of special concern to children, pregnant women, the elderly, and minority populations.

Part II: Health Concerns and Their Environmental Triggers provides readers with in-depth details on individual diseases with suspected environmental causes, including chemical sensitivity, cancer, respiratory problems, and certain viruses. It details the effects of the environment on fertility and pregnancy, and it explains how fetal and childhood exposures to some hazards can lead to disease later in life.

Part III: Outdoor Environmental Hazards: Air, Water, and Soil explores hazards, both natural and man-made, that are found in the outdoor environment. Readers will learn about pollution in air and water, as well as how chemicals and pesticides have spread through the food chain and how they can be avoided. It also explores hazards—such as noise and light pollution, smog and acid rain, and climate change—caused by the modern urban environment.

Part IV: Household and Indoor Hazards discusses the hazards people face in the environment where they spend up to 90% of their time—inside their homes, offices, and schools. These risks include indoor air contaminants, such as carbon monoxide, mold, asbestos, and lead, as well as unsafe indoor activities, such as smoking or inappropriately using chemicals and pesticides.

Part V: Foodborne Hazards includes facts about food safety regulations, potentially problematic food additives, and chemical contaminants in the food supply. It provides tips for avoiding the most common foodborne illnesses and for safely preparing food at home. Because most Americans rely on the industrial food chain for the majority of their food, it also discusses safety concerns related to food technologies, including genetic engineering, the use of antibiotics and hormones, and nanoparticles.

Part VI: Consumer Products and Medical Hazards tells readers about the health risks they face from consumer products, including everyday objects such as nonstick pans, hand soap, and plastics. It discusses the safety of imported goods, now found in virtually every home, and it describes concerns about the use of untested chemicals and additives in personal care products, such as cosmetics and sunscreens.

Part VII: Additional Resources includes a glossary of important terms and a directory of organizations providing information and advocacy on environmental health topics.

Bibliographic Note

This volume contains documents and excerpts from publications issued by the following U.S. government agencies: Centers for Disease Control and Prevention (CDC); Congressional Research Service; Consumer Product Safety Commission (CPSC); Department of Housing and Urban Development (HUD); Environmental Protection Agency (EPA); Federal Emergency Management Agency (FEMA); Food and Drug Administration (FDA); National Cancer Institute (NCI); National Institute of Allergy and Infectious Diseases (NIAID); National Institute of Environmental Health Sciences (NIEHS); U.S. Department of Agriculture (USDA); and U.S. Office of Air Quality and Radiation (AIRNow).

In addition, this volume contains copyrighted documents from the following organizations and publications: *American Journal of Preventive Medicine*; Asthma and Allergy Foundation of America; Autism Society of America; California Office of Environmental Health Hazard Assessment; Campaign for Safe Cosmetics; Center for Health, Environment, and Justice; Center for Science in the Public Interest; Cleveland Clinic; Collaborative on Health and the Environment; Environmental Justice and Health Union; Environmental Working Group; Food and Water Watch; Friends of the Earth; March of Dimes; Maryland Nurses Association; National Safety Council; Nemours Foundation; Pesticide Action Network North America; *Register-Herald* (Beckley, WV); Washington State Department of Health—Division of Environmental Health; and World Health Organization.

Full citation information is provided on the first page of each chapter or section. Every effort has been made to secure all necessary rights to reprint the copyrighted material. If any omissions have been made, please contact Omnigraphics to make corrections for future editions.

Acknowledgements

Thanks go to the many organizations, agencies, and individuals who have contributed materials for this *Sourcebook* and to medical consultant Dr. David Cooke and document engineer Bruce Bellenir. Special thanks go to managing editor Karen Bellenir and research and permissions coordinator Liz Collins for their help and support.

About the Health Reference Series

The *Health Reference Series* is designed to provide basic medical information for patients, families, caregivers, and the general public. Each volume takes a particular topic and provides comprehensive coverage. This is especially important for people who may be dealing with a newly diagnosed disease or a chronic disorder in themselves or in a family member. People looking for preventive guidance, information about disease warning signs, medical statistics, and risk factors for health problems will also find answers to their questions in the *Health Reference Series*. The *Series*, however, is not intended to serve as a tool for diagnosing illness, in prescribing treatments, or as a substitute for the physician/patient relationship. All people concerned about medical symptoms or the possibility of disease are encouraged to seek professional care from an appropriate health care provider.

A Note about Spelling and Style

Health Reference Series editors use *Stedman's Medical Dictionary* as an authority for questions related to the spelling of medical terms and the *Chicago Manual of Style* for questions related to grammatical structures, punctuation, and other editorial concerns. Consistent adherence is not always possible, however, because the individual volumes within the *Series* include many documents from a wide variety of different producers and copyright holders, and the editor's primary goal is to present material from each source as accurately as is possible following the terms specified by each document's producer. This sometimes means that information in different chapters or sections may follow other guidelines and alternate spelling authorities. For example, occasionally a copyright holder may require that eponymous terms be shown in possessive forms (Crohn's disease *vs.* Crohn disease) or that British spelling norms be retained (leukaemia *vs.* leukemia).

Locating Information within the Health Reference Series

The *Health Reference Series* contains a wealth of information about a wide variety of medical topics. Ensuring easy access to all the fact sheets, research reports, in-depth discussions, and other material contained within the individual books of the *Series* remains one of our highest priorities. As the *Series* continues to grow in size and scope, however, locating the precise information needed by a reader may become more challenging.

A Contents Guide to the Health Reference Series was developed to direct readers to the specific volumes that address their concerns. It presents an extensive list of diseases, treatments, and other topics of general interest compiled from the Tables of Contents and major index headings. To access *A Contents Guide to the Health Reference Series*, visit www.healthreferenceseries.com.

Medical Consultant

Medical consultation services are provided to the *Health Reference Series* editors by David A. Cooke, MD, FACP. Dr. Cooke is a graduate of Brandeis University, and he received his M.D. degree from the University of Michigan. He completed residency training at the University of Wisconsin Hospital and Clinics. He is board-certified in Internal Medicine. Dr. Cooke currently works as part of the University of Michigan Health System and practices in Ann Arbor, MI. In his free time, he enjoys writing, science fiction, and spending time with his family.

Our Advisory Board

We would like to thank the following board members for providing guidance to the development of this *Series*:

- Dr. Lynda Baker, Associate Professor of Library and Information Science, Wayne State University, Detroit, MI
- Nancy Bulgarelli, William Beaumont Hospital Library, Royal Oak, MI
- Karen Imarisio, Bloomfield Township Public Library, Bloomfield Township, MI
- Karen Morgan, Mardigian Library, University of Michigan-Dearborn, Dearborn, MI

- Rosemary Orlando, St. Clair Shores Public Library, St. Clair Shores, MI

Health Reference Series *Update Policy*

The inaugural book in the *Health Reference Series* was the first edition of *Cancer Sourcebook* published in 1989. Since then, the *Series* has been enthusiastically received by librarians and in the medical community. In order to maintain the standard of providing high-quality health information for the layperson the editorial staff at Omnigraphics felt it was necessary to implement a policy of updating volumes when warranted.

Medical researchers have been making tremendous strides, and it is the purpose of the *Health Reference Series* to stay current with the most recent advances. Each decision to update a volume is made on an individual basis. Some of the considerations include how much new information is available and the feedback we receive from people who use the books. If there is a topic you would like to see added to the update list, or an area of medical concern you feel has not been adequately addressed, please write to:

Editor
Health Reference Series
Omnigraphics, Inc.
P.O. Box 31-1640
Detroit, MI 48231
E-mail: editorial@omnigraphics.com

Part One

Understanding the Health Effects of Environmental Hazards

Chapter 1

Your Environment and Your Health

It's not too much of an exaggeration to say, your environment is your health. So to improve your health, see that your family's environment is a healthy one.

Of course, your environment isn't the only factor influencing your health. Genes play an important role, too, as your kids are sure to tell you. But, sorry, you can't choose your parents. You and your family can, on the other hand, do a lot about your personal environment—your surroundings, your exposures, your diet, and your health habits—to extend your life and to improve your fitness and appearance.

For an example of how society has improved health by environmental action, you have to look no further than our protected reservoirs and water disinfection plants. The purification of city water supplies has been the most significant reason that the average lifespan has very nearly doubled over the past century or so. Millions and millions of us live longer and better because of clean water and because our country and industries have reduced our exposures to lead and other substances.

In addition to the environments we share, each of us has his or her own personal environment. Our personal environments can greatly influence our lifespans and how healthy we feel and are. Here are simple but important steps that you and your family can take—health wise—about your environment....

"A Family Guide: 20 Easy Steps to Personal Environmental Health Now," National Institute of Environmental Health Sciences (www.niehs.nih.gov), 2000. Revised by David A. Cooke, MD, FACP, June 2009.

Read the Label on House and Garden Chemicals

Before you point that spray can, get your spectacles out and see if the directions or warnings have changed. They do, frequently. In fact, before you even buy a household or garden chemical, you can compare labels to be sure you're buying the safest product for your intended use. (You also may decide a bug-less, weed-less lawn isn't all that important.) Note whether a product is for inside or outside use, and what protections—rubber gloves, respirators, and such—are needed. What does the product do to birds, dogs, and barefoot children?

Read the labels for dry-cleaning solutions and other household chemicals, too. If a label says, "Open windows and ventilate," there's a reason. Likewise, read drug labels for warnings, and food labels for ingredients that don't agree with you, as well as to avoid excess calories and fat.

Labels have recently been added to some arts and craft supplies regarding ingredients posing a cancer risk. Charcoal has a new warning label.

Prescription and nonprescription drugs often get new warning labels when a new risk shows up during use.

Food labels were reformed in 1993 to be more informative about fats and calories. A reprint, "Food Label Close-Up," tells how to make best use of the new food label format. To have it sent to you, call your nearest Food and Drug Administration office listed in the U.S. section of your telephone book.

Turn Down the *!@# Volume

While occasional loud noises may just reduce your hearing temporarily, continuous exposures or very loud noises can cause permanent damage. Musicians know about efficient ear plugs that extend the life of their ears and perhaps their professional lives as well. You can buy them for your teens and for yourself. (You never know when your church is going to decide to do a production of *Jesus Christ, Superstar*.)

In addition to loud music, firecrackers and small arms fire, if close enough, can damage hearing, immediately or over time. That is, hearing may decline and/or there may be ringing, buzzing, or roaring in the ears or head. Additional information is available at the National Institute on Deafness and Other Communication Disorders Clearinghouse, 800-241-1044, or e-mail nidcd@aerie.com.

Your teens may relate to a story about a young rock musician's 40% hearing loss. "I was basically deaf for three years," says Kathy Peck of The Contractions. Her story is available at www.fda.gov/opacom/catalog/ots_ears.html.

Put a Carbon Monoxide Alarm in Your Home

Carbon monoxide from cars in garages, space heaters, and other home heating sources can be deadly. You need one or more smoke alarms, frequently checked of course, but they won't alert you to CO. For that, you need at least one carbon monoxide alarm. A few dollars, a trip to the hardware store, and a few minutes' installation are all you need to forestall a possible tragedy.

Grow Plants

Plants, including house plants, are not only nice to look at, there's evidence they clean pollutants from the air.

Put Drugs, Drain Openers, and Vitamins out of Kids' Reach

The iron-containing vitamins that many women take, as well as prescription and nonprescription drugs like aspirin or other pain relievers, can kill kids who think they're candy. Lock them up (we don't mean the kids) or put them out of reach. Same with paint thinners, detergents, drain openers, and other yard and home chemicals.

Look in your telephone book for your local Poison Control Center and ask for information and for "Mr. Yuk" telephone number stickers to place on your telephone for use in a poisoning emergency. Or you can get the location of your nearest center at www.poison.org/find_your_local_poison _center.htm.

Getting this information now, before an emergency happens, can be a good family lesson in prevention by planning ahead.

Know the Hazards of Your Job

Wherever you and your family members work there are risks. They may be physical, like falling off a ladder or lifting heavy packages, or chemical risks from petroleum products and solvents. In other occupations, computer use and other repetitive tasks pose risks of carpal tunnel syndrome. Identify the risks of your work and take the necessary precautions—whether a particular respirator, gloves, goggles, or a particular posture.

You say you work at home? Work is work. You can fall, spill corrosives on your skin, or breathe toxic fumes, if you're not careful—and there may not be anyone around to help. When it comes to work accidents, you're not home free.

See If That "Cold" Might Be an Allergy

You may think Johnny gets a lot of colds, but he may be allergic to dust mites, your cat, the pollen from trees, or cockroaches.

Plastic mattress and pillow covers, an exterminator, and the elimination of dust-holders like curtains and rugs in your bedroom may help. Or, if it's trees and pollen that get to you, air conditioning and air filters may provide relief.

The allergy may affect only one person in the family. (Being allergic means reacting to substances that don't bother most other people.) The substance you react to can be natural substances such as molds or various manufactured chemicals.

Asthma is often provoked by reactions to such substances.

Remember That Lakes and Streams Aren't Always Pure

A crystal-clear stream or lake may be a nice place to wade or swim but may harbor bacteria that can turn your stomach inside out. When you and your family walk in the wild, take along your own drinking water or a disinfection kit.

To avoid waterborne diseases in less-developed countries, you may need to avoid tap water (even ice cubes) and to stick to bottled water, to cooked foods, or to fruit that you peel yourself, such as bananas or oranges.

Watch for Lead, a Continuing Threat

A lot has been done to reduce our contact with the mind- and body-destroying lead in our environment. Lead-added paints and gasolines are a bad memory. (Lead content in paint was greatly reduced in the 1950s. Later, in 1978, the addition of lead was eliminated.) But there remain many deteriorating, pre-1950 buildings with flaking lead paint that contaminates the ground and ends up on children's hands and toys as dust. Your family may track in lead dust from a demolition site down the street.

If there's a chance a child in your family is being exposed to lead, a simple blood test can alert you before lead poisoning causes significant learning and behavior problems. More than one fifth of African American children living in housing built before 1946 have elevated blood lead levels.

Even low doses of lead can affect a child's development—causing problems with learning, remembering, and concentrating. Keep the toddlers away from lead by cleaning up the flakes and dust regularly and either carefully removing the source or walling it in.

Good nutrition, including plenty of milk products and other sources of calcium, may offer some protection from lead.

Occasional high-level lead poisonings still occur from craft-style lead-glazed pottery cups and dishes. Questionable products are best used for display, rather than food or drink.

Test for Radon

Radon is a gas you can't smell in your home, but you can test for it. A naturally occurring gas that seeps out of rocks and soils, it comes from uranium buried in the earth and is itself radioactive.

There is evidence of an elevated lung cancer risk among miners exposed to radon, especially miners who smoke. Radon also seeps into homes and collects in varying amounts. To assess the possible danger, the Institute of Medicine convened a panel of experts to review the data. These experts said the lung cancer risk from radon in homes is small compared to that from tobacco products. Of about 160,000 annual lung cancer deaths, radon-related deaths were estimated to probably total 15,400 to 21,800, mostly because of a synergism between smoking and radon. Fewer than 3,000 deaths were estimated as being radon-related among nonsmokers. But, say, smokers are people too.

The Harvard Center for Risk Analysis argues that the weight of evidence is that radon in homes may pose a greater risk to more people, mostly smokers, than die of accidental falls, poisonings, home fires and burns, or accidental discharges of firearms. Though the risk can be debated, it is clear that a radon test is cheap, and that, when found, high radon levels can often be turned into low levels by simple ventilation. For more information, call 800-SOS-RADON.

Don't Get Badly Overheated

Exercise is a way to keep fit, but when you or a family member competes or runs the dog in hot weather, try to do it in the cooler hours and/or have water handy and drink plenty of it. Keep some available for Fido and the cats, too.

Heat is a serious threat: Nearly 1,700 people lost their lives from heat-related illnesses in a big heat wave in 1980, and the forecast is for global warming. For more details on good health in the heat, visit www.cdc.gov/nceh/programs/emergenc/prevent/heat/heat.htm.

Know about Ozone

Ozone is a highly reactive form of oxygen—a linkage of three atoms of oxygen instead of the usual two—that occurs when there are a lot of vehicle exhaust and factory emissions. It accumulates when the air is stagnant.

Ozone can irritate and damage tissue in the lungs, nose, and throat, and can make breathing hard, especially if you exercise outdoors during its peaks. Watch for ozone and other air quality alerts in your newspaper, TV, and radio weathercasts. During alerts, jog in parks away from auto traffic, when possible. Especially if you have asthma, bronchitis, or emphysema, limit the time you spend outdoors when ozone levels are high.

Since evaporating gasoline adds to the ozone problem, when you service your car or mower, don't overfill the tank and spill the gasoline.

Wash Your Hands

Whether you've been sneezing, handling chicken or other raw poultry or meat…have been to the toilet or changed a diaper…or are preparing to deliver a baby or perform brain surgery, washing your hands and environs (such as your cutting board in the kitchen) is a most important way to prevent the spread of germs and infection. In many of these situations, it is the most important preventive measure you can take. It's as simple as that.

You may not be doing surgery, but more than 6.5 million cases of "tummy flu" or worse occur each year, often because hands and food implements aren't washed often enough, especially after handling poultry. To start youngsters out with good hand-washing habits, your closest FDA office (listed in the U.S. government pages of the telephone book) can provide the "Food Safety Coloring Book" for your kids. Or download it at www.foodsafety.gov/~dm/cbook.html.

In the past several years, "waterless" alcohol-based hand sanitizers have become widely available. These sanitizers are very helpful in promoting hand washing and reducing disease spread, as they are very quick and easy to use and don't require water or a sink. For some kinds of infections, they are actually better than soap and water. However, keep in mind that these cleaners work best when your hands are not visibly soiled. If you can see dirt, soap and water should be used.

Watch Pesticide Drift

If you spray your roses upwind of your tomatoes, you are likely to dose your family with unapproved pesticides. Some pesticides are for nonfood use only and have not been proved safe for foods.

Eat a Good Diet

Not just an apple but five or more servings of fruits and vegetables a day may help keep the doctor, and cancer and other disorders, away. For a booklet on the value of "five a day" or for other information on cancer and diet, call 800-4-CANCER.

Take a Vitamin

The federal government recommends all females of childbearing age take 400 micrograms (0.4 milligrams) of folic acid, one of the B vitamins, daily, to reduce the chances of having a child with a neural tube defect, a disorder in which the spine is open and easily damaged or even the child's brain is missing. The vitamin is needed regularly, before as well as during pregnancy, and it's hard to get the amount needed from an ordinary diet. But women and girls can get the additional folic acid they need by taking a multivitamin pill. Get more information at www.modimes.org.

You Can't Avoid All Accidents, But You Can Minimize the Results

Some good safety habits can save the lives and health of your family. Race car drivers know that wearing seat and shoulder belts can reduce risk by 45–50%. Other injury-preventing habits that athletes and regular folks alike take: wearing bike helmets and other protective athletic gear, looking ahead of time for the fire exits in a theater or hotel, checking your smoke and CO detectors at home to make sure they beep, locking hunting rifles and other firearms away from kids and others who might misuse them, and avoiding unlit and dangerous areas (and lit and dangerous people). Carry a first aid or snake bite kit when in the wild. Find a partner or two for climbing, swimming, or other exploits—someone to get you out of a tight spot or to go for help.

Respect Sex

More than 13 million Americans—two thirds of them under age 25—have sexually transmitted diseases, including HIV infections.

That's a pretty large monument to ignorance, as well as to youthful hormones and lack of restraint. For some young people, an infection may mean they'll never be able to have children. Other infections can lead to cervical cancer (cancer of the neck, of the uterus, or womb) or, in the case of HIV infections, early death.

Young people can only be 100% safe if they avoid sex—waiting until they're prepared to have a lasting relationship with another uninfected individual. But sexually active teens and young adults can gain considerable protection by correctly and consistently using a latex condom. That's the advice of federal health agencies. You should, er, discuss this with your kids before the fact—or at least see that they get responsible information. Some parents fear that they may promote sexual activity by discussing it. However, study after study shows that preparing children with good sex education does not promote earlier sex, and several studies suggest this preparation may delay the onset of sex.

Don't Puff or Chew

Just when some adults are getting a second wind, others of the same age are dying of tobacco-related lung cancer, or are crippled by other heart and lung problems.

New smokers—young people—may worry more about the smell of their breath, about their teeth getting dark, and about getting wrinkles than about dying.

Yet, smoking cigarettes, cigars, and pipe tobacco kills more people than AIDS, alcohol, drug abuse, car crashes, murders, suicides, and fires combined. For many, there's also a feeling of helplessness, of an addiction they can't break, at least alone. For help in quitting, call 800-4-CANCER, or the Office on Smoking and Health, 770-488-5705.

Watch out for the Sun and the Sunlamps

It's not just the temporary pain of a sunburn you need to worry about. A youngster's burns may mean not only wrinkles but serious trouble years later. Ordinary skin cancers can usually be surgically removed without difficulty, but melanomas (malignant moles) can kill, if not caught early.

Ultraviolet light from the sun or from sunlamps and sunbeds is also linked to cataracts that dim vision. Hats and other covers and ultraviolet-blocking sunglasses all can help.

For more on what melanomas look like call 800-4-CANCER.

Chapter 2

Health Risk Assessment: Determining Whether Environmental Substances Pose a Risk to Human Health

In recent years, the public has become increasingly aware of the presence of harmful chemicals in our environment. Many people express concerns about pesticides and other foreign substances in food, contaminants in drinking water, and toxic pollutants in the air. Others believe these concerns are exaggerated or unwarranted. How can we determine which of these potential hazards really deserve attention? How do we, as a society, decide where to focus our efforts and resources to control these hazards? When we hear about toxic threats that affect us personally, such as the discovery of industrial waste buried in our neighborhood or near our children's school, how concerned should we be?

Health risk assessment is a scientific tool designed to help answer these questions. Government agencies rely on risk assessments to help them determine which potential hazards are the most significant. Risk assessments can also guide regulators in abating environmental hazards. Members of the public who learn the basics of risk assessment can improve their understanding of both real and perceived environmental hazards, and they can work more effectively with decision makers on solutions to environmental problems.

This information in this chapter is excerpted from "A Guide to Health Risk Assessment," © 2001 California Office of Environmental Health Hazard Assessment. Reprinted with permission. For the complete text of this document, visit http://www.oehha.ca.gov/pdf/HRSguide2001.pdf. Reviewed by David A. Cooke, MD, FACP, June 2009.

The Four-Step Process of Risk Assessment

The risk assessment process is typically described as consisting of four basic steps: hazard identification, exposure assessment, dose-response assessment, and risk characterization. Each of these steps will be explained in the following text.

Step One: Hazard Identification

In the first step, hazard identification, scientists determine the types of health problems a chemical could cause by reviewing studies of its effects in humans and laboratory animals. Depending on the chemical, these health effects may include short-term ailments, such as headaches; nausea; and eye, nose, and throat irritation; or chronic diseases, such as cancer. Effects on sensitive populations, such as pregnant women and their developing fetuses, the elderly, or those with health problems (including those with weakened immune systems), must also be considered. Responses to toxic chemicals will vary depending on the amount and length of exposure. For example, short-term exposure to low concentrations of chemicals may produce no noticeable effect, but continued exposure to the same levels of chemicals over a long period of time may eventually cause harm. (See step three, "Dose-Response Assessment.")

An important step in hazard identification is the selection of key research studies that can provide accurate, timely information on the hazards posed to humans by a particular chemical. The selection of a study is based upon factors such as whether the study has been peer-reviewed by qualified scientists, whether the study's findings have been verified by other studies, and the species tested (human studies provide the best evidence). Some studies may involve humans that have been exposed to the chemical, while others may involve studies with laboratory animals.

Human data frequently are useful in evaluating human health risks associated with chemical exposures. Human epidemiologic studies typically examine the effects of chemical exposure on a large number of people, such as employees exposed to varying concentrations of chemicals in the workplace. In many cases, these exposures took place prior to the introduction of modern worker-safety measures.

One weakness of occupational studies is that they generally measure the effects of chemicals on healthy workers and do not consider children, the elderly, those with pre-existing medical conditions, or other sensitive groups. Since occupational studies are not controlled experiments, there may be uncertainties about the amount and duration of exposure or the influence of lifestyle choices, such as smoking or alcohol use, on the health of workers in the studies. Exposure of workers to other chemicals at the same time may also influence and complicate the results.

Laboratory studies using human volunteers are better able to gauge some health effects because chemical exposures can then be measured with precision. But these studies usually involve small numbers of people and, in conformance with ethical and legal requirements, use only adults who agree to participate in the studies. Moreover, laboratory studies often use simple measurements that identify immediate responses to the chemical but might miss significant, longer-term health effects. Scientists can also use physicians' case reports of an industrial or transportation accident in which individuals were unintentionally exposed to a chemical. However, these reports may involve very small numbers of people, and the level of exposure to the chemical could be greater than exposures to the same chemical in the environment. Nevertheless, human studies are preferred for risk assessment, so OEHHA [California Office of Environmental Health Hazard Assessment] makes every effort to use them when they are available.

Because the effects of the vast majority of chemicals have not been studied in humans, scientists must often rely on animal studies to evaluate a chemical's health effects. Animal studies have the advantage of being performed under controlled laboratory conditions that reduce much of the uncertainty related to human studies. If animal studies are used, scientists must determine whether a chemical's health effects in humans are likely to be similar to those in the animals tested. Although effects seen in animals can also occur in humans, there may be subtle or even significant differences in the ways humans and experimental animals react to a chemical. Comparison of human and animal metabolism may be useful in selecting the animal species that should be studied, but it is often not possible to determine which species is most like humans in its response to a chemical exposure. However, if seven similar effects were found in more than one species, the results would strengthen the evidence that humans may also be at risk.

Step Two: Exposure Assessment

In exposure assessment, scientists attempt to determine how long people were exposed to a chemical; how much of the chemical they were exposed to; whether the exposure was continuous or intermittent;

and how people were exposed—through eating, drinking water and other liquids, breathing, or skin contact. All of this information is combined with factors such as breathing rates, water consumption, and daily activity patterns to estimate how much of the chemical was taken into the bodies of those exposed.

People can be exposed to toxic chemicals in various ways. These substances can be present in the air we breathe, the food we eat, or the water we drink. Some chemicals, due to their particular characteristics, may be both inhaled and ingested. For example, airborne chemicals can settle on the surface of water, soil, leaves, fruits, vegetables, and forage crops used as animal feed. Cows, chickens, or other livestock can become contaminated when eating, drinking, or breathing the chemicals present in the air, water, feed, and soil. Fish can absorb the chemicals as they swim in contaminated water or ingest contaminated food. Chemicals can be absorbed through the skin, so infants and children can be exposed simply by crawling or playing in contaminated dirt. They can also ingest chemicals if they put their fingers or toys in their mouths after playing in contaminated dirt. Chemicals can also be passed on from nursing mothers to their children through breast milk.

To estimate exposure levels, scientists rely on air, water, and soil monitoring; human blood and urine samples; or computer modeling. Although monitoring of a pollutant provides excellent data, it is time consuming, costly, and typically limited to only a few locations. For those reasons, scientists often rely on computer modeling, which uses mathematical equations to describe how a chemical is released and to estimate the speed and direction of its movement through the surrounding environment. Modeling has the advantage of being relatively inexpensive and less time consuming, provided all necessary information is available and the accuracy of the model can be verified through testing.

Computer modeling is often used to assess chemical releases from industrial facilities. Such models require information on the type of chemicals released, facilities' hours of operation, industrial processes that release the chemicals, smokestack height and temperature, any pollution-control equipment that is used, surrounding land type (urban or rural), local topography and meteorology, and census data regarding the exposed population.

In all health risk assessments, scientists must make assumptions in order to estimate human exposure to a chemical. For example, scientists assessing the effects of air pollution may need to make assumptions about the time people spend outdoors, where they are more directly exposed to pollutants in the ambient air, or the time they spend in an area where the pollution is greatest. An assessment of soil contamination may require scientists to make assumptions about people's consumption of fruits and vegetables that may absorb soil contaminants.

To avoid underestimating actual human exposure to a chemical, scientists often look at the range of possible exposures. For example, people who jog in the afternoon, when urban air pollution levels are highest, would have much higher exposures to air pollutants than people who come home after work and relax indoors. Basing an exposure estimate on a value near the higher end of a range of exposure levels (closer to the levels experienced by the jogger than by the person remaining indoors) provides a realistic worst-case estimate of exposure. These kinds of conservative assumptions, which presume that people are exposed to the highest amounts of a chemical that can be considered credible, are referred to as "health-protective" assumptions.

Step Three: Dose-Response Assessment

In dose-response assessment, scientists evaluate the information obtained during the hazard identification step to estimate the amount of a chemical that is likely to result in a particular health effect in humans.

An established principle in toxicology is that "the dose makes the poison." For example, a commonplace chemical like table salt is harmless in small quantities, but it can cause illness in large doses. Similarly, hydrochloric acid, a hazardous chemical, is produced naturally in our stomachs but can be quite harmful if taken in large doses.

Scientists perform a dose-response assessment to estimate how different levels of exposure to a chemical can impact the likelihood and severity of health effects. The dose-response relationship is often different for many chemicals that cause cancer than it is for those that cause other kinds of health problems.

Cancer Effects: For chemicals that cause cancer, the general assumption in risk assessment has been that there are no exposures that have "zero risk" unless there is clear evidence otherwise. In other words, even a very low exposure to a cancer-causing chemical may result in cancer if the chemical happens to alter cellular functions in a way that causes cancer to develop. Thus, even very low exposures to carcinogens might increase the risk of cancer, if only by a very small amount.

Several factors make it difficult to estimate the risk of cancer. Cancer appears to be a progressive disease because a series of cellular transformations is thought to occur before cancer develops. In addition, cancer in humans often develops many years after exposure to a chemical. Also, the best information available on the ability of chemicals to cause cancer often comes from studies in which a limited number of laboratory animals are exposed to levels of chemicals that are much higher than the levels humans would normally be exposed to in the environment. As a result, scientists use mathematical models based on studies of animals exposed to high levels of a chemical to estimate the probability of cancer developing in a diverse population of humans exposed to much lower levels. The uncertainty in these estimates may be rather large. To reduce these uncertainties, risk assessors must stay informed of new scientific research. Data from new studies can be used to improve estimates of cancer risks.

Noncancer Effects: Noncancer health effects (such as asthma, nervous system disorders, birth defects, and developmental problems in children) typically become more severe as exposure to a chemical increases. One goal of dose-response assessment is to estimate levels of exposure that pose only a low or negligible risk for noncancer health effects. Scientists analyze studies of the health effects of a chemical to develop this estimate. They take into account such factors as the quality of the scientific studies, whether humans or laboratory animals were studied, and the degree to which some people may be more sensitive to the chemical than others. The estimated level of exposure that poses no significant health risks can be reduced to reflect these factors.

Step Four: Risk Characterization

The last step in risk assessment brings together the information developed in the previous three steps to estimate the risk of health effects in an exposed population. In the risk characterization step, scientists analyze the information developed during the exposure and dose-response assessments to describe the resulting health risks that are expected to occur in the exposed population. This information is presented in different ways for cancer and noncancer health effects, as explained here.

Cancer Risk: Cancer risk is often expressed as the maximum number of new cases of cancer projected to occur in a population of one million people due to exposure to the cancer-causing substance over a 70-year lifetime. For example, a cancer risk of one in one million means that in a population of one million people, not more than one additional person would be expected to develop cancer as the result of the exposure to the substance causing that risk.

An individual's actual risk of contracting cancer from exposure to a chemical is often less than the theoretical risk to the entire population calculated in the risk assessment. For example, the risk estimate for a drinking-water contaminant may be based on the health-protective assumption that the individual drinks two liters of water from a contaminated source daily over a 70-year lifetime. However, an individual's actual exposure to that contaminant would likely be lower due to a shorter time of residence in the area. Moreover, an individual's risk not only depends on the individual's exposure to a specific chemical but also on his or her genetic background (i.e., a family history of certain types of cancer); health; diet; and lifestyle choices, such as smoking or alcohol consumption.

Cancer risks presented in risk assessments are often compared to the overall risk of cancer in the general U.S. population (about 250,000 cases for every one million people) or to the risk posed by all harmful chemicals in a particular medium, such as the air. The cancer risk from breathing current levels of pollutants in California's ambient air over a 70-year lifetime is estimated to be 760 in one million.

Noncancer Risk: Noncancer risk is usually determined by comparing the actual level of exposure to a chemical to the level of exposure that is not expected to cause any adverse effects, even in the most susceptible people. Levels of exposure at which no adverse health effects are expected are called "health reference levels," and they generally are based on the results of animal studies. However, scientists usually set health reference levels much lower than the levels of exposure that were found to have no adverse effects in the animals tested. This approach helps to ensure that real health risks are not underestimated by adjusting for possible differences in a chemical's effects on laboratory animals and humans; the possibility that some humans, such as children and the elderly, may be particularly sensitive to a chemical; and possible deficiencies in data from the animal studies.

Depending on the amount of uncertainty in the data, scientists may set a health reference level 100 to 10,000 times lower than the levels of exposure observed to have no adverse effects in animal studies. Exposures above the health reference level are not necessarily hazardous, but the risk of toxic effects increases as the dose increases. If an assessment determines that human exposure to a chemical exceeds the health reference level, further investigation is warranted.

How Health Risk Assessment Is Used

Risk managers rely on risk assessments when making regulatory decisions, such as setting drinking water standards, or developing plans to clean up hazardous waste sites. Risk managers are responsible for protecting human health, but they must also consider public acceptance, as well as technological, economic, social, and political factors, when arriving at their decisions. For example, they may need to consider how much it would cost to remove a contaminant from drinking-water supplies or how seriously the loss of jobs would affect a community if a factory were to close due to the challenge of meeting regulatory requirements that are set at the most stringent level.

Health risk assessments can help risk managers weigh the benefits and costs of various alternatives for reducing exposure to chemicals. For example, a health risk assessment of a hazardous waste site could help determine whether placing a clay cap over the waste to prevent exposure would offer the same health protection as the more costly option of removing the waste from the site.

One of the most difficult questions of risk management is: How much risk is acceptable? While it would be ideal to completely eliminate all exposure to hazardous chemicals, it is usually not possible or feasible to remove all traces of a chemical once it has been released into the environment. The goal of most regulators is to reduce the health risks associated with exposure to hazardous pollutants to a negligibly low level.

Regulators generally presume that a one-in-one million risk of cancer from lifelong exposure to a hazardous chemical is an "acceptable risk" level because the risk is extremely low compared to the overall cancer rate. If a drinking water standard for a cancer-causing chemical were set at the level posing a "one-in-one million" risk, it would mean that not more than one additional cancer case (beyond what would normally occur in the population) would potentially occur in a population of one million people drinking water meeting that standard over a 70-year lifetime.

Actual regulatory standards for chemicals or hazardous waste cleanups may be set at less stringent risk levels, such as one in 100,000 (not more than one additional cancer case per 100,000 people) or one in 10,000 (not more than one additional cancer case per 10,000 people). These less stringent risk levels are often due to economic or technological considerations. Regulatory agencies generally view these higher risk levels to be acceptable if there is no feasible way to reduce the risks further.

For example, a regulatory agency may determine that the only water-treatment technology capable of reducing a given water contaminant to the one-in-one million risk level would be so prohibitively expensive that drinking-water suppliers would have to raise their rates to levels that their customers could not afford. At the same time, the regulatory agency may determine that several treatment technologies could economically reduce the contaminant to the "one-in-100,000" risk level. By setting the drinking-water standard at the one-in-100,000 level, the regulatory agency could reduce health risks to acceptable levels while ensuring that water rates remain affordable.

Chapter 3

Environmental Hazards for Children

Scientists are finding increasing evidence that exposure to some environmental factors jeopardizes children's health and may relate to large increases in the number of children diagnosed with asthma, attention deficit/hyperactivity disorder (ADHD), autism, and developmental impairment. Evidence is also strong that environmental health risks disproportionately affect children. Their nervous, immune, digestive, and other bodily systems are still developing while they receive disproportionately greater exposure to pollutants. They eat more food, drink more fluids, and breathe more air in relation to their body weight than adults do.

To address the increasingly evident disproportionate environmental health risks for children, President Bill Clinton signed Federal Executive Order 13045, Protection of Children from Environmental Health Risks and Safety Risks, on April 21, 1997 (62 FR 19883). This order mandated federal agencies to place a high priority on identifying and assessing risks affecting children and to ensure their policies, programs, activities, and standards address disproportionate risks to children.

In response, EPA's NCER [Environmental Protection Agency's National Center for Environmental Research] started a research program focusing on children's environmental health issues through its STAR grant program. In the 10 years since the executive order was

---

This section excerpted from "A Decade of Children's Environmental Health Research," Environmental Protection Agency (www.epa.gov), December 2007.

signed, NCER has developed a research portfolio of more than 100 individual projects the results of which have appeared in more than 1,000 peer-reviewed publications. Policymakers at state and local levels have used STAR grant research results to frame legislation and regulations. These results also have contributed to various approaches used to assess risk, and they have provided guidance to the public in creating safer, healthier environments.

In addition, NCER and NIEHS [National Institute of Environmental Health Sciences] have established the Centers for Children's Environmental Health and Disease Prevention Research ("Children's Centers"). This multidisciplinary research effort applies community-based, participatory research and innovative techniques in the investigation of environmental stressors on widespread childhood disorders such as asthma, autism, and learning disabilities. This research is also seeking effective strategies to reduce children's exposure to these environmental stressors.

The first eight Children's Centers, established in 1998, set out to study the effects of environmental factors such as pesticides and air pollution on childhood asthma and children's growth and development. In 2001, four more Children's Centers opened to study the basis of neurodevelopmental and behavioral disorders such as autism. Additional Children's Centers began investigations in 2004 and 2007 on how exposure to mixtures of chemicals affects children's health and which environmental pollutants cause disparities in birth outcomes. Since 1998, EPA has awarded 21 Children's Center grants that have fostered a collaborative network of pediatricians, basic scientists, epidemiologists, and community advocates across the United States, seeking to improve the health and environments of children.

This section highlights some important research findings from the STAR research grants, including the Children's Centers, during the past 10 years.

Summary of Relevant Research Findings across Life Stages

Prenatal

- Babies exposed before birth to higher levels of organophosphate (OP) insecticides have a shorter gestation period, smaller birth weight, shorter length, and decreased head circumference, and show delay in neurodevelopment up to age three. For example, babies exposed prenatally to chlorpyrifos and diazinon weighed less at birth by an average of 6.6 ounces, which is equivalent to that seen in babies born to women who smoked during pregnancy.

- Approximately 40% of babies exposed before their birth to a mixture of polycyclic aromatic hydrocarbons (PAHs) primarily from traffic sources and environmental tobacco smoke (ETS) have genetic damage that can be linked with increased cancer risk.
- Increases in maternal levels of dichlorodiphenyl trichloroethane (DDT), a pesticide, during pregnancy decrease scores on the Mental Development Index at two years of age. Each tenfold increase in DDT level is associated with a two- to three-point decrease in mental development.
- Prenatal exposure to lead or tobacco smoke has been implicated as a precursor of ADHD in children, possibly accounting for as many as one in three cases of ADHD in children.
- Maternal levels of ortho-substituted polychlorinated biphenyls (PCBs), one form of the class of compounds that compose PCBs, are associated with reduced weight gain up to 17 years of age in girls but not boys, suggesting that prenatal exposure to PCBs may affect female growth.

Neonatal: Birth to Less Than Three Months

- Human respiratory syncytial virus (RSV) infection in the first year of life increases the risk of asthmatic symptoms later in life. RSV affects the receptors in the airway that interact with environmental agents, which may explain why children with RSV-induced asthma are especially sensitive to their environment.
- Very low expression of the paraoxonase 1 (PON1) enzyme, an enzyme that facilitates the breakdown of pesticides into a less toxic form, is a major predictor of young children's susceptibility to the toxic effects of some OP insecticides. For example, decreases in the PON1 gene cause some newborns to be 26 to 50 times more susceptible to adverse health outcomes from exposure to certain OP pesticides than other newborns.
- Rat pups exposed to PCBs at the same level as babies breast-fed by mothers who live in high-PCB environments have developmental and auditory abnormalities, specifically, the ability for the brain to interpret auditory cues.

Infant/Crawler

- Children in farmworker families may be particularly vulnerable to pesticides because they often are exposed to these chemicals from multiple pathways such as pesticide drift from agricultural fields, take-home exposure from their parents, and breast milk from mothers who work or have worked in the fields.
- Children living within 75 meters of a major roadway have an increased risk of developing asthma. This effect was stronger in girls and in children without a family history of asthma.
- Early life exposures to traffic-related pollutants in urban environments appear to affect the immune system by increasing allergic responses, which can lead to respiratory symptoms in children as young as two years of age.
- Developmental exposure to noncoplanar PCBs, one of the many forms of compounds that compose the class of PCBs, increases the chance of a seizure. PCB exposure for autistic children is particularly dangerous because these children have a particularly high rate (about 30%) of seizure disorders.
- Placental tissues with higher concentrations of dichlorodiphenyl dichloroethene (DDE), a pesticide breakdown product, showed a correlation with increased levels of type 2 T-helper cells (Th2) cytokines. Elevated levels of these cells in very young children are a possible indicator for the development of asthma and other immune system disorders.

Toddler: One to Less Than Two Years

- About 30% of children with autistic spectrum disorder (ASD) exhibit loss of neurological and behavioral function during their first few years of life (12 to 30 months of age). This loss coincides with the onset of children's physical capacity to explore their environment, and, combined with repetitive behavior typical of ASD, it increases their exposure to environmental neurotoxicants. Autistic children also appear to have a different genetic or biochemical susceptibility.
- Toddlers in farmworker communities accumulate more pesticides on their clothing (socks and union suits) compared with younger, crawling children. In addition, toddlers show higher urinary metabolite levels than infants.

- Pesticide levels on children's hands are associated with pesticide metabolite levels in their urine, which means that their frequent hand-to-mouth behavior may cause them to ingest chemicals that they come in contact with.
- Exposure to lead during early childhood increases the risk of illegal behavior as an adult. There is a relationship between neuropsychological functioning in adolescence and police contacts in early adulthood, indicating a link between early lead exposure and adult antisocial activities.
- Children with iron deficiency retain more lead in their bodies. Childhood iron deficiency modifies behavior such as increasing pica (the desire to eat substances not normally eaten) and hand-to-mouth activity. These modified behaviors can increase children's exposure to environmental lead. Correlation between iron deficiency and blood lead levels is strongest among children aged one to two years.

Preschooler: Two to Less Than Six Years

- Mouse allergen exposure and asthma-related outcomes have a strong and consistent relationship. Children with high exposure to mouse allergens have more asthma-related unscheduled doctor visits, emergency department visits, and hospitalization than unexposed children.
- Elevated indoor particulate matter (PM) levels are associated with increased respiratory symptoms in preschool-aged children.
- Children with organic diets show lower median OP metabolite levels in their urine than children with conventional diets.
- Boys who spend the greatest amount of time playing outdoors have the highest pesticide exposure levels of any childhood group. Similarly, children who play extensively in laundry rooms and entryways exhibit higher rates of pesticide metabolites in urine than those who do not play, or play less, in these areas. Additionally, frequent hand washing does little to reduce children's pesticide exposures in households where chemical contamination is readily accessible.
- Floor dust appears to be the major source of exposure to OPs for young children (accounting for 68.8%), followed by solid food

(18.8%) and beverages (10.4%). Air and water contribute less than 2% to the total aggregate exposure.

- Autistic children showed higher levels of leptin (a hormone that affects the regulation of body weight, metabolism, and reproductive function, and influences the immune system) in their blood when compared to typically developing children.

School-Age: Six to Less Than Eleven Years

- An increased risk of respiratory-related school absences occurs in asthmatic and nonasthmatic children exposed to ETS.
- Placing air cleaners containing high-efficiency particulate air (HEPA) filters in inner-city asthmatic children's bedrooms can achieve a substantial, sustained improvement in indoor PM levels, one major cause of respiratory problems in children.
- Rural lifestyles may not protect children against developing asthma. Prevalence of asthma in rural areas is comparable to prevalence in large Midwestern cities.
- High levels of PM and ozone are associated with worsening pulmonary function and increased asthmatic symptoms among children from Detroit, Michigan, who have moderate to severe asthma.
- Disadvantaged asthmatic children in urban areas appear to be at increased risk for higher residential allergen levels, elevated air-pollution exposure, and higher levels of asthma triggers in the home.
- Children exposed to manganese and arsenic in the environment score lower on general intelligence tests and tests for memory.

Chapter 4

Environmental Hazards for Pregnant Women

There are more than 84,000 chemicals used in homes and businesses in this country, with little information on the effects of most of them during pregnancy.[1] However, a small number of chemicals are known to be harmful to an unborn baby. Most of these are found in the workplace, but certain environmental pollutants found in air and water, as well as chemicals used at home, also may pose a risk during pregnancy.

A pregnant woman can inhale these chemicals, ingest them in food or drink, or, in some cases, absorb them through the skin. For most hazardous substances, a pregnant woman would have to be exposed to a large amount for a long time in order for them to harm her baby.

Most workplaces have preventive measures to help reduce exposures to chemicals. However, because little is known about the effects of most chemicals on reproduction, a woman should discuss any chemical exposures in her workplace with her health care provider, preferably before pregnancy. She and her provider can determine whether additional on-the-job protections or alternative duty assignment is advisable. This is especially important for women who work in industries such as agriculture, manufacturing, dry cleaning, printing, pharmaceutical manufacturing, and health care. Pregnant women also can take steps to help protect themselves and their babies from pollutants and potentially risky chemicals used at home.

What are the risks of lead exposure during pregnancy?

Lead is a metal that was found for many years in gasoline, paint, and other products used in homes and businesses. Although lead is still present in the environment, the amounts have decreased greatly since the 1970s when the U.S. Environmental Protection Agency (EPA) banned its use in these products.

Lead poses health risks for everyone, but young children and unborn babies are at greatest risk. Exposure to high levels of lead during pregnancy contributes to miscarriage, preterm delivery, low birthweight, and developmental delays in the infant.[2] Lead is harmful even after birth. Children exposed to high levels of lead may develop behavioral and learning problems, slowed growth, and hearing loss.[3]

Women who live in older homes may be exposed to lead in deteriorating lead-based paint. Many homes built before 1978 were painted with lead-based paint. As long as paint is not crumbling or peeling, it poses little risk. However, crumbling paint can produce lead dust when the surface is disturbed, especially when it is sanded or scraped.

Children with pica, a pattern of eating non-food substances, such as paint, clay, dirt, and plaster, are at especially high risk of high blood lead levels if they dig peeling paint off walls and eat it, or chew on accessible areas, such as windowsills.

If lead-based paint needs to be removed from a home, pregnant women and children should stay out of the home until the project has been completed. Only experts should remove leaded paint, using proper precautions. For information on licensed lead-abatement contractors, visit the EPA website (www.epa.gov/lead).

A pregnant woman also can be exposed to significant amounts of lead in her drinking water if her home has lead pipes, lead solder on copper pipes, or brass faucets. A pregnant woman can contact her local health department or water supplier to find out how to get pipes tested for lead.

The EPA recommends running water for 15 to 30 seconds before using it for drinking or cooking to help reduce lead levels.[3] Water from the cold water pipe, which contains less lead than hot water, should be used for cooking and drinking during pregnancy, and for preparing baby formula. Many home filters do not remove lead, so a pregnant woman should look for a filter that is certified by NSF International (www.nsf.org) to remove lead.

Other possible sources of lead in the home include:

- Lead crystal glassware and some ceramic dishes. Pregnant women and children should avoid frequent use of these items. Commercial ceramics are generally safer than those made by craftspeople.

- Some arts and crafts materials (for example, oil paints, ceramic glazes, stained glass materials). A woman should use lead-free alternatives (such as acrylic or watercolor paints) during pregnancy and breastfeeding.
- Certain folk remedies for upset stomach, including those containing greta and azarcon.
- Vinyl mini-blinds imported from other countries.
- Lead solder in cans of food imported from other countries.
- Old painted toys.
- Cosmetics containing surma or kohl.

All people residing in the home who are exposed to lead on the job (for example, painters, plumbers, and those working in smelters, auto repair shops, battery manufacturing plants, or certain types of construction) should change their clothing (including shoes) and shower at work to avoid bringing lead into the home. They should wash contaminated clothing at work, if possible, or wash it at home separately from the rest of the family's clothing. The Occupational Safety and Health Administration (OSHA) requires that companies provide changing facilities for lead workers. For more information, visit the OSHA website (www.osha.gov/SLTC/lead/index.html).

Does mercury exposure pose a risk in pregnancy?

Mercury is a metal that is present in the environment. Elemental (pure) mercury and methylmercury are two forms of mercury that may pose risks in pregnancy.

Elemental mercury is used in thermometers, dental fillings, and some batteries. One recent study found a slightly increased risk of miscarriage in women working with amalgam in dental offices.[6] Amalgam is a silver-colored material used to fill cavities in teeth, containing elemental mercury, silver, and other metals. Some countries (Sweden and Canada) recommend that dentists avoid using dental amalgam in pregnant women as a precaution, although there is no evidence that it will harm their babies.[7]

Pregnant women who are concerned about the use of amalgam should discuss the use of alternative filling materials with their dentists. Women who work in industries that use mercury to manufacture products (including electrical, chemical, and mining industries) should discuss their workplace exposures with their health care providers and take all recommended precautions.

Mercury enters the environment from natural sources (such as volcanic activity) and man-made sources (such as coal-burning or other industrial pollution). Mercury in the air eventually is deposited in water where it is converted by bacteria to a more dangerous form (methylmercury), which accumulates in the tissues of fish. Eating fish is the main source of methylmercury exposure in humans.[4]

Trace amounts of mercury are present in many types of fish, but mercury is most concentrated in large fish that eat other fish. For this reason, the U.S. Food and Drug Administration (FDA) and the EPA advise pregnant women to avoid eating swordfish, shark, king mackerel, and tilefish, and to limit consumption of albacore (white) tuna to six ounces or less a week.[5] These fish may contain enough mercury to harm an unborn baby's developing nervous system, sometimes leading to learning disabilities. For additional guidance on eating fish during pregnancy, read "Food-borne Risks in Pregnancy" (www.marchofdimes.com/professionals/14332_1152.asp).

What other metals pose a risk in pregnancy?

Arsenic is another metal suspected of posing pregnancy risks. It enters the environment through natural sources (forest fires and weathering of rock) and man-made sources (mining and electronics manufacturing). Although arsenic is a well-known poison, the small amounts normally found in the environment are unlikely to harm a fetus.

However, certain women may be exposed to higher levels of arsenic that may pose an increased risk of pregnancy complications, including miscarriage and birth defects.

Women who may be exposed to higher levels of arsenic include those who:

- work at or live near metal smelters;
- live in agricultural areas where arsenic fertilizers (now banned) were used on crops;
- live near hazardous waste sites or incinerators;
- drink well water containing high levels of arsenic.

This can occur in the aforementioned locations, or in certain parts of the country with naturally high levels of arsenic in rock (including parts of New England, the Southwest, the Northwest, and Alaska).[8]

Women who live in areas that may have high arsenic levels can help protect themselves from arsenic exposure by limiting their contact with soil. Women who use well water should have their water tested for arsenic to determine whether it is safe to drink or drink bottled water. For more information, visit the EPA website (www.epa.gov/safewater/arsenic). Community water suppliers already test it for arsenic.

Until 2003, arsenic was included as part of a preservative in pressure-treated lumber that was used to build decks and outdoor play sets. The EPA recommends applying a penetrating stain or sealant to these structures at least once a year to reduce exposure to arsenic.[9] Anyone who works with arsenic (for example, in semiconductor manufacturing, metal smelting, or applying herbicides) should avoid bringing the metal home on clothing and shoes.

Can pesticides harm an unborn baby?

There is little proof that exposure to pest-control products at levels commonly used at home pose a risk to the fetus. However, all insecticides are to some extent poisonous. Some studies suggest that high levels of exposure to pesticides may contribute to miscarriage, preterm delivery, and birth defects.[10] Therefore, pregnant women should avoid pesticides whenever possible.

A pregnant woman can reduce her exposure to pesticides by controlling pest problems with less toxic products. For example, she can place sticky traps in areas inaccessible to children. If she must have her home or property treated with pesticides, a pregnant woman should:

- have someone else apply the chemicals and leave the area for the amount of time indicated on the package instructions;
- remove food, dishes, and utensils from the area before the pesticide is applied (afterwards, have someone open the windows and wash off all surfaces on which food is prepared);
- close all windows and turn off air conditioning when pesticides are used outdoors, so fumes aren't drawn into the house;
- wear rubber gloves when gardening to prevent skin contact with pesticides.

Pregnant women may be concerned about the safety of insect repellants during pregnancy. The insect repellant DEET (diethyltoluamide) is among the most effective at keeping insects, such as mosquitoes and ticks, from biting. Preventing insect bites is important during pregnancy because mosquito- and tick-borne infections, such as West Nile virus and Lyme disease, may be harmful in pregnancy. Because the safety of DEET during pregnancy has not been fully assessed, a pregnant woman should apply insect repellents with DEET mainly to her clothing, and only in small amounts to exposed skin, when necessary.[11] She can minimize her need for DEET by staying indoors during dawn and dusk, when mosquitoes are most likely to bite, and by wearing long pants and long sleeves.

What are organic solvents?

Solvents are chemicals that dissolve other substances. Organic solvents include alcohols, degreasers, paint thinners, and varnish removers. Lacquers, silk-screening inks, and paints also contain these chemicals. A 1999 Canadian study found that women who were exposed to solvents on the job during their first trimester of pregnancy were 13 times more likely than unexposed women to have a baby with a major birth defect, like spina bifida (open spine), clubfoot, heart defects, and deafness.[12] The women in the study included factory workers, laboratory technicians, artists, graphic designers, and printing industry workers.

Other studies have found that three workers in semiconductor plants exposed to high levels of solvents called glycol ethers were almost three times more likely to miscarry than unexposed women.[13] Glycol ethers also are used in jobs that involve photography, dyes, and silk-screen printing.

Pregnant women who work with solvents, including women who do arts and crafts at home, should minimize their exposure by making sure their workplace is well ventilated and by wearing appropriate protective clothing, including gloves and a face mask. They should never eat or drink in their work area. To learn more about the chemicals she works with, a woman can ask her employer for the Material Safety Data Sheets for the products she uses or contact the National Institute for Occupational Safety and Health.

Is drinking chlorinated tap water safe during pregnancy?

In recent years, media reports have raised concerns about possible pregnancy risks from by-products of chlorinated drinking water. Chlorine is added to drinking water to kill disease-causing microbes. However, when chlorine combines with other materials in water, it forms chemical by-products, including trihalomethanes (THMs). The level of THMs and other chlorification by-products in water supplies varies, although the EPA regulates the maximum level permitted in water supplies.

A 1998 California study suggested that women who consumed more than five glasses a day of cold tap water containing high levels of trihalomethanes had an increased risk of miscarriage.[14] However, a more recent North Carolina study found little or no increased risk from these chemicals.[15] Scientists continue to study the safety of these chemicals during pregnancy. Until we know more, pregnant women who are concerned about chlorination by-products may choose to drink bottled water.

Drinking water also can become contaminated with pesticides, lead, arsenic, and other metals. Women who suspect their water supply may be affected can have their water tested or drink bottled water.

Can air pollution harm the fetus?

Most women who live in areas with higher-than-average levels of air pollution have healthy babies. However, studies from the United States and other countries suggest that babies of pregnant women exposed to high levels of certain air pollutants (such as polycyclic aromatic hydrocarbons and small particle pollution, both of which result from vehicle exhaust and industrial sources) may be slightly more likely than babies of pregnant women living in less polluted areas to be small for their gestational age.[16, 17]

Air quality in many areas of the country has improved since the first Clean Air Act was passed in 1970. However, some pregnant women, including those living in large cities, are still exposed to unhealthful levels of pollution. Individuals can help limit their exposure to pollution by limiting outdoor activities, especially exercise, on days when air quality is expected to be poor.

Do household cleaning products pose a risk in pregnancy?

Although some household cleansers contain solvents, there are many safe alternatives. Pregnant women should read labels carefully and avoid products (such as some oven cleaners) with labels stating that they are toxic.

Products that contain ammonia or chlorine are unlikely to harm an unborn baby, although their odors may trigger nausea in a pregnant woman. A pregnant woman should open windows and doors and wear rubber gloves when using these products. She should never mix ammonia and chlorine products because the combination produces fumes that are dangerous for anyone.

A pregnant woman who is worried about household cleansers or bothered by their odors can substitute safe, natural products. For example, baking soda can be used as a powdered cleanser to scrub greasy areas, pots and pans, sinks, tubs, and ovens. A solution of vinegar and water can effectively clean many surfaces, such as countertops.

References

1. Lawson, C.C., et al. Workgroup Report: Implementing a National Occupational Reproductive Agenda: Decade One and Beyond. *Environmental Health Perspectives*, volume 114, number 3, March 2006, pages 435–441.
2. Agency for Toxic Substances and Disease Registry. Lead: CAS #7439-92-1. September 2005.
3. U.S. Environmental Protection Agency. Lead in Paint, Dust, and Soil. February 20, 2007.
4. U.S. Environmental Protection Agency. Mercury. May 2, 2007.
5. U.S. Department of Health and Human Services and U.S. Environmental Protection Agency. What You Need to Know about Mercury in Fish and Shellfish. March 2004.
6. Lindhohm, M.L., et al. Occupational Exposure in Dentistry and Miscarriage. *Occupational and Environmental Medicine*, volume 64, number 2, February 2007.
7. U.S. Food and Drug Administration. Questions and Answers on Dental Amalgam. October 31, 2006.
8. Agency for Toxic Substances and Disease Registry. Arsenic. January 2006.
9. U.S. Environmental Protection Agency. Chromated Copper Arsenate (CCA). May 11, 2005.
10. American Academy of Pediatrics Committee on Environmental Health. Pesticides. In: Etzel, R.A., ed., *Pediatric Environmental Health, 2nd edition*. Elk Grove Village, IL, American Academy of Pediatrics, 2003, pages 323–359.
11. Centers for Disease Control and Prevention (CDC). Natural Disasters and Special Populations: Effects on Pregnant Women–Environmental Exposures. July 5, 2007.

12. Khattak, S., et al. Pregnancy Outcome Following Gestational Exposure to Organic Solvents: A Prospective Controlled Study. *Journal of the American Medical Association*, volume 281, number 12, March 24/31, 1999, pages 1106–1109.

13. Correa, Adolfo, et al. Ethylene Glycol Ethers and Risks of Spontaneous Abortion and Subfertility. *American Journal of Epidemiology*, volume 143, number 7, 1996, pages 707–717.

14. Waller, K., et al. Trihalomethanes in Drinking Water and Spontaneous Abortion. *Epidemiology* 1998, volume 9, pages 134–140.

15. Savitz, D.A., et al. Drinking Water Disinfection By-Products and Pregnancy Outcome. AWWA Research Foundation/ Environmental Protection Agency Report, 2005.

16. Parker, J.D., et al. Air Pollution and Birth Weight among Term Infants in California. *Pediatrics*, volume 115, number 1, January 2005, pages 121–128.

17. Choi, H., et al. International Studies of Prenatal Exposure to Polycyclic Aromatic Hydrocarbons and Fetal Growth. *Environmental Health Perspectives*, volume 114, number 11, November 2006, pages 1744–1750.

Chapter 5

Environmental Hazards for the Elderly

Chapter Contents

Section 5.1

The Elderly and Hazards at Home

"Report: Elderly at Higher Risk from Hazards Found in Homes," by Ashley Morici, *Register-Herald* (WV), August 10, 2008.

According to AARP [American Association of Retired Persons] Services and the EPA [Environmental Protection Agency] Aging Initiative, older people are at a higher risk of suffering major health issues from hazards found around their homes.

Items that may cause illness or even premature death in the elderly include: household cleaners that have harmful chemicals in them, pesticides, paints and solvents, clothing, furniture, draperies, carpet pads, stuffing in furniture, and nonstick cooking pans. This information is provided by a recent AARP bulletin.

Household cleaners that may contain dangerous chemicals are ammonia, chlorine bleach, and glycol ethers that are found in substances that remove dirt and grime. Ammonia is a chemical that triggers asthma attacks. Chlorine bleach is a lung irritant and can be deadly if swallowed. And glycol ethers can be easily absorbed into the skin and eventually cause nerve damage.

Pesticides have been tied to Parkinson's disease. Anyone with a weakened heart or lungs should steer clear of pesticides because they can cause arrhythmia and possibly heart attacks.

Paints and solvents like mineral spirits, methanol, xylene, and turpentine can be used improperly and the fumes can put stress on lungs and heart, and eventually give the person an irregular heartbeat, says the EPA. Paints that can be harmful to older people especially include ones with Alkyd and oil bases to them because they tend to have higher amounts of volatile organic compounds, or VOCs, in them.

Some older fabrics used in clothing contain formaldehyde, which is an upper respiratory irritant. Clothing made from natural fibers like cotton is a safer bet.

Furniture, draperies, carpet pads, stuffing in furniture, and nonstick cooking pans all pose higher health risks to the elderly. It was not until 2000 that Scotchgard updated its formula in furniture and draperies to eliminate carcinogens found in its anti-stain treatments. Carpet pads and stuffing in older furniture and mattresses contain polybrominated diphenyl ethers, which are used as flame retardants in these products and have been shown to pose a risk to the thyroid gland and the nervous and reproductive systems in people.

Lastly, some nonstick cooking pans have been shown to release 15 different toxic chemicals, a few being carcinogens if the pans are left on a stove burner with no supervision, according to a study done by the Environmental Working Group, which is based in Washington and is a nonprofit research group.

There are ways to make sure the elderly person in your life does not become ill as a result of handling, inhaling, or touching these various household items. To aid air circulation, make sure to have indoor plants around the house because they have been known to help purify the air; also put a whole-house air purifier in the home to ensure the air quality in the house is at optimal levels, open windows around the house to maintain air circulation, and make sure to air out new appliances because they can send out tons of chemicals depending on how new they are.

Safer alternatives are available when it comes to pesticides. For ants people can use cinnamon, bay leaves, cayenne pepper, or even baby powder all around the house. In cases of cockroach infestation, using small amounts of part baking soda and part confectioner's sugar can relieve any household of the pests. If you have mice running around your house, put cotton-dipped peppermint oil in close proximity to troublesome areas around the house. And if your cat cannot seem to kill the mice around the house, use its litter box litter as a repellent as well.

Mosquitoes can be squashed by using two teaspoons of apple cider vinegar in a glass of water placed on any deck or balcony, and if that doesn't work then put lavender oil on wrists and elbows to ward off the critters. And finally, flies can be swatted away for good by putting small pouches of crushed mint all over the house, or a potted sweet basil plant will also do the trick.

The elderly are just as important as anyone else and so is their health. People need to make sure to check in on older people as often as possible, and help to ensure their lives continue to be fruitful, healthy, and prosperous.

Section 5.2

The Elderly and Outdoor Pollution

"Elderly Have Higher Risk for Cardiovascular, Respiratory Disease from Fine Particle Pollution," National Institute of Environmental Health Sciences (www.niehs.nih.gov), March 8, 2006.

New data from a four-year study of 11.5 million Medicare enrollees show that short-term exposure to fine particle air pollution from such sources as motor vehicle exhaust and power plant emissions significantly increases the risk for cardiovascular and respiratory disease among people over 65 years of age. The study, funded by the National Institute of Environmental Health Sciences (NIEHS), a component of the National Institutes of Health, is the largest ever conducted on the link between fine particle air pollution and hospital admissions for heart- and lung-related illnesses.

The study results show that small increases in fine particle air pollution resulted in increased hospital admissions for heart and vascular disease, heart failure, chronic obstructive pulmonary disease, and respiratory infection. "The data show that study participants over 75 years of age experienced even greater increases in admissions for heart problems and chronic obstructive pulmonary disease than those between 65 and 74 years of age," said National Institutes of Health Director Elias A. Zerhouni, MD.

The National Institute of Environmental Health Sciences and the U.S. Environmental Protection Agency provided funding to researchers at the Johns Hopkins Bloomberg School of Public Health for the study. The study results are published in the March 8, 2006, issue of the *Journal of the American Medical Association*.

According to the study, these findings document an ongoing threat from airborne particles to the health of the elderly, and provide a strong rationale for setting a national air quality standard that is as protective of their health as possible.

"These findings provide compelling evidence that fine particle concentrations well below the national standard are harmful to the cardiovascular and respiratory health of our elderly citizens," said NIEHS

Director David A. Schwartz, MD. "Now that the link between inhaled particles and adverse health effects has been established, we must focus our efforts on understanding why these particles are harmful, and how these effects can be prevented."

Fine particle air pollution consists of microscopic particles of dust and soot less than 2.5 microns in diameter—about 30 times smaller than the width of a human hair. These tiny particles primarily come from motor vehicle exhaust, power plant emissions, and other operations that involve the burning of fossil fuels. Fine particles can travel deep into the respiratory tract, reducing lung function and worsening conditions such as asthma and bronchitis.

The researchers based their fine particle analysis on 11.5 million Medicare enrollees who lived in 204 U.S. counties with populations larger than 200,000. Using billing records for 1999 to 2002, they tracked daily counts of hospital admissions for eight major outcomes—heart failure, heart rhythm disturbances, cerebrovascular events such as stroke or brain hemorrhage, coronary heart disease, peripheral vascular disease or narrowing of the blood vessels, chronic obstructive pulmonary disease, respiratory infection, and injury.

The investigators obtained daily measurements of fine particle concentrations from a network of air monitoring stations provided by the Environmental Protection Agency's Aerometric Information Retrieval Service. The average fine particle concentration for the 204 counties over the three-year period was 13.4 micrograms per cubic meter of air, slightly below the national air quality standard of 15 micrograms per cubic meter for an annual average.

"When we analyzed the data for heart failure, we observed a 1.28% increase in admissions for each 10 microgram per cubic meter increase in fine particle pollution," said Francesca Dominici, PhD, an associate professor of biostatistics with the Johns Hopkins Bloomberg School of Public Health and lead author on the study. "Most of these admissions increases occurred the same day as the rise in fine particle concentration, which suggests a short lag time between the change in pollution and the subjects' response."

The data also showed that the risk for air pollution-related cardiovascular disease was highest in counties located in the Eastern United States. "Identifying the various factors that might contribute to these differences between eastern and western regions is a very complex question that we must address," said Dominici.

According to Dominici, fine particles pose a significant health problem because they penetrate deep into the lungs, and some may even get into the bloodstream. "Now that we know that inhaled particles can affect cardiovascular and respiratory health, we must identify the specific characteristics of fine particles that produce these adverse health effects," she said. "In the meantime, these findings underscore the need for a national air quality standard that adequately protects the respiratory health of our citizens."

Chapter 6

Racial Disparities in Exposure to Environmental Hazards

Reports from local health, labor, and housing departments since the 1930s, and similar national agencies since the 1960s, indicate that environmental disease is a greater threat to low-income communities of color than other communities.

Low-income communities of color are limited by fewer environmental benefits (e.g., clean air, water, and land) and more environmental threats (e.g., hazardous chemicals and environmental illness). Such limits triggered the environmental justice movement. Environmental justice activists often find the limits so strong that they focus on a single issue. Environmental health professionals often do not sense these limits and sometimes blame the limits on the victims. Understanding how such limits are created, maintained, and interact to create environmental illness in low-income communities of color helps environmental justice activists and environmental health professionals develop better solutions.

Better health is a benefit often tied to more income, more education, and better jobs, as well as living in communities where more people have higher incomes and more education. However, race, class, and gender discrimination in the U.S. makes better health difficult to attain for people in poor minority communities. Limits on housing choice, education, income, and political power create environments for low-income

---

communities of color that trigger disease. The end result is that people in low-income communities of color have less healthy surroundings, less education, and less income to support their personal health, and to fight for better health care, than people in other communities. People residing in low-income communities of color also die sooner.

The environmental health consequences of such limitations are substantial. Exposure to toxins are greater in low-income communities of color because they are often located in or near polluting industrial areas and consist of cheap older housing where lead paint and pests are a threat. Employment in low-income communities of color is often limited to jobs with low pay, no health benefits, and, sometimes, severe workplace dangers. Low-income communities of color receive less treatment for environmental disease because health care resources are limited and environmental health expertise is rare. Finally, when environmental health threats are not eliminated, the harm jumps from generation to generation.

Lead

Lead poisoning is the most well-studied environmental disease in the United States. The cause and effect of lead poisoning on poor minority communities is known. Studies in northeastern cities dating back to the 1930s, and national studies since the 1970s, consistently showed that lead poisoning killed more children and produced more harm in poor minority communities than other communities. The removal of lead from gasoline, paint, solder for welding pipes, and water supplies has produced a very sharp decrease in lead poisoning in all communities. However, that benefit has not been evenly distributed. Questions remain about whether environmental health professionals have taken the best approach to preventing lead poisoning and, as they have been since the 1970s, poor minority communities nationwide remain at greatest risk for lead poisoning.

National data collected in 1994 indicates 890,000 children one to five years of age have elevated blood lead levels. 688,000 of those children are targeted in federal health care programs or enrolled in Medicaid or WIC [Special Supplemental Nutrition Program for Women, Infants, and Children], yet the majority are never screened for lead. 427,000 African American children (11.2% nationwide), 296,000 White children (2.3% nationwide), and 131,000 Latino children (4.8% nationwide) had elevated blood lead levels. However, while blood lead levels in African American and White children vary based on family income, location and culture minimize such differences among Latino children.

The blood lead levels of African American children were 80% greater than White children. Decreasing blood lead levels of African American children and Latino children to the levels of White children will result in more than $50 billion dollars of increased lifetime earnings.

Lead risks to children can be mapped at the community level. Children under six years are at increased risk for lead-based paint hazards in houses built before 1950. CDC [Centers for Disease Control and Prevention] has compiled U.S. Census data on housing age and population demographics at the ZIP code and census tract levels. Performing a "data query" will enable anyone to identify the risk of childhood lead poisoning in the community. State data on lead risks to workers is also available.

Occupational lead exposure also remains a problem. The Occupational Safety and Health Administration and the National Institute of Occupational Safety and Health provide information on worker exposure to lead. While most workers are not tested, of 20,000 that were recently tested, about 20% had high blood lead levels.

Asthma

Asthma and deaths due to asthma have rapidly increased since 1980. Though the exact cause of asthma remains uncertain, environment very likely plays a key role. Research is heavily focused on indoor environmental triggers for asthma instead of the contribution of outdoor environmental triggers. Asthma prevention, as a result, is focused more on the habits of parents than the possible harmful effect of industry and traffic on air quality in poor minority communities.

Health centers around the country conduct asthma research and treatment. Efforts focused on poor minority communities are overseen by several Department of Health and Human Services agencies including the National Institute of Environmental Health Sciences. Research, though, on industrial triggers for asthma is primarily supported by the National Institute of Occupational Safety and Health.

While numerous nonprofit environmental health groups focus on asthma, relatively few actually work as partners with poor minority communities. The American Academy of Allergy Asthma & Immunology [AAAAI], through Academy CAN! (Consulting Allergist Network), places volunteer allergists in community health care centers where they consult with center clinicians and training staff on the latest diagnosis and management of allergies and asthma. In partnership with the Congress of National Black Churches, the AAAAI has also created educational materials about asthma. The Asthma and Allergy

Foundation of America has numerous local chapters, some of which partner with poor minority communities to fight asthma.

A survey of state health departments in 1996 found that no state had an asthma control program. Yet, recent studies estimate the cost of childhood asthma from household triggers to exceed $800 million per year. The cost of occupational asthma is estimated to be $1.6 billion. Poor minority communities, and the health care systems that serve them, bear the brunt of these costs. Comprehensive models to eliminate childhood asthma have been proposed but have yet to be implemented.

PCBs and Dioxins

Dioxin triggers cancer at a smaller dose than any other chemical. PCBs (polychlorinated biphenyls) are a closely related chemical that also likely cause cancer. PCBs, when burned, can become dioxin. PCBs and dioxin contribute to numerous other illnesses in people. However, the pathway from exposure to PCBs and dioxin to disease is not well understood. Researchers suspect the large amounts of chlorine in PCBs and dioxins are responsible for the illness.

National PCB studies were performed in the 1970s as part of the National Human Adipose Tissue Survey (NHATS). Local and early NHATS results found PCB levels in African American populations may have been greater than those of White populations. Later studies supported those results, but found that the percentage of the population with high PCB levels had begun to decrease in 1977, the year PCB production was banned in the United States. The PCBs in the Great Lakes and the Arctic pose the greatest threat to Native American communities.

Summary of Environmental Exposures in Non-Hispanic Blacks Identified in "Environmental Exposure and Racial Disparities"

- Dioxin and PCBs: 40 chemicals examined. 21 of the 40 are not detected. The remaining 19 are not widely found. The highest levels of 18 of the 19 are in non-Hispanic Blacks. The remaining 1 is found at the highest level in Mexican Americans.

- Phthalates: 7 chemicals measured. Of the 7, 4 are widely found. The mean level of 3 of the 4 widely found is higher in non-Hispanic Blacks. The mean level of the remaining 1 widely found is higher in Mexican Americans. However, the highest levels of each of the 7 are detected in non-Hispanic Whites.

- Tobacco smoke: 1 chemical measured. It is not widely found and is detected in highest levels in non-Hispanic Blacks.
- Limited exposure: 5 chemicals (3 types of dioxins and PCBs, the pesticide Mirex, and the herbicide 2,4-Dichlorophenoxyacetic acid) are only detected in non-Hispanic Blacks.

Summary of Environmental Exposures in Mexican Americans Identified in "Environmental Exposure and Racial Disparities"

- Pesticides: 26 chemicals examined. 6 of the 26 are not detected. Of the remaining 20, 6 are widely found. The mean level of 2 of the 6 is higher in Mexican Americans while the mean level of the remaining 4 is highest in non-Hispanic Whites. Of the 14 that are not widely found, the highest levels of 7 are in Mexican Americans.
- Herbicides and pest repellants and disinfectants: 9 chemicals examined. 4 of the 9 are not found in any person. Of the remaining 5, 3 are widely found and had a mean level highest in Mexican Americans. The 2 that are not widely found are detected in highest levels in non-Hispanic Blacks.
- Limited exposure: 1 chemical (3-hydroxychrysene) is only detected in Mexican Americans.

Summary of Environmental Exposures in Non-Hispanic Whites Identified in "Environmental Exposure and Racial Disparities"

- Metals: 13 chemical examined. 2 of the 13 are not detected. The remaining 11 are widely found. The mean level of 7 of the 11 is higher in non-Hispanic Whites. The highest levels for 6 of the 11 are in non-Hispanic Whites.
- PAHs [Polycyclic aromatic hydrocarbons]: 14 chemical examined. 2 of the 14 are not detected. Of the 7 that are widely found, the mean level in non-Hispanic Whites is higher in 5. The highest levels for 6 of the 12 that are detected are found in non-Hispanic Whites.

- Phytoestrogens: 6 chemicals examined. The mean level in non-Hispanic Whites is higher in 5 of the 6. The highest level for 4 of the 6 is in non-Hispanic Whites.
- Limited exposure: No chemicals are only found in non-Hispanic Whites.

Part Two

Health Concerns and Their Environmental Triggers

Chapter 7

Human Health Problems with Environmental Causes

The air, the water, the sun, the dust, plants and animals, and the chemicals and metals of our world...They support life. They make it beautiful and fun. But, as wonderful as they are...They can also make some people sick. Here are some diseases that are related to your environment from *A* to *Z* and some ideas for preventing or caring for them.

Allergies and Asthma

Slightly more than half of the 300 million people living in the U.S. are sensitive to one or more allergens. They sneeze, their noses run, and their eyes itch from pollen, dust, and other substances. Some suffer sudden attacks that leave them breathless and gasping for air. This is allergic asthma. Asthma attacks often occur after periods of heavy exercise or during sudden changes in the weather. Some can be triggered by pollutants and other chemicals in the air and in the home. Doctors can test to find out which substances are causing reactions. They can also prescribe drugs to relieve the symptoms.

"Environmental Diseases from A to Z," National Institute of Environmental Health Sciences (www.niehs.nih.gov), June 2007. This document with full references is available online at http://www.niehs.nih.gov/health/docs/enviro-a-z.pdf.

Birth Defects

Sometimes, when pregnant women are exposed to chemicals or drink a lot of alcohol, harmful substances reach the fetus. Some of these babies are born with an organ, tissue, or body part that has not developed in a normal way. Aspirin and cigarette smoking can also cause birth problems. Birth defects are the leading cause of death for infants during the first year of life. Many of these could be prevented.

Cancer

Cancer occurs when a cell or group of cells begins to multiply more rapidly than normal. As the cancer cells spread, they affect nearby organs and tissues in the body. Eventually, the organs are not able to perform their normal functions. Cancer is the second leading cause of death in the U.S., causing more than 500,000 deaths each year. Some cancers are caused by substances in the environment: cigarette smoke, asbestos, radiation, natural and manmade chemicals, alcohol, and sunlight. People can reduce their risk of getting cancer by limiting their exposure to these harmful agents.

Dermatitis

Dermatitis is a fancy name for inflamed, irritated skin. Many of us have experienced the oozing bumps and itching caused by poison ivy, oak, and sumac. Some chemicals found in paints, dyes, cosmetics, and detergents can also cause rashes and blisters. Too much wind and sun make the skin dry and chapped. Fabrics, foods, and certain medications can cause unusual reactions in some individuals. People can protect themselves from poison ivy by following a simple rule: "Leaves of three, leave them be." Smart folks know their poisons.

Emphysema

Air pollution and cigarette smoke can break down sensitive tissue in the lungs. Once this happens, the lungs cannot expand and contract properly. This condition is emphysema. About two million Americans have this disease. For these people, each breath is hard work. Even moderate exercise is difficult. Some emphysema patients must breathe from tanks of oxygen.

Fertility Problems

Fertility is the ability to produce children. However, one in eight couples has a problem. However, more than 10% of couples cannot conceive after one year of trying to become pregnant. Infertility can be caused by infections that come from sexual diseases or from exposure to chemicals on the job or elsewhere in the environment. Researchers at the National Institute of Environmental Health Sciences (NIEHS) have shown that too much caffeine in the diet can temporarily reduce a woman's fertility.

Goiter

Sometimes people don't get enough iodine from the foods they eat. This can cause a small gland called the thyroid to grow larger. The thyroid can become so large that it looks like a baseball sticking out of the front of your neck. This is called goiter. Since the thyroid controls basic functions like growth and energy, goiter can produce a wide range of effects. Some goiter patients are unusually restless and nervous. Others tend to be sluggish and lethargic. Goiter became rare after public health officials decided that iodine should be added to salt.

Heart Disease

Heart disease is the leading cause of death in the United States and is a major cause of disability. Almost 700,000 Americans die of heart disease each year. While these may be due in part to poor eating habits and/or lack of exercise, environmental chemicals also play a role. While most chemicals that enter the body are broken down into harmless substances by the liver, some are converted into particles called free radicals that can react with proteins in the blood to form fatty deposits called plaques, which can clog blood vessels. A blockage can cut off the flow of blood to the heart, causing a heart attack.

Immune Deficiency Diseases

The immune system fights germs, viruses, and poisons that attack the body. It is composed of white blood cells and other warrior cells. When a foreign particle enters the body, these cells surround and destroy this "enemy." We have all heard of AIDS [acquired immunodeficiency syndrome] and the harm it does to the immune system. Some chemicals and drugs can also weaken the immune system by damaging its specialized cells. When this occurs, the body is more vulnerable to diseases and infections.

Job-Related Illnesses

Every job has certain hazards. Even a writer can get a paper cut. But did you know that about 137 workers die from job-related diseases every day? This is more than eight times the number people of who die from job-related accidents. Many of these illnesses are caused by chemicals and other agents present in the workplace. Factories and scientific laboratories can contain poisonous chemicals, dyes, and metals. Doctors and other health workers have to work with radiation. People who work in airports or play in rock concerts can suffer hearing loss from loud noise. Some jobs involve extreme heat or cold. Workers can protect themselves from hazards by wearing special suits and using goggles, gloves, ear plugs, and other equipment.

Kidney Diseases

About 7.5 million adults have some evidence of chronic kidney disease. These diseases range from simple infections to total kidney failure. People with kidney failure cannot remove wastes and poisons from their blood. They depend on expensive kidney machines in order to stay alive. Some chemicals found in the environment can produce kidney damage. Some nonprescription drugs, when taken too often, can also cause kidney problems. Be sure to read the label and use drugs as directed.

Lead Poisoning

Sometimes, infants and children will pick up and eat paint chips and other objects that contain lead. Lead dust, fumes, and lead-contaminated water can also introduce lead into the body. Lead can damage the brain, kidneys, liver, and other organs. Severe lead poisoning can produce headaches, cramps, convulsions, and even death. Even small amounts can cause learning problems and changes in behavior. Doctors can test for lead in the blood and recommend ways to reduce further exposure.

Mercury Poisoning

Mercury is a silvery metal that is extremely poisonous. Very small amounts can damage the kidneys, liver, and brain. Years ago, workers in hat factories were poisoned by breathing the fumes from mercury used to shape the hats. Remember the "Mad Hatter" in *Alice in Wonderland*? Today, mercury exposure usually results from eating contaminated fish and other foods that contain small amounts of mercury compounds. Since the body cannot get rid of mercury, it gradually builds up inside the tissues. If it is not treated, mercury poisoning can eventually cause pain, numbness, weak muscles, loss of vision, paralysis, and even death.

Nervous System Disorders

The nervous system, which includes the brain, spinal cord, and nerves, commands and controls our thoughts, feelings, movements, and behavior. The nervous system consists of billions of nerve cells. They carry messages and instructions from the brain and spinal cord to other parts of the body. When these cells are damaged by toxic chemicals, injury, or disease, this information system breaks down. This can result in disorders ranging from mood changes and memory loss to blindness, paralysis, and death. Proper use of safety devices such as seat belts, child restraints, and bike helmets can prevent injuries and save lives.

Osteoporosis

Over 10 million Americans have osteoporosis, while 18 million others have lost bone mass and are likely to develop osteoporosis in the future. About 25 million Americans suffer from some kind of bone thinning. As people get older, back problems become more common, and bones in the spine, hip, and wrists break more easily. Young people can lower their chances of getting osteoporosis in later years by exercising and eating calcium-rich foods like milk and yogurt.

Pneumoconiosis

Ordinary house and yard dusts do not pose a serious health hazard. But some airborne particles can be very dangerous. These include fibers from asbestos, cotton, and hemp, and dusts from such compounds as silica, graphite, coal, iron, and clay. These particles can damage sensitive areas of the lung, turning healthy tissue into scar tissue. This condition is called pneumoconiosis, or black lung. Chest pains and shortness of breath often progress to bronchitis, emphysema, and/or early death. Proper ventilation and the use of protective masks can greatly reduce the risk of lung disease.

Queensland Fever

People do not usually get diseases from farm animals. However, those who work with hides and animal products can get sick from breathing the infected dust around them. This illness is called Queensland fever because it was first discovered among cattle ranchers and dairy farmers in Queensland, Australia. It is caused by a tiny organism that infects livestock and then spreads to the milk and feces. Symptoms include fever, chills, and muscle aches and pains. Researchers have developed vaccines to protect livestock workers from this illness.

Reproductive Disorders

Beginning in the late 1940s, many women who were in danger of losing their unborn babies were prescribed a synthetic female hormone called DES (diethylstilbestrol). In 1971, scientists discovered that some of the daughters of these women were developing a very rare cancer of the reproductive organs. Since then, the use of DES and other synthetic hormones during pregnancy has been discontinued. NIEHS and other agencies are studying the possibility that some natural chemicals and manmade pesticides may cause similar problems. They are finding that some of these chemicals are so similar to female estrogen that they may actually "mimic" this important hormone. As a result, they may interfere with the development of male and female reproductive organs. This can lead to an increased risk of early puberty, low sperm counts, ovarian cysts, and cancer of the breast or testicles.

Sunburn and Skin Cancer

Almost everyone has stayed in the sun too long and been burned. Too much sunlight can also produce the most common type of cancer—skin cancer. Some skin cancers are easy to treat because they do not spread beyond the surrounding tissue. Others, like melanoma, are much more dangerous because they spread to other parts of the body. Deaths due to melanoma are increasing by 4% each year. More than 7,800 people died from melanomas of the skin in 2003.

Tooth Decay

In the 1930s, health experts noticed that people who lived in areas where the water contained natural chemicals called fluorides had fewer cavities. Today, all U.S. residents are exposed to fluoride to some degree, and its use has resulted in a significant decline in tooth decay. National surveys report that the incidence of tooth decay among children 12 to 17 years of age has declined from 90% in 1971 to 67% in 1988. Dentists can also protect young teeth by applying special coatings called sealants.

Uranium Poisoning

Uranium is a dangerous element because it is radioactive. This means it gives off high-energy particles that can go through the body and damage living tissue. A single high dose of radiation can kill. Small doses over a long period can also be harmful. For example, miners who are exposed to uranium dust are more likely to get lung cancer. Uranium poisoning can also damage the kidneys and interfere with the body's ability to fight infection. While most people will never come in contact with uranium, those who work with medical x-rays or radioactive compounds are also at risk. They should wear lead shields and follow recommended safety guidelines to protect themselves from unnecessary exposure.

Vision Problems

Our eyes are especially sensitive to the environment. Gases found in polluted air can irritate the eyes and produce a burning sensation. Tiny particles from smoke and soot can also cause redness and itching of the eyes. Airborne organisms like molds and fungus can cause infections of the eyes and eyelids. Too much exposure to the sun's rays can eventually produce a clouding of the lens called a cataract.

Waterborne Diseases

Even our clearest streams, rivers, and lakes can contain chemical pollutants. Heavy metals like lead and mercury can produce severe organ damage. Some chemicals can interfere with the development of organs and tissues, causing birth defects. Others can cause normal cells to become cancerous. Some of our waterways also contain human and animal wastes. The bacteria in the wastes can cause high fever, cramps, vomiting, and diarrhea.

Xeroderma Pigmentosa

Xeroderma is a rare condition that people inherit from their parents. When these people are exposed to direct sunlight, their skin breaks out into tiny dark spots that look like freckles. If this condition is not treated, the spots can become cancerous. These areas must then be removed by a surgeon.

Yusho Poisoning

In 1968, more than 1,000 people in western Japan became seriously ill. They suffered from fatigue, headache, cough, numbness in the arms and legs, and unusual skin sores. Pregnant women later delivered babies with birth defects. These people had eaten food that was cooked in contaminated rice oil. Toxic chemicals called PCBs (polychlorinated biphenyls) had accidentally leaked into the oil during the manufacturing process. Health experts now refer to this illness as "Yusho," which means "oil disease."

For years, PCBs were widely used in the manufacturing of paints, plastics, and electrical equipment. When scientists discovered that low levels of PCBs could kill fish and other wildlife, their use was dramatically reduced. By this time, PCBs were already leaking into the environment from waste disposal sites and other sources. Today, small amounts of these compounds can still be found in our air, water, soil, and some of the foods we eat.

Zinc Deficiency/Poisoning

Zinc is a mineral that the body needs to function properly. In rare cases, people can be poisoned if there is too much zinc in their food or water. However, most people can take in large quantities without any harmful effects. In areas where nutrition is a problem, people may not get enough zinc from their diet. This can lead to retarded growth, hair loss, delayed sexual maturation, eye and skin lesions, and loss of appetite.

Chapter 8

Chemical Sensitivity (Multiple Chemical Sensitivity Syndrome)

A variety of vague and hard-to-pinpoint symptoms are experienced by an undetermined, but possibly sizable, number of adults and children. Occasionally, they may suggest allergy or asthma, but most often the symptoms are much wider in scope.

Not much is currently known about what is referred to as "chemical sensitivity," but it is a subject that is often mentioned as a growing problem in the popular media. Since there are considered to be a variety of adverse health effects from so-called "chemical sensitivities," the public and their health care providers are rightly confused about what it is all about.

Why are chemical sensitivities gaining so much interest?

There are several reasons, among which are:

- a greater number of complex chemical compounds (polymers) in our natural environment than in the past;
- less indoor air exchange in more highly insulated houses and buildings;
- greater media coverage of news and opinions about chemical sensitivities and their possible ill effects on our health.

A few physicians who refer to themselves as "ecologically oriented" have proposed diagnoses such as the "Twentieth Century Disease," "Chemical AIDS," "multiple chemical sensitivities," or "Candida hypersensitivity." Intriguing as these labels may be to some whose symptoms seem to frustrate the attempts of a medical diagnosis and treatment, no single test or combination of tests has yet to clearly identify the causes of these symptoms.

Nevertheless, caring physicians are sensitive to patients with vague complaints. They endeavor to keep them from seeking in desperation care and "cures" that lack a medical-scientific basis or require much more study.

What are considered chemical sensitivities?

There are four general ways that we can classify chemical sensitivity:

Annoyance Reactions: These result from a heightened sensitivity to unpleasant odors, called olfactory awareness, in some susceptible individuals. Your ability to cope with offensive—but mostly nonirritating—odors has a lot to do with genetic or acquired factors, among which are infection and inflammation of the mucous membranes or polyps (growths of the nasal or sinus membranes) and abuse of tobacco and nasal decongestants.

Irritational Syndromes: These are caused by significant exposure to irritating chemicals that are more likely than others to penetrate the mucous membranes. These types of reactions can affect certain nerve endings and cause burning sensations in the nose, eyes, and throat. They usually come and go, and can be reversed.

Immune Hypersensitivity: This is the basis of allergic diseases, such as allergic rhinitis (hay fever) and asthma. They are generally caused by naturally occurring organic chemicals found in pollens, molds, dust, and animals. At present, only a relatively few industrial chemicals are known to have the capability of provoking a true immune system response. Among them are acid anhydrides and isocyanates and other chemicals that are able to bond to human proteins.

Intoxication Syndrome: In some cases, long-term exposure to noxious chemicals may cause serious illness, or even death. Permanent damage to health may be the outcome of such reactions, which are dependent on the nature and extent of the chemical exposure. Toxic pollutants are given off by a number of building products, such as furniture, cleaning fluids, pesticides, and paints.

How does pollution affect my health?

Most people who believe they have symptoms from chemical sensitivity are concerned that they are related to their exposure to pollution, either outdoors or indoors. Outdoor pollution may result from natural causes (the eruption of volcanoes, dust storms, forest fires), or man-made causes (vehicle exhaust, fossil fuel combustion, petroleum refining). Other pollutants that may cause respiratory illness include:

Sulfur Dioxide: Substantial scientific evidence has linked specific air pollutants to increased respiratory illness and decreased pulmonary function, especially in children. People prone to allergy, especially those with allergic asthma, can be extremely sensitive to inhaled sulfur dioxide, for example. Symptoms may include bronchospasm, hives, gastrointestinal disorders, and inflammation of the blood vessels (vasculitis-related disorder).

Ozone and Nitrogen Dioxide: Temporary or perhaps permanent bronchial hypersensitivity has been connected to inhaled ozone and nitrogen dioxide. Long-term exposure to nitrogen dioxide has been associated with the increased occurrence of respiratory illness.

Significant exposure to airborne pollution occurs inside homes, offices, and nonindustrial buildings. These settings have not received nearly the attention by pollution control agencies that they deserve.

Cigarette Smoke: One of the most disagreeable and potentially dangerous indoor pollutants is cigarette smoke. It is made up of a complex mixture of gases and particles that contain numerous chemicals. Indoor tobacco smoking substantially increases levels of carbon monoxide, formaldehyde, nitrogen dioxide, acrolein, polycyclic aromatic hydrocarbons, hydrogen cyanide, and many other substances and inhaled particles found in the air.

Formaldehyde is not only found indoors from cigarette smoke, but also outdoors from gasoline and diesel combustion. Data indicates that formaldehyde is capable of acting as a respiratory irritant. It also is known to cause an allergic skin rash. However, there is no convincing evidence that this pollutant is able to sensitize the respiratory system.

Wood-Burning Stoves: There are more than 11 million wood-burning units in American homes today. Wood burning usually occurs in cold, oxygen-poor conditions that heighten the emission of carbon monoxide and other inhaled chemicals and particles. Increased use of wood as a heating fuel has raised concern because of its ability to contaminate a home. Poorly ventilated stoves give off increased levels of carbon monoxide, nitrogen and sulfur oxides, formaldehyde, and benzopyrene.

Building-Related Illness: Poor air quality in today's tightly insulated homes and other buildings has been associated with a variety of syndromes, or group of symptoms. The term "building-related illness" or "sick-building syndrome" is applied to an office building in which one or more occupants develop a generally accepted, well-defined syndrome for which a specific cause related to the building is found.

There are a variety of illnesses broadly known as hypersensitivity pneumonitis—in which one or more organic dusts can create complex immune system reactions and symptoms, including mucous membrane irritation, coughing, chest tightness, headache, and fatigue. These are well-defined, and there are validated tests for diagnosing these conditions. Building occupants with these symptoms have been identified as having "multiple chemical sensitivities" or other forms of environmental illness.

One study, however, showed that the majority of nonspecific complaints by office workers had developed before the worker began working in the building suspected of causing their symptoms. Collaboration between the physician, industrial hygienist, and building engineer may be necessary to clearly establish a cause-and-effect relationship between any indoor air quality level and disease.

How is chemical sensitivity diagnosed?

There are strategies that can produce reliable diagnoses with relatively low costs, reliable diagnoses at significant costs, or questionable diagnoses at great expense. Obviously, the first alternative is preferable. It includes:

- a careful patient medical history that includes a review of all previous medical records and, when symptoms may be related to potentially hazardous substances in the workplace, reviewing a Materials Safety Data Sheet supplied by the employer;
- upper respiratory tract and selective skin tests and a neurological examination;
- routine laboratory studies, including nasal smear;
- lung function measurements (spirometry and peak flow monitoring).

If these diagnostic procedures do not produce a definite diagnosis, more expensive—but worthwhile—evaluations may help. They include an industrial hygiene evaluation of the workplace, an evaluation of the home environment, and psychiatric evaluations.

Diagnostic approaches are expensive and not effective in explaining suggested chemical sensitivity such as the RAST test [radioallergosorbent test], and tests for the Epstein-Barr virus, autoimmune disease, food allergies, and evaluations to determine airborne molds and bacteria.

Chapter 9

Cancer and Environmental Concerns

Chapter Contents

Section 9.1

Environmental Causes of Cancer

"The Majority of Cancers Are Linked to the Environment," National Cancer Institute (www.cancer.gov), June 17, 2004. Reviewed by David A. Cooke, MD, FACP, June 2009.

One of the hopeful messages from cancer research is that most of the cases of cancer are linked to environmental causes and, in principle, can be prevented. Together, the National Cancer Institute (NCI) and the National Institute of Environmental Health Sciences (NIEHS) have recently published a new booklet titled "Cancer and the Environment," which focuses on the agents in the environment that cause cancer and what we can do to lower our cancer risk. Environmental causes include both lifestyle factors such as smoking and diet, as well as exposure to agents in the air and water. The following interview with Aaron Blair, PhD, the chief of the Occupational Epidemiology Branch in NCI's Division of Cancer Epidemiology and Genetics, will address the contribution of various agents to our overall cancer burden.

As far back as the 1960s, several studies have concluded that by acting on what we know about the causes of cancer, we could prevent the majority of cancers. Some reports even estimate that we could reduce the incidence of cancer by as much as 80–90%. What is your reaction to these assessments?

Most epidemiologists and cancer researchers would agree that the relative contribution from the environment toward cancer risk is about 80–90%. When I use the word *environmental*, I mean it in a broad sense to include both lifestyle factors such as diet, tobacco, and alcohol, as well as radiation, infectious agents, and substances in the air, water, and soil.

This information comes from studies that have been around for a long time. For example, if you look at migrant studies you find that people who migrate from an area of high cancer risk to an area of low cancer risk, or the reverse, within their lifetime take on the cancer rates of the country to which they move. Since the gene pool changes only after many generations, this means that these changes must be environmental, not genetic. And so, the migrant studies very clearly tell us that the wide range of cancer rates is largely driven by environmental causes.

Epidemiologic studies on risk factors tell us the same thing. For decades, scientists have been conducting epidemiological investigations looking at a variety of environmental and host genetic risk factors. And, almost always, the cancer burden is much greater for environmental causes than just the hereditable genetic factors.

There are several categories of agents in the environment that we know cause cancer—tobacco, alcohol, infectious agents, diet, medical drugs, occupational exposures, and ionizing radiation. Over the years, epidemiologists have made estimates as to the percentage of new cancer cases and cancer deaths caused by these agents (see Table 9.1). For example, the estimates for cancer deaths attributable to tobacco have been consistently around 30% and the proportion of cancers due to occupations, air and water pollution, medicines, and medical procedures are individually much smaller—most are less than 5%. Which of these estimates do we know with the most certainty?

We know with considerable certainty the estimates for tobacco. It is a single agent, many studies have been done, and we can fully and completely document that tobacco is a major contributor to cancer. One other factor that falls into the certain category is ionizing radiation. We really know a lot about the cancer risks associated with exposure to ionizing radiation. This includes radiation from many sources—cosmic rays, radon, X-rays, atomic bombs, and above ground nuclear bomb tests. So, the estimates for tobacco and ionizing radiation are very solid. However, the total contribution from all the other causes of cancer, such as diet, occupational exposures, or air and water pollution, may be correct, but we are less certain. This is because they are just so much harder to study. There are many more components to consider in studies of diet, medicines, or industrial products, for example. For these categories, we never know if we have really identified all the potential factors that contribute to the cancer risk in the population.

Although the proportion of cancer deaths caused by dietary factors account for the highest percentage, they also seem to be the least reliable data. Do you agree? Why is this data so uncertain?

The estimates made by two English epidemiologists, Richard Doll and Richard Peto, in the early 1980s are still reasonable (see Table 9.1). Tobacco is a major contributor. Diet probably is a major contributor. But our knowledge and certainty about diet is much less firm than tobacco.

It's undergoing a state of flux now. Things in the diet that we thought 10 years ago were very clearly linked with increases of cancer—low fiber intake, for example—are less certain now. They haven't gone away, but there are changes in thinking and contradictory findings in studies have confused the picture. But I think the estimate that diet may contribute 30–35% is probably right. But the certainty about this is not great. That's because it's really hard to figure out what the diet is. All diets are very complex, and it's hard to determine exactly what people have eaten over time and the amount of micronutrients. So, tobacco and diet are major contributors. The other causes of cancer (medicinal, occupational, viral, radiation) fall in about the same range of 10% less.

It is known that dietary factors have a strong influence on cancer cases and death, but, at the same time, no single dietary factor aside from alcohol shows a strong and consistent enough effect to establish it unequivocally as an important carcinogen or anti-carcinogen. Is this because it is inherently difficult to tease out which factors in the diet have a strong influence on health or that there are no dietary factors that have a strong effect on cancer risk?

The major limitation is that it is so difficult to characterize a person's diet over time. Typically it's not the diet today that is important for the cancer diagnosed today. We need to know what people ate in the past, and that is really hard to determine. Investigators are getting better at this. The interviews are getting better. There are now some molecular and biological probes that provide us some information that can be useful. Progress is being made. But, it's still a hard road.

What are some success stories where the environmental causes of cancer have been controlled and resulted in lower cancer rates?

Tobacco is a major success story. The proportion of the U.S. population that smoke has been going down for several decades, and just within the last decade, lung cancer rates have also started to go down. There is still room for improvement, but we can look with some pride at our successes in the tobacco arena.

There are a number of occupational exposures where we have been successful in decreasing harmful exposures. It's a little hard to document exactly what the reduction in cancer risk has been, but there is evidence that it has occurred. It's very clear that by understanding the relationship between occupational exposures and cancer, there have been real reductions in exposure to several toxic substances—

arsenic, asbestos, and benzidine, for example. There are quite a number of chemicals that are under regulation in most countries around the world and there is some evidence that rates are decreasing for some cancers that are related to these exposures.

Table 9.1 Proportion of Cancer Deaths Caused By Different Avoidable Cancers

Causes	Percent 1981 (U.S.)*	Percent 1998 (U.K.)**
Tobacco	25–40	29–31
Diet	10–70	20–50
Medicines	0.3–1.5	<1
Infection: parasites, bacteria, viruses	10 best estimate	10–20
Ionizing and UV light	2–4	5–7
Occupation	2–8	2–4
Pollution: air, water, food	<1–5	1–5
Physical inactivity		1–2

*Doll R and Peto R. The causes of cancer: quantitative estimates of avoidable risks of cancer in the United States today. *Journal of the National Cancer Institute* 1981;66:1191–1308.

**Doll R. Epidemiological evidence of the effects of behavior and the environment on the risk of human cancer. *Recent Results in Cancer Research* 1998;154:3–21.

Today, for men, more than half of the new cancer cases and deaths are from prostate, lung, and colorectal cancers. For women, over half of the new cancer cases and deaths are due to breast, lung, and colorectal cancer. Do environmental factors account for most of these cancers? What is the evidence for this? Besides tobacco, are there any strong environmental contenders linked to these cancers?

There is very solid evidence that environmental factors are the major cause of cancer, although the specific environmental factors involved differ by tumor. Tobacco smoke is the major cause of lung cancer. But there is a long list of other chemicals that cause lung cancer—arsenic, asbestos, PAHs (polyaromatic hydrocarbons), and chromium, to name a few. For breast cancer, hormone use is one of the major factors affecting risk. Prostate cancer has nothing that reaches the level of evidence of lung or breast cancer, although there are a number of strong leads. Physical inactivity is strongly linked to colorectal cancer, as well as a number of dietary factors—low fiber is probably implicated.

In the nearly 25 years since Doll and Peto wrote their seminal analysis of the avoidable causes of cancer (1981), what new data has emerged to modify their estimates?

The estimates are still pretty solid, however, a few things have changed. When Doll and Peto wrote their article, there was very little information on viruses and bacteria. Since then, we have a lot of information. We now know that HIV [human immunodeficiency virus] and HPV [human papillomavirus] are significant risk factors for certain cancers, and the bacterium *H. pylori* is an important risk factor in stomach cancer. There was a suspicion in the early 1980s that viruses were linked to cancer, but there was very little conclusive human data. Another area where strong information has emerged since the 1980s are the health effects of physical activity and obesity—two environmental conditions also tied to diet. For example, physical inactivity is now pretty clearly related to cancers of the colon, breast, and prostate, and associations with additional cancer sites are likely to be made in the future.

A recent report estimated that, in the United States, 14% of deaths from cancer in men and 20% of deaths in women were due to obesity and being overweight. As you alluded to in the previous answer, obesity and being overweight were not mentioned in Doll and Peto's 1981 report. Is there any other environmental/lifestyle factor that you would predict may emerge as a significant cause of cancer deaths within the next decade or two that only accounts for a small percentage of cancer deaths now?

My hunch is that general environmental exposures (pollutants in air and water) will be understood to be more important in the future decades. These won't account for as large a percentage of cancers as tobacco, although they could rise above the 2–5% range because of the large numbers of people exposed. They were on Doll and Peto's list, but there was very little information to back up their estimates (see Table 9.1). Doll and Peto assumed that several environmental exposures in the industrial arena were the same as in the general population. Researchers are beginning to focus on potentially hazardous substances in the water and air. This is a difficult research area and is every bit as hard to study as diet. My suspicion is that we will have much more solid information in the next couple of decades about how these things may contribute to cancer. Now we're reasoning by analogy rather than from real data.

There is currently a lot of information on obesity, but it may be that physical inactivity will turn out to be every bit as important as obesity. Obesity has gotten more attention, in part, because it's easier to study. People remember their weight more easily than they remember physical activity patterns. In addition, to take a good physical activity history involves a much longer questionnaire than required for obesity, and even then there can be considerable misclassification. Weight is just a lot easier to study. However, weight and physical activity are tied together. It's not exactly clear which one is the most important. Probably both contribute to cancer risk. I think in the next few decades we will get much of this sorted out. There is some evidence that people who are physically fit, but overweight, have lower total mortality rates than people who are thin and not fit. That tells you that fitness may be important for general health, and I suspect this will be the case for cancer, too. We also keep adding to the cancer sites which appear to be linked with physical activity. It's very clear that colorectal and breast cancers are linked to physical activity, and prostate, lung, ovarian, and endometrial cancers are probably linked, too.

It is estimated that there are over 100,000 chemicals commonly used by Americans in household cleaners, solvents, pesticides, food additives, lawn care, and other products. And every year, another 1,000 or so are introduced. However, our National Toxicology Program only tests between 5–20 suspected carcinogens every year. For some people, our ignorance about most of the products in the environment is alarming; others are encouraged by the benefits that have already been demonstrated from the control of known causes of cancer. What is your reaction to these statistics?

Our ability to identify hazardous chemicals in the environment is better than these numbers suggest. There is actually a pyramid effect here. It's true that not many bioassays are done every year—these cost millions of dollars to do and take a long time. But there are many experimental steps undertaken prior to launching bioassays that help identify the chemicals or classes of chemicals that have the best chance of being a health problem. The bioassays are, therefore, only carried out on chemicals that have already gone through a number of tests that indicate that we ought to be concerned about them. It is correct that many chemicals have not been put through a standard bioassay, but they are usually the ones for which there are no other data to suggest they might be hazardous. So I think we're doing a lot better than the numbers would suggest. Of course, there will be some that we miss. For example, some substance may not cause genetic alterations—one of the laboratory tests we use to screen for possible cancer-causing substances—but may cause cancer through some immune system activity. So, it will test negative and would not be considered as a candidate for a bioassay. However, another reassuring observation is that many substances that we suspected would cause cancer in animals actually do not. Of course, it is possible that they do cause cancer in humans, but, in fact, our experience has shown us that most of the chemicals we have tested don't cause cancer.

Section 9.2

Carcinogens

This section excerpted from "Cancer and the Environment," U.S. Department of Health and Human Services (hhs.gov), 2003. Reviewed by David A. Cooke, MD, FACP, June 2009.

What Substances in the Environment Are Known to Cause or Are Likely to Cause Cancer in Humans?

Every two years, scientists from a wide range of government agencies and educational institutions collaborate with scientists from the National Toxicology Program (NTP) in Research Triangle Park, North Carolina, to publish the *Report on Carcinogens*. The report identifies substances that are either known to cause or suspected of causing cancer in humans and to which a significant number of people in the United States are exposed. It is the source for the agents listed in this section.

This section does not include all of the more than 200 agents listed in the *Report on Carcinogens*. Those discussed here are those for which there is a great deal of public interest.

Tobacco

Exposure to the carcinogens in tobacco products accounts for about one-third of all cancer deaths in the United States each year. Cigarette, cigar, and pipe smoking; chewing tobacco; snuff; and exposure to environmental tobacco smoke (ETS or secondhand smoke) are all linked to increased cancer risks. Cigarette, cigar, and pipe smoking have been associated with cancers of the lung, mouth, bladder, colon, kidney, throat, nasal cavity, voice box, esophagus, lip, stomach, cervix, liver, and pancreas, and with leukemia; smokeless tobacco has been linked to cancers of the mouth; and ETS has been implicated in lung cancer. Cigarette smoke contains more than 100 cancer-causing substances. The risk for cancers of the mouth, voice box, and esophagus is further increased among smokers who also drink more than two drinks/day.

Diet/Weight/Physical Inactivity

Because there are few definite relationships between food and cancer, the *Report on Carcinogens* does not refer to the cancer-related effects of specific foods. However, several studies show that heavy consumption of red and preserved meats, salt-preserved foods, and salt probably increase the risk of colorectal and stomach cancers. There is also evidence that a diet rich in fruits and vegetables may decrease the risks of esophageal, stomach, and colorectal cancers.

Being overweight or obese appears to be one of the most important modifiable causes of cancer, after tobacco. Large population studies show a consistent association between obesity and certain kinds of cancer. The strongest links are with breast cancer in older women, and cancers of the endometrium, kidney, colon, and esophagus.

There is strong evidence that physical inactivity increases the risk for colon and breast cancer. The beneficial effect of exercise is greatest among very active people. Together, it is estimated that inactivity and obesity account for 25 to 30% of the cases of several major cancers—colon, breast (postmenopausal), endometrial, kidney, and cancer of the esophagus.

Alcoholic Drinks

Heavy drinkers (more than two drinks/day) have an increased risk of cancer, particularly among those who also smoke. Cancers associated with heavy drinking include cancers of the mouth, throat, voice box, liver, and esophagus. There is also some evidence linking alcohol and cancer of the breast.

Ultraviolet Radiation

Ultraviolet (UV) radiation from the sun, sunlamps, or tanning beds causes premature aging of the skin and DNA damage that can lead to melanoma and other forms of skin cancer. The incidence of skin cancers is rapidly increasing.

Viruses and Bacteria

Infectious agents such as viruses and bacteria clearly contribute to the development of several types of cancer. A sexually transmitted virus called human papillomavirus (HPV) is the primary cause of cervical and anal cancer. Women who begin sexual intercourse at age 16 or younger or have many sexual partners have an increased risk of infection. Infection with HPV is increasingly common. However, even though infection with HPV is the primary cause of cervical cancer, most infections do not result in cancer.

Hepatitis B (HBV) and hepatitis C (HCV) viral infections are major causes of liver cancer. In Asia and Africa, HBV is usually acquired in childhood and it carries a high risk of liver cancer. HBV infection is less common in the United States. Risk factors for HBV include occupational exposure to blood products, injection drug use, and high-risk sexual behavior (unprotected sex with multiple partners). A vaccine is available to prevent infection with HBV. The rising incidence of liver cancer in the United States is thought to be due to HCV. The strongest risk factor for HCV infection is injection drug use, but sexual transmission is also possible. People who received a blood transfusion prior to 1989 may also be infected with this virus. Currently, there is no vaccine for HCV.

Almost all adults are infected with Epstein-Barr virus (EBV), which is linked to some types of lymphoma. EBV is the virus that causes mononucleosis. Another type of virus called Kaposi's sarcoma–associated herpesvirus (KSHV), also known as human herpesvirus 8 (HHV-8), is linked to a particular type of sarcoma called Kaposi's sarcoma. KSHV infection only occurs through close person-to-person contacts. In Mediterranean and African countries, KSHV infection in childhood is common. In the U.S., KSHV infection is most common in homosexual men. The risk of cancer for people infected with either KSHV or EBV is low, except for those whose immune systems are weakened, such as people infected with HIV, the virus that causes acquired immunodeficiency syndrome (AIDS).

Infection with *Helicobacter pylori*, a bacterium, is widespread and is the primary cause of peptic ulcers and chronic gastritis (inflammation of the stomach). *H. pylori* contributes to the development of stomach cancer. Most *H. pylori* infections, however, result in neither symptoms nor cancer.

Ionizing Radiation

Ionizing radiation is invisible, high-frequency radiation that can damage the DNA or genes inside the body.

Everyone is exposed to very small doses of ionizing radiation from cosmic rays (rays that enter the earth's atmosphere from outer space). Radiation from this source may account for a very small percentage (about 1%) of our total cancer risk.

Some homes have elevated levels of radon, a naturally occurring radioactive gas found at low levels in most soil. Radon is produced by the breakdown of uranium, which naturally releases low levels of ionizing radiation. Higher levels of radon can be found in certain types of rocky soil. The health effects of radon were first seen in the elevated levels of lung cancer found in underground uranium miners in the United States and around the world. Radon gas seeps into homes from the surrounding soil through cracks and other openings in the foundation. About 1 out of 20 homes has elevated levels of radon. Even though the cancer risks for radon exposure in the home are much lower than for radon-exposed miners, it is estimated that about 20,000 lung cancer deaths every year are caused by radon exposure in homes. There are various strategies for reducing residential radon exposure.

Another source of ionizing radiation is the radioactive substances released by atomic bombs or nuclear weapons known as "fallout." The doses of ionizing radiation received by the atomic bomb survivors in Japan resulted in increased risks of leukemia and cancers of the breast, thyroid, lung, stomach, and other organs. Radioactive substances were also released in the aboveground atomic bomb testing conducted by the U.S. government in the late 1950s and early 1960s in Nevada. People exposed, especially as children, to one radioactive form of iodine, called Iodine-131 or I-131, which collects in the thyroid gland, may have an increased risk of thyroid disease, including thyroid cancer. For more information visit cancer.gov/i131.

People are also exposed to ionizing radiation during certain medical procedures. Some patients who receive radiation to treat cancer or other conditions may be at increased cancer risk. For example, persons treated with radiation in childhood to treat acne, ringworm, and other head and neck conditions have been shown to be at increased risk for thyroid cancer and other tumors of the head and neck. X-rays used to diagnose or screen for a disease are also forms of ionizing radiation. The dose of radiation from procedures used to diagnose or screen for a disease is much lower than the dose received to treat a disease. Most studies on the long-term effects of exposure to radiation used to diagnose or screen for cancers or other diseases have not shown an elevated cancer risk, but it is possible that there is a small risk associated with this exposure. One exception is children whose mothers received diagnostic X-rays during pregnancy. These children were found to have increased risks of childhood leukemia and other types of cancer, which led to the current ban on diagnostic X-rays in pregnant women. Several other studies of women who received small weekly X-ray doses to the chest over extended periods to monitor treatment for tuberculosis showed a radiation-related increased risk of breast cancer.

Pesticides

Of the nearly 900 active ingredients in registered pesticides in the United States, about 20 have been found to be carcinogenic in animals, although not all have been tested. In the United States, a number of pesticides have been banned or their use has been restricted. These include ethylene oxide, amitrole, some chlorophenoxy herbicides, DDT [dichlorodiphenyltrichloroethane], dimethylhydrazine, hexachlorobenzene, hexamethylphosphoramide, chlordecone, lead acetate, lindane, mirex, nitrofen, and toxaphene. Studies of people with high exposures to pesticides, such as farmers, pesticide applicators, crop duster pilots, and manufacturers, have found high rates of blood and lymphatic system cancers, cancers of the lip, stomach, lung, brain, and prostate, as well as melanoma and other skin cancers. So far, human studies do not allow researchers to sort out exactly which pesticides are linked to which cancers. Therefore, most of these pesticides are still listed in the *Report on Carcinogens* as likely to be cancer causing, rather than as known carcinogens. For more information, visit www.aghealth.org.

Medical Drugs

Some drugs used to treat cancer (e.g., cyclophosphamide, chlorambucil, melphalan) have been shown to increase the occurrence of second cancers, including leukemia. Others that are used as immunosuppressants, such as cyclosporin and azathioprine for patients having organ transplants, also are associated with increased cancer risks, especially lymphoma. However, the Food and Drug Administration has determined that the life-saving benefits of these drugs outweigh the additional cancer risks years later. It is recommended that people weigh the risks and benefits concerning the use of a drug with the help of a physician or other health care specialist. Some medicines have been linked to reduced risk of cancer. For example, some studies find a reduced risk of colon cancer in persons who regularly take aspirin or other nonsteroidal anti-inflammatory medicines. Evidence for protection of other cancers such as breast cancer or prostate cancer is inconsistent.

Estrogens used to treat symptoms of menopause and other gynecological conditions have been shown to increase the incidence of endometrial cancer. In addition, some studies have shown an increased risk of breast cancer with estrogen use, but a reduced risk of colon cancer. Progesterone, another hormone now taken in combination with estrogen for hormone replacement therapy in older women, helps to protect against the increased endometrial cancer risk with estrogen alone. However, increased risks of breast cancer, heart disease, stroke, and blood clots have recently been shown to be associated with the use of estrogen plus progestin, a synthetic form of progesterone. Long-term users of combination oral contraceptives have substantially reduced risks of endometrial and ovarian cancers, but may experience increases in early-onset breast cancers and liver cancer. The amount of estrogen and progesterone in oral contraceptives is substantially less than in previous years, which means that the risk of the current formulations is likely to be less than those used in the past.

Increased risks of endometrial cancer as well as increased risks of stroke and blood clots are also associated with tamoxifen use. Tamoxifen is a synthetic hormone used to prevent the recurrence of breast cancer after breast cancer surgery. It is also used to prevent breast cancer in women at high risk for the disease because of family history or other factors. Again, it is recommended that people weigh the risks and benefits concerning the use of a drug with the help of a physician or other health care specialist.

Diethylstilbestrol (DES) is a synthetic form of estrogen prescribed to pregnant women from the early 1940s to 1971. It was found that their daughters who were exposed to DES before birth have an increased chance of developing a rare type of cervical and vaginal cancer. In addition, women who took DES during pregnancy may have a slightly higher risk for developing breast cancer. Based on these findings, DES is no longer prescribed, and its use as a cattle feed additive has been banned.

Solvents

Several solvents used in paint thinners, paint and grease removers, and in the dry cleaning industry are known or suspected of being cancer causing in animal studies. These include benzene, carbon tetrachloride, chloroform, dichloromethane (methylene chloride), tetrachloroethylene, and trichloroethylene. Human studies are suggestive, but not conclusive, except for benzene. Therefore, with the exception of benzene, these substances are listed as likely to be cancer causing in humans.

Benzene is known to cause leukemia in humans. It has widespread use as a solvent in the chemical and drug industries and as a gasoline component. After 1997, its use as an ingredient in pesticides was banned. Workers employed in the petrochemical industry, pharmaceutical industry, leather industry, rubber industry, gas stations, and in the transportation industry are exposed to benzene. Inhaling contaminated air is the primary method of exposure. Because benzene is present in gasoline, air contamination occurs around gas stations and in congested areas with automobile exhaust. It is also present in cigarette smoke. It is estimated that half of the exposure to benzene in the United States is from cigarette smoking. About half of the U.S. population is exposed to benzene from industrial sources, and virtually everyone in the country is exposed to benzene in gasoline.

Fibers, Fine Particles, and Dust

Exposures to various fibers, fine particles, and dust occur in several industrial settings and are associated with increased cancer risks. Exposure can also occur in nonindustrial settings. Asbestos fibers and all commercial forms of asbestos are human carcinogens. Increased rates of mesothelioma, a rare cancer of the lining of the lung and abdominal cavity, and cancer of the lung have been consistently observed in a variety of occupations involving asbestos exposure. Asbestos exposures account for the largest percent of occupational cancer, with the greatest risks among workers who smoke. Asbestos fibers are released into the environment from the use and deterioration of more than 5,000 asbestos products, including roofing, thermal, and electrical insulation; cement pipe and sheet; flooring; gaskets; plastics; and textile and paper products. Workers in asbestos insulation, brake maintenance and repair, and building demolition jobs are exposed to high levels of asbestos. The entire population may have been exposed to some degree because asbestos has been so widely used. Because the use of asbestos has been greatly restricted in the United States, exposure to the general population has decreased. Nonetheless, workers employed in construction trades, electricians, and carpenters can still experience high levels of asbestos exposures through renovations, repairs, and demolitions. Ceramic fibers are now used as insulation materials and are a replacement for asbestos. Because they can withstand high temperatures, they are used to line furnaces and kilns. These fibers cause lung cancer in experimental animals. Silica dusts are associated with an excess risk of lung cancer in humans and are found in industrial and occupational settings such as coal mines, mills, granite quarrying and processing, crushed stone and related industries, and sandblasting operations. Wood dust, associated with cancers of the nasal cavities and sinuses, is a known carcinogen for unprotected workers who are exposed regularly from sanding operations and furniture manufacturing.

Dioxins

Dioxins are unwanted byproducts of chemical processes that contain chlorine and hydrocarbons (substances that contain both hydrogen and carbon). There are at least 100 different kinds of dioxins. They are not intentionally manufactured by industry. They are produced by paper and pulp bleaching; incineration of municipal, toxic, and hospital wastes; certain electrical fires; and smelters (plants where metal is extracted from ores). They are also found as a contaminant in some insecticides, herbicides, and wood preservatives. Dioxins are widespread environmental contaminants. They accumulate in fats and break down slowly. A particular dioxin that is likely to be carcinogenic to humans is called TCDD (2,3,7,8-tetrachlorodibenzo-p-dioxin). TCDD is highly carcinogenic in animals, and, in highly exposed workers, increased overall cancer death rates have been reported. Fortunately, modifications of industrial processes such as bleaching and incineration have resulted in reduced dioxin emissions and have lowered dioxin levels in people. The general population is exposed to low levels of TCDD primarily from eating dairy products, fish, and meat, including poultry.

Polycyclic Aromatic Hydrocarbons (PAHs)

A number of studies show increased incidence of cancer (lung, skin, and urinary cancers) in humans exposed to mixtures of polycyclic aromatic hydrocarbons (PAHs). The primary source of PAHs is from burning carbon-containing compounds. PAHs in air are produced by burning wood and fuel for homes. They are also contained in gasoline and diesel exhaust, soot, coke, cigar and cigarette smoke, and charcoal-broiled foods. In addition, they are the byproducts of open fires, waste incinerators, coal gasification, and coke oven emissions. Foods that contain small amounts of PAHs include smoked, barbecued, or charcoal-broiled foods, roasted coffees, and sausages.

Metals

Arsenic compounds are associated with many forms of skin, lung, bladder, kidney, and liver cancers, particularly when high levels are consumed in drinking water. In addition, occupational exposure to inhaled arsenic, especially in mining and copper smelting, has been consistently associated with an increased risk of lung cancer. Arsenic is also used in wood preservatives, glass, herbicides, insecticides (ant killers), and pesticides, and it is a general environmental contaminant of air, food, and water.

Beryllium compounds are known to cause lung cancer based primarily on studies of workers in beryllium production facilities. These compounds are used as metals for aerospace and defense industries; for electrical components, X-ray tubes, nuclear weapons, aircraft brakes, rocket fuel additives, light aircraft construction, and the manufacture of ceramics; and as an additive to glass and plastics, dental applications, and golf clubs. Industry is also increasingly using beryllium for fiber optics and cellular network communication systems. Workers can be exposed through jobs related to the aforementioned activities, as well as through recycling of computers, cell phones, and other high-tech products. Outside of these industries, beryllium exposure occurs primarily through the burning of coal and fuel oil. The general population can be exposed to trace amounts of beryllium by inhaling air and consuming food contaminated with beryllium residues. Small concentrations have been reported in drinking water, food, and tobacco.

Studies of groups of workers show that cadmium metal and cadmium compounds are associated with an increased risk of lung cancer. Workers with the highest exposures are those involved in removing zinc and lead from minerals, producing cadmium powders, welding cadmium-coated steel, and working with solders that contain cadmium. Cadmium metal is primarily used to coat metals to prevent corrosion. Other uses are in plastic and synthetic products, in batteries, as stabilizers for polyvinyl chloride, and in fungicides. The industrial processes involved in making these products release cadmium into the air, surface water, ground water, and topsoil where it can be taken up by both land and water plants and, in turn, transferred to animals. Contaminated topsoil that allows uptake into tobacco plants may be indirectly responsible for the greatest nonoccupational human exposure to cadmium—smoking. Food is the main source of human exposure to cadmium for nonsmokers.

Some chromium compounds are known to cause lung cancer. The steel industry is the major consumer of chromium. It is used for protection against corrosion of metal accessories, including automotive parts, as well as for electroplating, layering one metal over another. Electroplating converts chromium 6, the carcinogenic form, to a noncarcinogenic form of chromium. This means that workers who handle chromium 6 are at greater risk than the general population. Other uses include nuclear and high-temperature research; the textile and leather-tanning industry; pigments for floor covering products, paper, cement, and asphalt roofing; and creating an emerald color in colored glass. Chromium is widely distributed in the air, water, soil, and food, and the entire population is probably exposed to some of these compounds. The highest exposure occurs in occupations related to stainless steel production, welding, chrome plating, and leather tanning. Typical levels in most fresh foods are low.

Lead acetate and lead phosphate are likely to be human carcinogens based on the evidence of kidney and brain tumors in animal studies. Lead acetate is used in cotton dyes; as a coating for metals; as a drier in paints, varnishes, and pigment inks; as a colorant in certain permanent hair dyes (progressive dyes); in explosives; and in washes to treat poison ivy. Lead phosphate is used as a stabilizer in certain plastics and specialty glass. Primary exposures are through skin contact, eating, and inhaling.

Nickel and nickel compounds are associated with several kinds of cancers in rats and mice. Studies in human populations link nickel exposure to cancers of the nasal cavity, lung, and possibly the larynx (voice box). Nickel is used in steel, dental fillings, copper and brass, permanent magnets, storage batteries, and glazes. Because nickel is present in the air, water, soil, food, and consumer products in the United States, we are exposed through eating, breathing, and skin contact.

Diesel Exhaust Particles

The particles in diesel exhaust are suspected of being carcinogens because of the elevated lung cancer rates found in occupational groups exposed to diesel exhaust, such as railroad workers, mine workers, bus garage workers, trucking company workers, car mechanics, and people who work around diesel generators. Cancer risks from lower exposures in day-to-day living are not known.

Toxins from Fungi

Aflatoxins are cancer-causing substances produced by certain types of fungi growing on food. Grains and peanuts are the most common foods on which these fungi grow. Meat, eggs, and milk from animals that eat aflatoxin-contaminated feed are other sources of exposure. Agricultural workers are potentially at risk if they inhale contaminated airborne grain dust. Exposure to high levels of aflatoxins increases the risk of liver cancer. Peanuts are screened for aflatoxin in most countries, including the United States, before processing. The risk of aflatoxin exposure is higher in developing countries where there is no screening for the fungus.

Vinyl Chloride

Vinyl chloride, a colorless gas, is a human carcinogen associated with lung cancers and angiosarcomas (blood vessel tumors) of the liver and brain. It is used almost exclusively in the United States by the plastics industry in manufacturing many consumer products, including containers, wrapping film, electrical insulation, water and drain pipes, hosing, flooring, windows, and credit cards. Human exposure can occur primarily in workers in the plastic industry, not by using the end products such as vinyl siding or hosing. The major source of releases of vinyl chloride into the environment is believed to be from the plastics industries. People living near a plastics plant are exposed by breathing contaminated air, but the exposure of the general population away from the plant is essentially zero.

Benzidine

Benzidine was one of the first chemicals recognized as being associated with increased cancer risk in humans. As early as 1921, increased cases of bladder cancer were reported to be associated with benzidine, a compound used in the production of more than 250 benzidine-based dyes for textiles, paper, and leather products. Human exposure to either benzidine or benzidine-based dyes is now known to be carcinogenic. The dyes break down into benzidine once inside the body. In most cases, dyes that metabolize to benzidine are hazards only in the vicinity of dye and pigment plants where wastes may escape or be discharged.

Section 9.3

Cancer Clusters

"Cancer Clusters," National Cancer Institute (www.cancer.gov), October 5, 2006.

Defining Disease Clusters

A disease cluster is the occurrence of a greater than expected number of cases of a particular disease within a group of people, a geographic area, or a period of time. Clusters of diseases have concerned scientists for centuries. Some recent disease clusters include the initial cases of a rare type of pneumonia among homosexual men in the early 1980s that led to the identification of HIV and AIDS; the outbreak in 2003 of a respiratory illness, later identified as severe acute respiratory syndrome (SARS), caused by a previously unrecognized virus; and periodic outbreaks of food poisoning caused by eating food contaminated with bacteria.

Cancer clusters may be suspected when people report that several family members, friends, neighbors, or co-workers have been diagnosed with the same or related cancer(s). In the 1960s, one of the best-known cancer clusters emerged, involving many cases of mesothelioma (a rare cancer of the lining of the chest and abdomen). Researchers traced the development of mesothelioma to exposure to asbestos, a fibrous mineral that was used heavily in shipbuilding during World War II and has also been used in manufacturing industrial and consumer products. Working with asbestos is the major risk factor (something that may increase the chance of developing a disease) for mesothelioma.

Facts about Cancer

Some concepts about cancer that can be helpful when trying to understand suspected cancer clusters are the following:

- Cancer is the uncontrolled growth and spread of abnormal cells anywhere in the body. However, cancer is not just one disease; it is actually an umbrella term for at least 100 different but related diseases.

- Each type of cancer has certain known and/or suspected risk factors associated with it.
- Cancer is not caused by injuries, nor is it contagious. It cannot be passed from one person to another like a cold or flu virus.
- Cancer is almost always caused by a combination of factors that interact in ways that are not yet fully understood.
- Carcinogenesis (the process by which normal cells are transformed into cancer cells) involves a series of changes within cells that usually occur over many years. More than 10 years can go by between the exposure to a carcinogen (any substance that causes cancer) and a diagnosis of cancer, which makes it difficult to pinpoint the cause of that cancer.
- Cancer is more likely to occur as people get older; because people are living longer, more cases of cancer can be expected in the future. This increased life expectancy may create the impression that cancer is becoming much more common, even though an increase in the number of cases of cancer is related in large part to the growing number of elderly people in the population.
- Some racial and ethnic groups have higher rates of cancer than other racial and ethnic groups. Such differences may be due to multiple factors, such as late stage of disease at diagnosis, barriers to health care access, history of other diseases, biologic and genetic differences, health behaviors, and other risk factors.
- Cancer, in general, is common. More than 17 million new cases of cancer have been diagnosed since 1990.

Facts about Cancer Clusters

Reported disease clusters of any kind, including suspected cancer clusters, are investigated by epidemiologists (scientists who study the frequency, distribution, causes, and control of diseases in populations). Epidemiologists use their knowledge of diseases, environmental science, lifestyle factors, and biostatistics to try to determine whether a suspected cluster represents a true excess of cancer cases.

Epidemiologists have identified certain circumstances that may lead them to suspect a potential common source or cause of cancer among people thought to be part of a cancer cluster. A suspected cancer cluster is more likely to be a true cluster, rather than a coincidence, if it involves one or more of the following factors:

- A large number of cases of one type of cancer, rather than several different types
- A rare type of cancer, rather than common types
- An increased number of cases of a certain type of cancer in an age group that is not usually affected by that type of cancer

Before epidemiologists can assess a suspected cancer cluster accurately, they must determine whether the type of cancer involved is a primary (original) cancer or a cancer that has metastasized (spread from another organ). This is important to know because scientists consider only the primary cancer when they investigate a possible cancer cluster. Epidemiologists also try to establish whether the suspected exposure has the potential to cause the reported cancer, based on what is known about that cancer's likely causes and about the cancer-causing potential of the exposure.

After developing a case definition (the guidelines that determine whether the cases being investigated are related to the cluster), epidemiologists must identify the time period of concern and the population at risk. They then calculate the expected number of cases and compare that number with the observed number of cases. Epidemiologists must show that the number of cancer cases that have occurred is significantly greater than the expected number of cases, given the age, gender, and racial distribution of the group of people at risk of developing the disease.

Epidemiologists must also determine if the cancer cases could have occurred by chance. They often test for "statistical significance," which is a mathematical measure of the difference between groups. The difference is said to be statistically significant if it is greater than what would be expected to happen by chance alone. In common practice, a statistically significant finding means that the probability that the observed number of cases could have happened by chance alone is 5% or less. For instance, if one examines the number of cancer cases in 100 neighborhoods, and cancer cases are occurring by chance alone, one should expect to find about five neighborhoods with a statistically significant elevation in the number of cancer cases. In other words, some amount of clustering within the same family or neighborhood may occur simply by chance.

Accurately defining the group of people who should be considered "at risk" is important when investigating a possible cancer cluster. One of the greatest problems in defining clusters is the tendency to expand the geographic borders of the cluster to include additional cases of the suspected disease as they are discovered. The tendency to define the borders of a cluster on the basis of where known cases are located, rather than to first define the population and geographic area and then determine if the number of cancers is excessive, creates many "clusters" that are not real.

Epidemiologists must also consider that a confirmed cancer cluster may not be the result of any single, external cause or hazard. A cancer cluster could be the result of chance, an error in the calculation of the expected number of cancer cases, or differences in the case definition between observed and expected cases. Moreover, because people change where they live from time to time, it can be difficult for epidemiologists to identify previous exposures and find the medical records that are needed to determine the kind of cancer a person had—or if it was cancer at all.

Because a variety of factors often work together to create the appearance of a cluster where nothing abnormal is occurring, most reports of suspected cancer clusters are not shown to be true clusters. Many reported clusters do not include enough cases for epidemiologists to arrive at any conclusions.

Sometimes, even when a suspected cluster has enough cases for study, a greater than expected number of cases cannot be demonstrated. Other times, epidemiologists find a true excess of cases, but they cannot find an explanation for it. For example, a suspected carcinogen may cause cancer only under certain circumstances, making its impact difficult to detect.

Genetics and Environment

Because most cancers are thought to be caused by a combination of factors related to genetics and environment (including behavior and lifestyle), studies of suspected cancer clusters usually focus on these two issues. Genetic factors are inherited, that is, passed from parents to children. However, establishing a genetic-environmental interaction (significant and valid evidence that a specific genetic factor leads to an increased chance that a particular environmental exposure will result in cancer) requires studies of large populations over long periods of time. Researchers are just beginning to learn about the roles genetics and environmental exposures play in carcinogenesis. Some of their discoveries are outlined here:

Genetics

- All cancers develop because of genetic alterations of one kind or another. An alteration is a change or mutation in the physical structure of a gene that interferes with the gene's normal functions.

- Some genetic alterations that increase the risk of cancer are present at birth in the genes of all cells in the body, including reproductive cells. These changes, which are called germline mutations, can be passed from parent to child. This type of alteration is known as an inherited susceptibility; most cancers are not due to an inherited susceptibility.
- Most cancers result from genetic changes that occur after birth during one's lifetime. Genetic changes can occur in any cell that divides. These genetic changes are called somatic alterations.
- Familial cancer clusters (cancer that occurs in families more often than would be expected by chance) have been reported for many types of cancer. Because cancer is a common disease, it is not unusual for several cases to occur within a family. Familial cancer clusters are sometimes linked to inherited susceptibility, but environmental factors and chance may also be involved.
- Having an inherited susceptibility for a type of cancer does not necessarily mean that the individual will be diagnosed with the cancer; it means the chance of developing cancer increases if other factors that promote the development of cancer are present or are encountered later.

Environment

- The term environment includes not only air, water, and soil, but also substances and conditions in the home and workplace. It also includes diet; the use of tobacco, alcohol, or drugs; exposure to chemicals; and exposure to sunlight and other forms of radiation.
- People are exposed to a variety of environmental factors for varying lengths of time, and these factors interact in ways that are still not fully understood. Further, individuals have varying levels of susceptibility to these factors.
- Hazardous substances are often found in higher levels in the workplace than in the general environment. For this reason, some workers may have greater and longer exposures to such substances than the general population. Findings of higher than expected numbers of cancer cases among workers in particular occupations or industries provide important leads regarding causes of cancer among the general public. In fact, occupational studies (studies of specific groups of workers) have identified many specific cancer-causing substances and have provided

the motivation to find ways to reduce or eliminate exposures in the workplace and elsewhere.

Reporting Suspected Cancer Clusters

A suspected cancer cluster may be reported to a state or local health department or state cancer registry. State and local health departments and cancer registries use established criteria to investigate reports of cancer clusters. When a suspected cancer cluster is first reported, the investigating department or agency gathers information and gives the inquirer general information about cancer clusters. Although investigators may use different processes, most follow a basic procedure in which increasingly specific information is obtained and analyzed in stages. Investigators are likely to request the following:

- Information about the potential cluster: type(s) of cancer, number of cases, suspected exposure(s), and geographic area/ time period of concern
- Information about each person with cancer in the potential cluster: name, address, telephone number, gender, race, age, occupation(s), as well as area(s) lived in/length of time
- Information about each case of cancer: type of cancer, date of diagnosis, age at diagnosis, possible causes, metastatic sites, and physician contact

Most reports of suspected cancer clusters are resolved at this initial contact because concerned individuals realize that what seemed like a cancer cluster is not a true cluster. If further evaluation is needed, epidemiologists will take the following steps to investigate a possible cancer cluster:

- Attempt to verify the reported cases by contacting patients and relatives and obtaining medical records
- Compare the number of cases in the suspected cancer cluster with information in census data and cancer registries to determine if there is a higher than expected number of cases
- Review the scientific literature to establish whether the reported cancer(s) has been linked to the suspected exposure
- Work with federal agencies, if necessary, to gather additional information to help decide whether to conduct a comprehensive epidemiological study

Chapter 10

Respiratory Problems with Environmental Triggers

Chapter Contents

Section 10.1

Asthma and Air Pollution

"You Can Control Your Asthma," Centers for Disease Control and Prevention (www.cdc.gov), 2006.

What is asthma?

Asthma is a disease that affects your lungs. It is the most common long-term disease of children, but adults have asthma, too. Asthma causes repeated episodes of wheezing, breathlessness, chest tightness, and nighttime or early morning coughing. If you have asthma, you have it all the time, but you will have asthma attacks only when something bothers your lungs.

We know that if someone in your family has asthma, you are also more likely to have it. In most cases, we don't know what causes asthma, and we don't know how to cure it. You can control your asthma by knowing the warning signs of an attack, staying away from things that trigger an attack, and following the advice of your health care provider. When you control your asthma, you won't have symptoms like wheezing or coughing, you'll sleep better, you won't miss work or school, you can take part in all physical activities, and you won't have to go to the hospital.

How is asthma diagnosed?

Asthma can be hard to diagnose, especially in children under five years of age. Regular physical checkups that include checking your lung function and checking for allergies can help your health care provider make the right diagnosis.

During a checkup, the health care provider will ask you questions about whether you cough a lot, especially at night, and whether your breathing problems are worse after physical activity or during a particular time of year. Health care providers will also ask about other symptoms such as chest tightness, wheezing, and colds that last more than 10 days. They will ask you whether your family members have or have had asthma, allergies, or other breathing problems, and they will ask you questions about your home. The health care provider will also ask you about missing school or work and about any trouble you may have doing certain activities.

A lung function test, called spirometry, is another way to diagnose asthma. A spirometer measures the largest amount of air you can exhale, or breathe out, after taking a very deep breath. The spirometer can measure airflow before and after you use asthma medicine.

What is an asthma attack?

An asthma attack happens in your body's airways, which are the paths that carry air to your lungs. As the air moves through your lungs, the airways become smaller, like the branches of a tree are smaller than the tree trunk. During an asthma attack, the sides of the airways in your lungs swell, and the airways shrink. Less air gets in and out of your lungs, and mucus that your body produces clogs up the airways even more. The attack may include coughing, chest tightness, wheezing, and trouble breathing. Some people call an asthma attack an "episode."

What causes an asthma attack?

An asthma attack can occur when you are exposed to things in the environment such as house dust mites and tobacco smoke. These are called asthma triggers. Some of the most important triggers are listed later in this section.

How is asthma treated?

You can control your asthma and avoid an attack by taking your medicine exactly as your health care provider tells you to do and by avoiding things that can cause an attack.

Not everyone with asthma takes the same medicine. Some medicines can be inhaled, or breathed in, and some can be taken as a pill. Asthma medicines come in two types—quick-relief and long-term control. Quick-relief medicines control the symptoms of an asthma attack. If you need to use your quick-relief medicines more and more, you should visit your health care provider to see if you need a different medicine. Long-term control medicines help you have fewer and milder attacks, but they don't help you if you're having an asthma attack.

Asthma medicines can have side effects, but most side effects are mild and soon go away. Ask your health care provider about the side effects of your medicines.

The important thing to remember is that you can control your asthma. With your health care provider's help, make your own asthma management plan so that you know what to do based on your own symptoms. Decide who should have a copy of your plan and where he or she should keep it. You can learn more about asthma management plans from the American Academy of Family Physicians (familydoctor.org/x2272.xml). Take your long-term control medicine even when you don't have symptoms.

What are some important asthma triggers?

Environmental Tobacco Smoke (Secondhand Smoke): Environmental tobacco smoke is often called "secondhand smoke" because it is smoke that is breathed in not by a smoker but by a second person nearby. Parents, friends, and relatives of children with asthma should try to stop smoking and should never smoke around a person with asthma. They should only smoke outdoors and not in the family home or car. They should not allow others to smoke in the home, and they should make sure their child's school is smoke-free.

Dust Mites: Dust mites are in almost everybody's home, but they don't cause everybody to have asthma attacks. If you have asthma, dust mites may be a trigger for an attack. To help prevent asthma attacks, use mattress covers and pillow case covers to make a barrier between dust mites and yourself. Don't use down-filled pillows, quilts, or comforters. Remove stuffed animals and clutter from your bedroom.

Outdoor Air Pollution: Pollution caused by industrial emissions and automobile exhaust can cause an asthma attack. Pay attention to air quality forecasts on radio and television and plan your activities for when air pollution levels will be low if air pollution aggravates your asthma.

Cockroach Allergen: Cockroaches and their droppings may trigger an asthma attack. Get rid of cockroaches in your home and keep them from coming back by taking away their food and water. Cockroaches are usually found where food is eaten and crumbs are left behind. Remove as many water and food sources as you can because cockroaches need food and water to survive. Vacuum or sweep areas that might attract cockroaches at least every two or three days. You can also use roach traps or gels to decrease the number of cockroaches in your home.

Pets: Furry pets may trigger an asthma attack. When a furry pet is suspected of causing asthma attacks, the simplest solution is to find the pet another home. If pet owners are too attached to their pets or are unable to locate a safe, new home for the pet, they should keep the pet out of the bedroom of the person with asthma.

Pets should be bathed weekly and kept outside as much as possible. People with asthma are not allergic to their pet's fur, so trimming your pet's fur will not help your asthma. If you have a furry pet, vacuum often to clean up anything that could cause an asthma attack. If your floors have a hard surface, such as wood or tile, and are not carpeted, damp mop them every week.

Mold: When mold is inhaled or breathed in, it can cause an asthma attack. Get rid of mold in all parts of your home to help control your asthma attacks. Keep the humidity level in your home between 35% and 50%. In hot, humid climates, you may need to use an air conditioner or a dehumidifier or both. Fix water leaks, which allow mold to grow behind walls and under floors.

Other Triggers: Strenuous physical exercise; some medicines; bad weather such as thunderstorms, high humidity, or freezing temperatures; and some foods and food additives can trigger an asthma attack.

Strong emotional states can also lead to hyperventilation and an asthma attack.

Learn what triggers your attacks so that you can avoid the triggers whenever possible and be alert for a possible attack when the triggers cannot be avoided.

Remember, *you can control your asthma!*

Section 10.2

Airborne Allergies

"What Can I Do to Reduce Airborne Allergens?" © 2009 The Cleveland Clinic Foundation, 9500 Euclid Avenue, Cleveland, OH 44195. All rights reserved. Reprinted with permission. Additional information is available from the Cleveland Clinic Health Information Center, 216-444-3771, toll-free 800-223-2273 extension 43771, or at http://my.cleveland clinic.org/health.

General Suggestions to Reduce Exposure to Airborne Allergens

- Keep windows and doors closed.
- Avoid using window or attic fans that draw in outside air.
- Use air conditioning.
- Refrain from outside activities, if possible, during times of high pollen counts (if you are sensitive to pollens). Note that peak pollination occurs at different times of the day for different plants (e.g., ragweed in the late morning, grasses in the afternoon).
- Shower or bathe and change clothes following outdoor activity.
- Dry clothes in vented dryer, not outside.

Specific Suggestions to Reduce Exposure to Mold and Fungus Allergens

Outdoor Exposure

- Do not walk through uncut fields, work with compost or dry soil, or rake leaves.
- Keep windows and doors closed.
- Avoid using window or attic fans that draw in outside air.
- Use air conditioning.

Indoor Exposure

- Clean moldy surfaces.
- Wash swamp coolers.
- Fix all water leaks.
- Use air conditioning and a dehumidifier to reduce indoor humidity to < 50%, if possible.

Specific Suggestions to Reduce Exposure to House Dust Mite Allergens

"Must Do" Actions

- Encase mattress, pillow, and box springs in an allergen-impermeable cover.
- Wash bedding weekly in hot water (130° F).
- Reduce indoor humidity to 50%, if possible.
- Remove stuffed toys from the bedroom.

"Should Do" Actions

- Remove carpets from the bedroom and carpets laid on concrete from all rooms.
- Reduce the number of upholstered furniture pieces in the home.
- Use HEPA filters. Electrostatic filters can be used, but note that although they are less efficient than HEPA filters, they still remove particles that can be inhaled.

Specific Suggestions to Reduce Exposure to Animal Allergens

- Remove the pet from the home.
- If removal of the animal is not acceptable, then:
    - keep the pet out of the bedroom and bathroom by closing the door;
    - do not allow the pet on upholstered furniture and carpets;
    - wash the pet weekly to decrease the amount of dander and dried saliva (the evidence to support this recommendation had not been firmly established);

- use a HEPA-type air cleaner in the bedroom and elevate the cleaner off the floor;
- close the air ducts in the bedroom.

Specific Suggestions to Reduce Exposure to Tobacco Smoke and Wood Smoke

While tobacco smoke and wood smoke are not true allergens, they can cause nasal symptoms in patients with inhalant allergies.

- Inform the family that there should be no smoking:
    - around the patient;
    - in the patient's home;
    - in the patient's car.
- Help family members and/or caregivers stop smoking.
- Limit the use of wood-burning stoves and fireplaces. (Encourage use of airtight stove/fireplace if wood must be burned.)

Common Allergen Sources

- Bedding
- Upholstered furniture
- Pets
- Water damage
- Carpet
- Moldy air conditioners, refrigerators, humidifiers, dehumidifiers
- Kitchens or bathrooms without vents or windows; laundry rooms without vented dryers
- Crawl spaces
- Pollens from trees and grasses
- Molds

Section 10.3

Chronic Obstructive Pulmonary Disease (Emphysema and Chronic Bronchitis)

"Facts about Chronic Obstructive Pulmonary Disease (COPD)," Centers for Disease Control and Prevention (www.cdc.gov), 2003. Reviewed by David A. Cooke, MD, FACP, June 2009.

What is chronic obstructive pulmonary disease (COPD)?

Chronic obstructive pulmonary disease, or COPD, refers to a group of diseases that cause airflow blockage and breathing-related problems. It includes emphysema, chronic bronchitis, and in some cases asthma.

COPD is a leading cause of death, illness, and disability in the United States. In 2000, 119,000 deaths, 726,000 hospitalizations, and 1.5 million hospital emergency department visits were caused by COPD. An additional eight million cases of hospital outpatient treatment or treatment by personal physicians were linked to COPD in 2000.

What causes COPD?

In the United States, tobacco use is a key factor in the development and progression of COPD, but asthma, exposure to air pollutants in the home and workplace, genetic factors, and respiratory infections also play a role. In the developing world, indoor air quality is thought to play a larger role in the development and progression of COPD than it does in the United States.

Who has COPD?

In the United States, an estimated 10 million adults had a diagnosis of COPD in 2000, but data from a national health survey suggest that as many as 24 million Americans are affected.

From 1980 to 2000, the COPD death rate for women grew much faster than the rate for men. For U.S. women, the rate rose from 20.1

deaths per 100,000 women to 56.7 deaths per 100,000 women over that 20-year span, while for men the rate grew from 73.0 deaths per 100,000 men to 82.6 deaths per 100,000 men.

U.S. women also had more COPD hospitalizations (404,000) than men (322,000) and more emergency department visits (898,000) than men (551,000) in 2000. Additionally, 2000 marked the first year in which more women (59,936) than men (59,118) died from COPD.

However, the proportion of the U.S. population aged 25–54, both male and female, with mild or moderate COPD has declined over the past quarter century, suggesting that increases in hospitalizations and deaths might not continue.

Why are women's COPD rates rising so much faster than men's?

These increases probably reflect the increase in smoking by women, relative to men, since the 1940s. In the United States, a history of currently or formerly smoking is the risk factor most often linked to COPD, and the increase in the number of women smoking over the past half-century is mirrored in the increase in COPD rates among women. The decreases in rates of mild and moderate COPD in both men and women aged 25–54 in the past quarter century reflect the decrease in overall smoking rates in the United States since the 1960s.

How can COPD be prevented?

Early detection of COPD might alter its course and progress. A simple test can be used to measure pulmonary function and detect COPD in current and former smokers aged 45 and over and anyone with respiratory problems. Avoiding tobacco smoke, home and workplace air pollutants, and respiratory infections are key to preventing the initial development of COPD.

How is COPD treated?

Treatment of COPD requires a careful and thorough evaluation by a physician. The most important aspect of treatment is avoiding tobacco smoke and removing other air pollutants from the patient's home or workplace. Symptoms such as coughing or wheezing can be treated with medication. Respiratory infections should be treated with antibiotics, if appropriate. Patients who have low blood oxygen levels in their blood are often given supplemental oxygen.

Chapter 11

Viruses Spread through Hazards in the Environment

Chapter Contents

Section 11.1

Avian Influenza (Bird Flu)

This section excerpted from "Avian Influenza," Food Safety Research Information Office, U.S. Department of Agriculture (fsrio.nal.usda.gov), March 2008. The full document and references are available online at http://fsrio.nal.usda.gov/document_fsheet.php?product_id=207.

The highly pathogenic avian influenza H5N1 virus has killed millions of poultry in a growing number of countries throughout Asia, Europe, and Africa. Although avian influenza viruses are essentially animal diseases, the highly pathogenic H5N1 is able to infect and kill humans. Health experts are concerned that the co-existence of human flu viruses and avian flu viruses (especially H5N1) will provide an opportunity for genetic material to be exchanged between species-specific viruses, possibly creating a new virulent influenza strain that is easily transmissible and lethal to humans.

In addition to human health concerns, if H5N1 is introduced into the United States by migratory birds or other means, it could have a very significant impact on the North American poultry industry and the safety and stability of the food supply. In an effort to protect our commercial flocks and prevent infected birds from reaching the farm-to-table continuum, scientists, epidemiologists, and animal health experts from industry, government, and academia are developing avian influenza control measures in the areas of biosecurity, surveillance, intervention, and inspection. If, however, H5N1 infected birds should enter the U.S. food supply, commercial food processing interventions currently used to reduce microbial pathogens (i.e., *Salmonella*) would further help to eliminate the virus.

Type A Influenza Viruses and Avian Influenza

Avian influenza (AI) or "bird flu" is a type A influenza virus. Type A influenza viruses are also found in mammals including humans, pigs, horses, and marine mammals. Waterfowl and seabirds provide a natural reservoir for all known influenza A viruses and scientific evidence suggests that mammalian influenza viruses could have evolved from avian influenza viruses even though a significant species barrier exists making avian-to-mammalian transmission inefficient and limited. In May of 1997, when the first influenza A H5N1 subtype was isolated from a child in Hong Kong, it became clearer that, in spite of a host-range restriction, AI can cause zoonotic disease and should be closely monitored.

Influenza A viruses are categorized into subtypes on the basis of two glycoproteins or surface antigens: hemagglutinin (HA) and neuraminidase (NA). Hemagglutinin attaches the virion [complete infectious virus particle] to the host cell receptor for cell entry and neuraminidase facilitates the spread of the progeny virus. There are 16 different HA subtypes, H1 to H16, and 9 different NA subtypes, N1 to N9, allowing for many different combinations of HA and NA proteins. These subtypes are further classified into strains.

There are genetic differences between the influenza A subtypes that infect birds and the subtypes that infect both people and birds. There are three HA subtypes (H1–H3) of influenza A viruses that are known to only infect humans, such as influenza A virus H1N1, which caused the Spanish Flu Epidemic in 1918. The three HA subtypes of the avian influenza A viruses that are known to infect both birds and humans are H5, H7, and H9. The H5 and H7 subtypes cause a highly pathogenic form of AI such as H7N7, H7N3, and H5N1 viruses.

Type A influenza viruses are very unstable and dynamic, evolving through either of two processes: antigenic drift or antigenic shift.

- Antigenic drift happens frequently through point mutations in the two genes that produce the surface antigens HA and NA, causing minor gradual changes in these glycoproteins.
- Antigenic shift is not frequent and represents an abrupt, large change resulting in a new influenza A subtype that has never circulated among humans. Antigenic shift can occur during direct animal-to-human transmission or through genetic reassortment, a process that occurs when human and animal influenza A virus genes exchange genetic material in a host co-infected with both strains. This process can result in a novel human influenza A virus that is lethal and highly transmissible between persons. Some experts suggest that genetic reassortment could have preceded the influenza pandemics of 1918, 1957, and 1968.

The avian influenza A (H5N1) virus currently being spread by migratory birds across Asia, Europe, and Africa, causing poultry outbreaks and mortality in both poultry and humans, is an example of the instability of the type A viruses. According to some scientists, "several lines of evidence indicate that the currently circulating influenza A (H5N1) viruses have in fact evolved to more virulent forms since 1997, with a higher mortality among human cases, different antigenic properties, a different internal gene constellation, and an expanded host range."

As a matter of fact, researchers at the United States Department of Agriculture's (USDA) Agricultural Research Service (ARS) have compared the relationships between H5N1 viruses from multiple countries over several years. The study found that most of the H5N1 isolates from humans were antigenically homogeneous and distinct from viruses circulating before the end of 2003, and some of the 2005 isolates showed evidence of antigenic drift.

Transmission

Avian species differ in their susceptibility to the type A influenza virus, but domestic chickens and turkeys are most susceptible, and large outbreaks have previously been initiated by direct or indirect contact with waterfowl. Generally, wild waterfowl are both natural and silent reservoirs of avian influenza viruses since they carry and transmit the virus to domestic birds and are asymptomatic because the virus is often nonpathogenic to them. However, since late 2002, H5N1 outbreaks in Asia have resulted in severe, systemic disease and mortality among waterfowl, especially young ducks.

Natural carriers (waterfowl, seabirds) shed the AI virus in their feces, nasal secretions, and saliva, transmitting it to domestic flocks of chickens and turkeys. Once the virus has infected one domestic bird in a flock, it quickly spreads because of the following:

- Infected birds shed the virus in their oral secretions and feces for up to 10 days.
- The virus can live for long periods of time (several weeks) in the feces shed from sick birds.
- Poultry are kept in close quarters facilitating further spread of the virus.

According to the World Health Organization (WHO), "susceptible birds become infected when they have contact with contaminated secretions or excretions or with surfaces that are contaminated with secretions or excretions from infected birds. Domesticated birds may become infected with avian influenza virus through direct contact with infected waterfowl or other infected poultry, or through contact with surfaces (such as dirt or cages) or materials (such as water or feed) that have been contaminated with the virus."

Food Safety and Highly Pathogenic (Mainly H5N1) Avian Influenza Viruses

Researchers are evaluating the risk of highly pathogenic avian influenza viruses being transmitted to humans via poultry products in the food chain. The transmission of highly pathogenic avian influenza viruses to humans, mainly H5N1, is not clearly understood and exploring all possible sources of infection and routes of transmission will help determine the public health risk. "The exact entry route(s) of the virus in humans is (are) not known but it is generally accepted that respiratory and/or oropharyngeal tissues are the entry sites."

Current evidence suggests that humans can become infected with H5N1 avian influenza virus following direct contact with live or dead infected birds, and the greatest risk of exposure is for those individuals who handle and slaughter infected birds. It is possible that handling or ingesting "uncooked" or "improperly cooked" poultry products, such as raw chicken meat and eggs, could be a possible transmission route.

Handling and Consumption of Poultry Products

Virus quantities present in infected food of avian origin is quite variable and depends on several factors: virus strain; avian species; type of organ; stage of infection at which the food product was collected; the degree of viremia; physical or chemical treatments on the food (heating, cooking, freezing); and pH changes in meat after slaughter. Refrigeration and freezing can actually help the virus to survive on fresh contaminated poultry meat; therefore, it can be spread during food marketing, distribution, and preparation, making good hygiene practices essential to avoid cross contamination.

Since the H5N1 virus is present in the meat and eggs of infected poultry, some experts are concerned about advising the public that it is safe to eat poultry meat and eggs. These experts have raised the issue that although thorough cooking can kill the virus, people don't always follow the guidelines for safe handling of food. In addition, although evidence doesn't prove that the human intestinal tract is a portal of entry for infection or that the virus replicates in the gut, evidence also doesn't prove against it. Some mammals (felines, ferrets, mice) have already become infected by eating raw infected bird meat.

The WHO clearly states that the key to preventing avian influenza in food consumption is to properly cook the meat product(s). "To date, no epidemiological data suggests that the disease can be transmitted to humans through properly cooked food (even if contaminated with the virus prior to cooking). However, in a few instances, cases have been linked to consumption of dishes made of raw contaminated poultry blood."

The Food Standards Agency (FSA) of the United Kingdom is also advising its consumers that avian flu does not pose a food safety risk and is emphasizing the importance of proper food handling during poultry preparation. Following recent risk assessment advice from its independent expert scientific body, the Advisory Committee on Microbiological Safety of Food (ACMSF), the FSA has suggested that even if the AI virus is present after cooking, several other factors exist in humans that will prevent or limit infection following ingestion. The human factors include: saliva, gastric acid, and the lack of appropriate receptors in the gut needed for the virus to enter the body.

The European Food Safety Authority (EFSA)'s published scientific risk assessment report released in February 2006 titled "Food as a Possible Source of Infection with Highly Pathogenic Avian Influenza Viruses for Humans and other Mammals" also agrees that no direct evidence implicates poultry products in the transmission of H5N1 avian influenza virus to humans. The report reviews the science regarding the fate of highly pathogenic avian influenza viruses in avian species, and the food chain, as a potential vehicle of transmission. It states that no evidence currently exists to prove that the human intestinal tract is a portal of entry or a target organ for the H5N1 virus, but that the existence of an undisclosed virus entry site in the intestinal tract can not be ruled out at this time. The report recommended that experimental inoculation studies be conducted on animal models (i.e., pigs, cats, ferrets) to examine different inoculation routes and virus replication in different tissues along the course of infection.

EFSA's current position statement is, "on present evidence, humans who have acquired the infection have been in direct contact with infected live or dead birds. There is no epidemiological evidence to date that avian influenza can be transmitted to humans through consumption of food, notably poultry and eggs. EFSA and other organizations such as the WHO generally support longstanding food safety advice that chicken and eggs be properly cooked in order to protect consumers from possible risks of food poisoning. Thoroughly cooking poultry meat and eggs also eliminates viruses, thereby providing further safety assurance in the unlikely event that H5N1 virus maybe present in raw poultry products entering the food chain."

Cooking poultry products (chicken, duck, goose, turkey, and guinea fowl) thoroughly and to the proper temperature (at or above 70° C in all parts of the product) is essential to kill the H5N1 virus and prevent transmission from food.

Avian Influenza (H5N1) and Humans

Since the first avian influenza outbreak occurred in 1997, there has been an increasing number of HPAI H5N1 bird-to-human transmissions leading to clinically severe and fatal human infections. However, because there is a significant species barrier that exists between birds and humans, the virus does not easily cross over to humans, and currently there is no evidence that human-to-human transmission is occurring. Although millions of birds have become infected with the virus since its discovery, 206 humans have died from the H5N1 in 12 countries according to WHO data as of November 2007. For more information use the following resources:

- View the cumulative number of human cases reported to WHO (www.who.int/csr/disease/avian_influenza/country/en/).
- Access the most recent avian influenza situation updates by country at the WHO's Epidemic and Pandemic Alert and Response (www.who.int/csr/disease/avian_influenza/updates/en/index.html).

More research is necessary to understand the pathogenesis and epidemiology of the H5N1 virus in humans. Exposure routes and other disease transmission characteristics such as genetic and immunological factors that may increase the likelihood of infection are not clearly understood. To date, the majority of humans infected with the H5N1 lived or worked in small family farms with backyard flocks, and/or are poultry workers that handled or butchered infected birds in wet markets or live animal markets.

Other possible exposure routes are direct contact with poultry feces or swimming in water contaminated with carcasses or feces of infected birds. In a few cases, children were thought to become sick because they had contact with contaminated feces of free-ranging chickens while playing. In some cases, no exposure route was identified, suggesting unknown environmental factors may act as disease vectors.

Clinical Signs and Symptoms in Humans

According to the WHO, the highly pathogenic H5N1 virus has an aggressive course with rapid clinical deterioration and high fatality rates. Current data for H5N1 infection in humans suggests it may be longer than the seasonal influenza (two to three days) with an incubation period anywhere from two to eight days or as long as 17 days.

Initial symptoms included below have been reported in some, not all, infected H5N1 patients. The spectrum of clinical symptoms may be broader than those mentioned.

- High fever, usually with a temperature higher than 38° C and influenza-like symptoms
- Influenza-like symptoms
- Diarrhea, vomiting, abdominal pain, chest pain, and bleeding from the nose and gums
- Watery diarrhea without blood
- Respiratory symptoms
- Development of manifestations in the lower respiratory tract

Other clinical features three or more days post symptom onset are the following:

- Difficulty breathing, respiratory distress, a hoarse voice, and a crackling sound when inhaling are commonly seen
- Sputum production is variable and sometimes bloody
- Blood-tinted respiratory secretions
- Pneumonia (primary viral pneumonia)
- Multi-organ dysfunction
- Common laboratory abnormalities: leukopenia (mainly lymphopenia), mild-to-moderate thrombocytopenia, elevated aminotransferases, and with some instances of disseminated intravascular coagulation

These clinical features could change given the tendency of this virus to evolve quickly and unpredictably.

Section 11.2

Severe Acute Respiratory Syndrome (SARS)

This section includes excerpts from "Basic Information about SARS" and "Guidance about Severe Acute Respiratory Syndrome (SARS) for Persons Traveling to Areas Where SARS Cases Have Been Reported," Centers for Disease Control and Prevention (www.cdc.gov), May 3, 2005.

Severe acute respiratory syndrome (SARS) is a viral respiratory illness caused by a coronavirus, called SARS-associated coronavirus (SARS-CoV). SARS was first reported in Asia in February 2003. Over the next few months, the illness spread to more than two dozen countries in North America, South America, Europe, and Asia before the SARS global outbreak of 2003 was contained.

The SARS Outbreak of 2003

According to the World Health Organization, a total of 8,098 people worldwide became sick with SARS during the 2003 outbreak. Of these, 774 died. In the United States, only eight people had laboratory evidence of SARS-CoV infection. All of these people had traveled to other parts of the world with SARS. SARS did not spread more widely in the community in the United States. For an update on SARS cases in the United States and worldwide as of December 2003, see "Revised U.S. Surveillance Case Definition for Severe Acute Respiratory Syndrome (SARS) and Update on SARS Cases—United States and Worldwide," December 2003 (www.cdc.gov/mmwr/preview/mmwrhtml/mm5249a2.htm).

Symptoms of SARS

In general, SARS begins with a high fever (temperature greater than 100.4° F). Other symptoms may include headache, an overall feeling of discomfort, and body aches. Some people also have mild respiratory symptoms at the outset. About 10% to 20% of patients have diarrhea. After two to seven days, SARS patients may develop a dry cough. Most patients develop pneumonia.

How SARS Spreads

The main way that SARS seems to spread is by close person-to-person contact. The virus that causes SARS is thought to be transmitted most readily by respiratory droplets (droplet spread) produced when an infected person coughs or sneezes. Droplet spread can happen when droplets from the cough or sneeze of an infected person are propelled a short distance (generally up to three feet) through the air and deposited on the mucous membranes of the mouth, nose, or eyes of persons who are nearby. The virus also can spread when a person touches a surface or object contaminated with infectious droplets and then touches his or her mouth, nose, or eye(s). In addition, it is possible that the SARS virus might spread more broadly through the air (airborne spread) or by other ways that are not now known.

What Does "Close Contact" Mean?

In the context of SARS, close contact means having cared for or lived with someone with SARS or having direct contact with respiratory secretions or body fluids of a patient with SARS. Examples of close contact include kissing or hugging, sharing eating or drinking utensils, talking to someone within three feet, and touching someone directly. Close contact does not include activities like walking by a person or briefly sitting across a waiting room or office.

Guidance about SARS for Persons Traveling to Areas Where SARS Cases Have Been Reported

The following guidance is provided for persons (other than health care workers or household contacts) who are traveling to areas where SARS cases have been reported. These recommendations are based on the experience to date and may be revised as more information becomes available.

Before You Leave

- Assemble a travel health kit containing basic first aid and medical supplies. Be sure to include alcohol-based hand rub for hand hygiene.
- Inform yourself and others who may be traveling with you about SARS. Information about SARS is provided on CDC's SARS website (www.cdc.gov/ncidod/sars/index.htm).

- Be sure you are up to date with all of your shots, and see your health care provider at least four to six weeks before travel to get any additional shots or information you may need. Information on CDC's health recommendations for international travel is provided on CDC's Travelers' Health website (www.cdc.gov/travel/).
- You may wish to check your health insurance plan or get additional insurance that covers medical evacuation in the event of illness. Information about medical evacuation services is provided on the website of the U.S. Department of State (www.travel.state.gov/medical.html).
- Identify in-country health care resources in advance of your trip.

While You Are in An Area Where SARS Cases Have Been Reported

- As with other infectious illnesses, one of the most important and appropriate preventive practices is careful and frequent hand washing. Cleaning your hands often using either soap and water or a waterless, alcohol-based hand rub removes potentially infectious materials from your skin and helps prevent disease transmission.
- To minimize the possibility of infection, observe precautions to safeguard your health. This includes avoiding settings where SARS is most likely to be transmitted, such as health care facilities caring for SARS patients.
- On the basis of limited available data, it would be prudent for travelers to China to avoid visiting live food markets and to avoid direct contact with civets and other wildlife from these markets. Although there is no evidence that direct contact with civets or other wild animals from live food markets has led to cases of SARS, viruses very similar to SARS-CoV—the virus that causes SARS—have been found in these animals. In addition, some persons working with these animals have evidence of infection with SARS-CoV or a very similar virus.
- CDC does not recommend the routine use of masks or other personal protective equipment while in public areas.

After Your Return

- Persons returning from an area where SARS cases have been reported should monitor their health for 10 days.

- Anyone who becomes ill with fever or respiratory symptoms during this 10-day period should consult a health care provider. Before your visit to a health care setting, tell the provider about your symptoms and recent travel so that arrangements can be made to prevent potential transmission to others in the health care setting.
- Close contacts of a person with known or possible SARS should follow the recommendations for SARS patients and their close contacts.

Section 11.3

West Nile Virus

"West Nile Virus: Questions and Answers," Centers for Disease Control and Prevention (www.cdc.gov), September 12, 2006.

What is West Nile virus (WNV)?

West Nile virus is a flavivirus commonly found in Africa, West Asia, and the Middle East. It is closely related to St. Louis encephalitis virus, which is also found in the United States. The virus can infect humans, birds, mosquitoes, horses, and some other mammals.

How long has West Nile virus been in the U.S.?

It is not known how long it has been in the U.S., but CDC scientists believe the virus has probably been in the eastern U.S. since the early summer of 1999, possibly longer.

I understand West Nile virus was found in "overwintering" mosquitoes in the New York City area in early 2000. What does this mean?

One of the species of mosquitoes found to carry West Nile virus is the *Culex* species, which survive through the winter, or "overwinter," in the adult stage. That the virus survived along with the mosquitoes was documented by the widespread transmission the summer of 2000.

Is West Nile virus now established in the Western Hemisphere?

The continued expansion of West Nile virus in the United States indicates that it is permanently established in the Western Hemisphere.

Is the disease seasonal in its occurrence?

In the temperate zone of the world (i.e., between latitudes 23.5° and 66.5° north and south), West Nile encephalitis cases occur primarily in the late summer or early fall. In the southern climates where temperatures are milder, West Nile virus can be transmitted year round.

Transmission

How do people get infected with West Nile virus?

The main route of human infection with West Nile virus is through the bite of an infected mosquito. Mosquitoes become infected when they feed on infected birds, which may circulate the virus in their blood for a few days. The virus eventually gets into the mosquito's salivary glands. During later blood meals (when mosquitoes bite), the virus may be injected into humans and animals, where it can multiply and possibly cause illness.

Additional routes of human infection became apparent during the 2002 West Nile epidemic. It is important to note that these other methods of transmission represent a very small proportion of cases. Investigations have identified WNV transmission through transplanted organs and through blood transfusions (see /www.cdc.gov/ncidod/dvbid/westnile/qa/transfusion.htm).

There is one reported case of transplacental (mother-to-child) WNV transmission. This case is detailed in *MMWR (Morbidity and Mortality Weekly Report)* December 20, 2002 (www.cdc.gov/mmwr/preview/mmwrhtml/mm5150a3.htm). There is also one reported case of transmission of WNV through breast-milk. See www.cdc.gov/ncidod/dvbid/westnile/qa/breastfeeding.htm for more information on this topic.

If I live in an area where birds or mosquitoes with West Nile virus have been reported and a mosquito bites me, am I likely to get sick?

No. Even in areas where the virus is circulating, very few mosquitoes are infected with the virus. Even if the mosquito is infected, less than 1% of people who get bitten and become infected will get severely ill. The chances you will become severely ill from any one mosquito bite are extremely small.

Can you get West Nile encephalitis from another person?

No. West Nile encephalitis is *not* transmitted from person to person. For example, you cannot get West Nile virus from touching or kissing a person who has the disease, or from a health care worker who has treated someone with the disease.

Is a woman's pregnancy at risk if she gets infected with West Nile virus?

There is one documented case of transplacental (mother-to-child) transmission of WNV in a human. Although the newborn in this case was infected with WNV at birth and had severe medical problems, it is unknown whether the WNV infection itself caused these problems or whether they were coincidental. More research will be needed to improve our understanding of the relationship—if any—between WNV infection and adverse birth outcomes.

Nevertheless, pregnant women should take precautions to reduce their risk for WNV and other arboviral infections by avoiding mosquitoes, using protective clothing, and using repellents containing DEET. When WNV transmission is occurring in an area, pregnant women who become ill should see their health care provider, and those whose illness is consistent with acute WNV infection should undergo appropriate diagnostic testing.

Can you get West Nile virus directly from birds?

There is no evidence that a person can get the virus from handling live or dead infected birds. However, persons should avoid bare-handed contact when handling any dead animals and use gloves or double plastic bags to place the carcass in a garbage can.

Can you get WNV from eating game birds or animals that have been infected?

There is no evidence that WNV virus can be transmitted to humans through consuming infected birds or animals. In keeping with overall public health practice, and due to the risk of known foodborne pathogens, people should always follow procedures for fully cooking meat from either birds or mammals.

How does West Nile virus actually cause severe illness and death in humans?

Following transmission by an infected mosquito, West Nile virus multiplies in the person's blood system and crosses the blood-brain barrier to reach the brain. The virus interferes with normal central nervous system functioning and causes inflammation of brain tissue.

How long does the West Nile virus remain in a person's body after they are infected?

There is no scientific evidence indicating that people can be chronically infected with West Nile virus. What remain in a person's body for long periods of time are antibodies and "memory" white blood cells (T-lymphocytes) that the body produces to the virus. These antibodies and T-lymphocytes last for years, and may last for the rest of a person's life. Antibodies are what many diagnostic tests look for when clinical laboratories testing is performed. Both antibodies and "memory" T-lymphocytes provide future protection from the virus.

If a person contracts West Nile virus, does that person develop a natural immunity to future infection by the virus?

It is assumed that immunity will be lifelong; however, it may wane in later years.

Symptoms

What are the symptoms of WNV infection?

Infection with WNV can be asymptomatic (no symptoms), or can lead to West Nile fever or severe West Nile disease.

It is estimated that about 20% of people who become infected with WNV will develop West Nile fever. Symptoms include fever, headache, tiredness, and body aches, occasionally with a skin rash (on the trunk of the body) and swollen lymph glands. While the illness can be as short as a few days, even healthy people have reported being sick for several weeks.

The symptoms of severe disease (also called neuroinvasive disease, such as West Nile encephalitis or meningitis or West Nile poliomyelitis) include headache, high fever, neck stiffness, stupor, disorientation, coma, tremors, convulsions, muscle weakness, and paralysis. It is estimated that approximately 1 in 150 persons infected with the West

Nile virus will develop a more severe form of disease. Serious illness can occur in people of any age; however, people over age 50 and some immunocompromised persons (for example, transplant patients) are at the highest risk for getting severely ill when infected with WNV.

Most people (about four out of five) who are infected with West Nile virus will not develop any type of illness (an asymptomatic infection), however you cannot know ahead of time if you'll get sick or not when infected.

What is the incubation period in humans (i.e., time from infection to onset of disease symptoms) for West Nile disease?

Usually 2 to 15 days.

How long do symptoms last?

Symptoms of West Nile fever will generally last a few days, although even some healthy people report having the illness last for several weeks. The symptoms of severe disease (encephalitis or meningitis) may last several weeks, although neurological effects may be permanent.

What is meant by West Nile encephalitis, West Nile meningitis, West Nile poliomyelitis, "neuroinvasive disease," and West Nile fever?

The most severe type of disease due to a person being infected with West Nile virus is sometimes called "neuroinvasive disease," because it affects a person's nervous system. Specific types of neuroinvasive disease include: West Nile encephalitis, West Nile meningitis, West Nile meningoencephalitis and West Nile poliomyelitis. Encephalitis refers to an inflammation of the brain, meningitis is an inflammation of the membrane around the brain and the spinal cord, meningoencephalitis refers to inflammation of the brain and the membrane surrounding it, and poliomyelitis refers to an inflammation of the spinal cord.

West Nile fever is another type of illness that can occur in people who become infected with the virus. It is characterized by fever, headache, tiredness, aches, and sometimes rash. Although the illness can be as short as a few days, even healthy people have been sick for several weeks.

If I have West Nile fever, can it turn into West Nile encephalitis?

When someone is infected with West Nile virus they will typically have one of three outcomes: No symptoms (most likely), West Nile fever (WNF in about 20% of people), or severe West Nile disease, such as meningitis or encephalitis (less than 1% of those who get infected). If you develop a high fever with severe headache, consult your health care provider.

West Nile fever is characterized by symptoms such as fever, body aches, headache, and sometimes swollen lymph glands and rash. West Nile fever generally lasts only a few days, though in some cases symptoms have been reported to last longer, even up to several weeks. West Nile fever does not appear to cause any permanent health effects. There is no specific treatment for WNV infection. People with West Nile fever recover on their own, though symptoms can be relieved through various treatments (such as medication for headache and body aches, etc.).

Some people may develop a brief, WNF-like illness (early symptoms) before they develop more severe disease, though the percentage of patients in whom this occurs is not known.

Occasionally, an infected person may develop more severe disease such as West Nile encephalitis, West Nile meningitis, or West Nile meningoencephalitis. Although there is no treatment for WNV infection itself, the person with severe disease often needs to be hospitalized.

Care may involve nursing IV fluids, respiratory support, and prevention of secondary infections.

Prevention

What can I do to reduce my risk of becoming infected with West Nile virus?

Protect yourself from mosquito bites.

- Apply insect repellent to exposed skin. Generally, the more active ingredient a repellent contains the longer it can protect you from mosquito bites. A higher percentage of active ingredient in a repellent does not mean that your protection is better—just that it will last longer. Choose a repellent that provides protection for the amount of time that you will be outdoors.

- Repellents may irritate the eyes and mouth, so avoid applying repellent to the hands of children.
- Whenever you use an insecticide or insect repellent, be sure to read and follow the manufacturer's directions for use, as printed on the product.
- For detailed information about using repellents, see the "Insect Repellent Use and Safety" questions (www.cdc.gov/ncidod/dvbid/westnile/qa/insect_repellent.htm).

- Spray clothing with repellents containing permethrin or another EPA-registered repellent since mosquitoes may bite through thin clothing. Do not apply repellents containing permethrin directly to exposed skin. Do not apply repellent to skin under your clothing.
- When weather permits, wear long-sleeved shirts and long pants whenever you are outdoors.
- Place mosquito netting over infant carriers when you are outdoors with infants.
- Consider staying indoors at dawn, dusk, and in the early evening, which are peak mosquito biting times.
- Install or repair window and door screens so that mosquitoes cannot get indoors.

Help reduce the number of mosquitoes in areas outdoors where you work or play by draining sources of standing water. In this way, you reduce the number of places mosquitoes can lay their eggs and breed.

- At least once or twice a week, empty water from flower pots, pet food and water dishes, birdbaths, swimming pool covers, buckets, barrels, and cans.
- Check for clogged rain gutters and clean them out.
- Remove discarded tires, and other items that could collect water.
- Be sure to check for containers or trash in places that may be hard to see, such as under bushes or under your home.

Note: Vitamin B and "ultrasonic" devices are NOT effective in preventing mosquito bites.

Chapter 12

Reproductive Issues and the Environment

Chapter Contents

Section 12.1

Fertility

"The Vallombrosa Consensus Statement on Environmental Contaminants and Human Fertility Compromise," October 2005. © Collaborative on Health and the Environment (www.healthandenvironment.org). Reprinted with permission.

Introduction

A recent national survey indicates that 12% of the reproductive age population in the United States, or 7.3 million couples, reports experiencing difficulty conceiving and/or carrying a pregnancy to term. This is precisely termed impaired fecundity, but commonly referred to, as a general experience, as infertility. Proximate causes of infertility vary widely; for example, from impaired sperm quality or reproductive tract abnormalities, to fallopian tube obstruction, hormone/menstrual cycle irregularities and anovulation, to implantation difficulties and recurrent miscarriage. Some seek medical intervention to help them conceive, and the number of people doing so has risen sharply over the last two decades. In 2002, an estimated $2.9 billion was spent on infertility treatments in the United States. Now, some 46,000 (or 1 in 100) babies born to Americans each year are conceived as a result of the most advanced assisted reproductive technologies (ART).

These increasingly effective medical procedures have helped hundreds of thousands of couples around the world achieve successful pregnancies. They can, however, also be a hardship emotionally and/or financially, and often the financial costs place these interventions beyond the reach of couples who need them.[1] For those who can pursue such assistance, despite its great promise, success is not a given: An estimated one fifth or more of treated couples do not end up with a baby after a course of ART cycles. Too, other medical and/or mental health conditions can be associated with infertility in the couple experiencing it (and research is ongoing as to whether there are increased health risks that attend treatment or conception via ART). In light of all these considerations, a high value should be placed on minimizing preventable causes of infertility as well as on the treatment of it.

Multiple interacting factors are likely to contribute to biological fertility challenges, including age, heredity, lifestyle, underlying disease, reproductive tract infections, and nutritional status. Demographers have identified voluntary delays in first pregnancy as a major factor. Yet, data from the U.S. Centers for Disease Control and Prevention show that impaired fecundity over the last two decades appears to have increased in all reproductive age groups, but most sharply in younger women (under age 25). These data, together with a growing body of epidemiological literature and many experimental research results showing male and female fertility-related impairment in laboratory animals caused by a wide array of modern chemicals, implicate environmental factors also as possible contributors to human infertility.

Scientific understanding of the relationship between environment and human health is advancing rapidly. It reveals that a larger portion of health problems, including infertility, may be caused by environmental exposures than thought possible even a decade ago. These exposures include but are not limited to occupational sources. For some environmental agents known to have adverse effects in experimental animal studies or wildlife, impacts on human reproductive health are being found as well, and at exposure levels within the range humans commonly experience (termed "environmentally relevant"). If involuntary infertility is actually on the rise, and troubling insights from animal studies accurately predict human impacts, then the personal and societal costs of fertility compromise could become increasingly burdensome and significant shifts in reproductive health and norms at the level of whole populations could occur. This has profound implications for public health and strongly suggests that a more comprehensive, coordinated research agenda must be developed and funded—because adverse effects caused by environmental exposures are, in principal, preventable.

Responding to these concerns, a multidisciplinary group of experts gathered at the Vallombrosa Center, Menlo Park, California, February 27–March 1, 2005, to assess what is known about the contribution of environmental contaminants, specifically synthetic compounds and heavy metals, to human infertility and associated health conditions. Workshop organizers chose this focus because critical recent discoveries in the field have raised many new, intriguing scientific questions and heightened interest in environmental risk factors within patient organizations and reproductive medicine/science professional societies. This was the first time researchers in reproductive epidemiology, biology, toxicology, and clinical medicine convened with representatives of relevant professional societies as well as infertility support, women's health, and reproductive advocacy organizations from the United States to review the state of environmental health science as it pertains to infertility.

The purposes of the meeting were:

- To review findings from diverse research disciplines concerning environmental contaminants and the biological basis of compromised fertility, with special attention to critical recent discoveries in related basic sciences;
- To identify conclusions that could be drawn with confidence from existing data;
- To identify critical knowledge gaps and areas of uncertainty;
- To establish key elements of a coherent research agenda to help fill these gaps and resolve uncertainties;
- To consider recommendations for educational initiatives and preventive interventions if and where warranted.

Rapid advances and critical recent discoveries:

- Even very low doses of some biologically active contaminants can alter gene expression important to reproductive function.
- Exposures during fetal development can adversely affect health of the individual in adulthood, including reproductive health.
- Humans are exposed to complex mixtures of chemicals that can interact to cause increased effects.
- People differ in susceptibility to exposures. Not identifying and studying susceptible subgroups can result in failure to detect even very high risk.

Over the course of the meeting, the following core points of consensus were identified, which we offer to help scientists, medical professionals, and public health advocates understand, in broad brush, the current state of scientific understanding in the field and to identify important research areas that will be crucial to further advances:

A. Based on existing evidence, we are confident of the following:

1: In the United States today, at least 12% of the reproductive age population reports experiencing impaired fecundity. This appears to be a rising trend, most markedly in women under 25 years old.

2: Human biological characteristics relevant to fertility vary geographically and over time. For example, semen quality varies within and between men and geographically among populations. Hypospadias, cryptorchidism, and testicular cancer are increasing in some areas but not in others. Other fertility-related diseases, for example endometriosis and polycystic ovarian syndrome (PCOS), are diagnosed more frequently now, which may result from an increase in prevalence, better detection, or both. Current data are inadequate to analyze global trends conclusively.

3: Specialists can identify proximate (or apparent) cause or risk factors in the male, female, or couple in the majority of infertility cases. Within this "explained" category, however, sometimes ultimate (or underlying) causes and mechanisms are understood, but very often they are not. In up to 10% of cases, absolutely no reason for the infertility can be discovered at all—and in a much higher percentage than that, only minor abnormalities that are not severe enough to account for the infertility are identified. These cases are termed "unexplained." It is biologically plausible that environmental factors could be contributing to (or a component of) ultimate causation of infertility, in both the explained and unexplained case categories.

It is helpful to distinguish between "proximate" and "ultimate" causes of infertility. A proximate cause might be reduced sperm quality, hormone imbalances, endometriosis, etc. It is a factor preventing successful conception or pregnancy. But what causes the proximate cause? Why is sperm quality reduced, for example? An ultimate cause is the factor (or factors) responsible for the proximate cause.

4: Considerable data from experimental animal and human studies demonstrate adverse effects of cigarette smoke on a spectrum of sensitive reproductive endpoints in both men and women. Cigarette smoke contains thousands of chemicals, some of which are thought to be involved in its impact on reproduction. These compounds are also encountered elsewhere in the environment, and there is no a priori reason to eliminate these exposure pathways from concerns about reproductive health. Effects of other environmental mixtures are likely to be similarly diverse and complex.

Potential effects of exposure to cigarette smoke include menstrual abnormalities, longer time to pregnancy, increased risk of pregnancy loss, earlier menopause, shortened gestation, intrauterine growth restriction, lower IVF [in vitro fertilization] success rates. In males, smoking is associated with impotence, subfertility, reduced semen quality, and damage to sperm DNA. Sons of mothers who smoke while pregnant have been reported to have lower sperm counts.

5: Considerable experience with the pharmaceutical diethylstilbestrol (DES) clearly demonstrated that prenatal exposure to a synthetic estrogen can adversely affect reproductive physiology and impair fertility later in life, with many endpoints altered. This compound serves as a model for environmental agents that are hormonally active, in other words, endocrine disruptors. Laboratory experiments with DES-exposed animals have repeatedly demonstrated causal effects that are congruent with data on DES offspring, particularly DES daughters. While doses of DES ingested by pregnant women were much greater than those that come from exposure to environmental estrogens, many underlying mechanisms of action appear to be similar.

6: Moreover, environmental contaminant concentrations and/or potency can be amplified because of persistence (biomagnification and bioaccumulation) and because they always occur in mixtures.

7: A wide range of wildlife populations has been shown to be adversely affected by exposure to endocrine-disrupting contaminants. Well-documented effects include: decreased fertility and increased reproductive tract abnormalities in birds, fish, shellfish, and mammals; feminization and demasculinization in male fish, birds, mammals, and reptiles; masculinization and defeminization in female fish, birds, mammals, and reptiles.

8: Some environmental contaminants at high, occupational exposure levels were shown decades ago to impair human fertility, for example lead and the fumigant dibromochloropropane. These types of exposures, however, are unlikely to explain more than a small fraction of the infertility observed in today's population. More recently, considerable data support the contention that exposure to certain agricultural pesticides at moderate or environmentally relevant exposure levels are associated with adverse reproductive outcomes in men and women working on or living near farms (male subfertility and sperm damage; menstrual alterations, increased time to pregnancy, and spontaneous miscarriage rates).

9: Recent research with animals has demonstrated effects on specific aspects of reproductive system development at very low levels of exposure to environmental contaminants (levels within ranges experienced by the general public). This is a finding that may ultimately alter how human safety thresholds are established. In animal and cell culture experiments using these low-dose exposure levels, some contaminants, for example bisphenol A and dioxin, have been shown to interfere with cellular signaling pathways that are important to fertility and reproduction. Proposed mechanisms through which such chemicals may act include perturbation of nuclear hormone signaling, inappropriate activation or inactivation of transcription factors, and alterations in hormone metabolism. For some contaminants, nonmonotonic dose-response curves have been observed when responses are examined across a wide range of exposure levels.

10: Very few relevant data from epidemiological studies are available to investigate the possible associations suggested by these studies between low-level environmental exposures and reproductive health. Much more work in this area must be done given the import if animal data on low-dose effects translate to humans.

11: Genetic signaling mechanisms are highly similar across vertebrate classes, particularly with respect to the structure of key signaling molecules such as steroid hormones and their receptors. Animal models of reproductive toxicity thus offer useful guidance for identifying potential reproductive toxicants in humans. For some compounds, especially DES, there has been remarkable concordance of responses between humans and other vertebrates. A similar pattern is emerging in studies of phthalates. Although differences do exist, consistency of impact across multiple species (especially if the species are from diverse vertebrate classes, e.g. birds and mammals and fish) increases the utility of animal data for identifying human reproductive toxicants.

12: Single contaminants can affect multiple endpoints in more than one tissue through alterations in the expression of multiple genes affecting multiple pathways. Some contaminants have been shown to alter the expression of hundreds of genes, and effects can vary with timing and dose. Different contaminants can affect the same physiological endpoint by acting on the same signaling pathway.

13: Genetic variation, or DNA polymorphisms, within populations (humans, wildlife, and laboratory animals) can result in greater sensitivity to specific contaminants in some individuals. While such variation/sensitivity has been linked to increased risk of specific problems such as, for example, bladder cancer and fetal alcohol syndrome, it has yet to be discovered whether there are genetic polymorphisms that affect response to environmental toxicants and cause or contribute to infertility.

14: Recent measurements of contaminants in people show that humans are exposed, starting at conception, to at least hundreds of chemicals simultaneously—and some at levels within ranges known individually (chemical by chemical) in cell culture and/or animal studies to affect physiological processes relevant to reproduction.

15: The effects of a single chemical exposure have been shown in laboratory studies to differ from the effects of the same chemical in a mixture. Experiments with single chemicals can significantly underestimate effects of the same chemical in mixtures.

16: Exposures during different stages of life (pre- and periconceptional, fetal, perinatal, peripubertal, and adult) have different impacts, because developmental processes create discreet windows of vulnerability for specific effects. The consequences of exposure can manifest on different time scales, some involving long latency. For example, prenatal exposures can cause abnormalities at birth or later that have impacts on adult reproductive function (e.g., as shown with DES). The abnormalities may involve structural or functional alterations, or enhanced sensitivity to subsequent endogenous or exogenous exposures.

17: To date few if any epidemiological studies have successfully incorporated the full complement of these considerations (assessing mixtures, life stage of exposure, the possibility of differential individual genetic susceptibility, etc.) into study design. Epidemiological research that does not factor in these biological considerations will be more likely to conclude erroneously that a study is "negative" and less likely to confirm adverse impacts. Facing these limitations, when epidemiological studies do report positive associations, they should be taken seriously.

18: New scientific methods and tools can and should be developed to further scientific understanding of environmental contributions to human infertility and identify opportunities for preventive interventions. However, a current lack of adequate research funding in the field is a significant impediment.

B. We consider the following to be likely but requiring confirmation:

1: It is likely that gene-environment interactions are involved in the etiology of many reproductive problems including impaired sperm quality; PCOS; endometriosis; uterine fibroids; premature puberty, ovarian failure, and menopause; and reproductive cancers. Further, it is possible that environmental (i.e., low-level ambient) exposures having the biggest impact are those that occur before conception, in utero and neonatally.

2: A cluster of abnormalities of the male reproductive tract is associated in what is termed "testicular dysgenesis syndrome" (TDS), which is hypothesized to originate from a common causal pathway of developmental errors in the fetal testis. TDS can produce a range of outcomes including cryptorchidism and hypospadias at birth, and reduced sperm quality and testicular cancer in adulthood. Semen quality in specific populations has declined (though with no geographic uniformity), and several recent epidemiological studies suggest this may be related to environmental agents. The mechanisms have not been established.

3: It is likely that environmental endocrine disruptors contribute to some manifestations of TDS in humans. In the etiology of TDS, some evidence points to interference with testosterone metabolism mediated by disruption of genetic signaling. Given the well-known, multiple effects of DES on male and female reproductive tract development, it is likely that a syndrome analogous to TDS involving interference with estrogen signaling by environmental chemicals will be identified.

4: It is likely that a broad spectrum of women's reproductive health endpoints is affected by environmental agents including heavy metals, polychlorinated biphenyls (PCBs), and other hormonally active chemicals. Attributing risk of adverse reproductive effects from these exposures is challenging, but several female-factor secular trends in some populations lend biological plausibility to such an association and support the need for further research. For example, increases in the incidence of reproductive cancers may reflect nonhereditary genetic factors, lifestyle, and/or environmental factors or exposures. Age at onset and progression of puberty have been reported to be decreasing over time in several developed countries, suggesting environmental etiology inclusive of lifestyle and diet. Similarly, as prevalence of endometriosis is reported to be increasing, earlier ages at diagnosis are also noted. While greater access to medical care may account for some of these temporal patterns, accumulating evidence suggests an etiologic role for environmental contaminants.

5: Current data contradict the assumption that "weak" environmental estrogens are not a concern because of their low estrogenic potential compared to the endogenous estrogen, estradiol. Studies of mixtures in cell cultures and animals indicate that multiple "weak" estrogens can combine to have effects even when present at levels at which singly they would have no impact. Additionally, some "weak" estrogens affect cellular signaling through recently discovered cell membrane receptors as well as through "traditional" nuclear hormone receptor mediated pathways. In the former case, "weak" estrogens like bisphenol A can be equally as powerful as estradiol at provoking cellular responses.

Contaminants of concern:

Contaminants implicated by research as having effects on fertility/reproductive health fall into a wide range of chemical types. Some are persistent; some are not. Common sources of exposure include a vast array of consumer products (e.g., beauty, personal, and home care, as well as home furnishing and decorating products), food and water, hobbies, arts and crafts. Exposures can happen at home, work, school, play—and in utero. Certain occupations put employees at greater risk of toxic chemical exposures, for instance work that involves solvents (e.g., nail salons, laboratory work, mechanics), pesticides (agricultural work, applicators), plastics manufacturing/dismantling, welding, painting, etc. Exposure pathways are multiple and vary from compound to compound. Common routes are through air, water (drinking and bathing), food, soil, and household dust—via ingestion, inhalation, and/or absorption through the skin.

Examples of chemicals and heavy metals of concern:

Persistent: Dioxins/furans, polychlorinated biphenyls, polybrominated diphenyl ethers, organochlorine pesticides, lead, perfluorinated compounds.

Not Persistent: Triazine herbicides (e.g., atrazine); organophosphate pesticides; solvents including toluene, xylene, styrene, and perchloroethylene; methyl mercury; phthalates; bisphenol A; tobacco smoke.

C. Research on a wide array of fertility-related endpoints suggests several broad themes which we believe should be pursued in future scientific investigations:

1: Information about rates of infertility/subfecundity and specific contributing health conditions in the general population is very limited. For most fertility/fecundity-related endpoints, we have no population data and must rely on women, men, or couples seeking medical treatment. These data are unlikely to be representative of the total population of couples of reproductive age. For this reason, the magnitude of fertility/fecundity impairments has not been fully described and quantified. This poses a challenge to scientists when attempting to assess trends or environmental influences on human reproductive health. Standardizing definitions, identifying consistent endpoints that can be compared across studies, and better public health tracking of fertility/fecundity-related endpoints would strengthen the investigation of environmental associations with reproductive health compromise. More research into geographic variations and factors contributing to differences among populations would also be highly useful.

2: Highly reproducible effects in animal studies indicate that today's framework for evaluating environmental chemical risks to reproductive health is inadequate. Study designs should explicitly incorporate the complex causal framework that has emerged from animal research, including long latencies (of effect following preconceptional, in utero, neonatal, and peripubertal exposures) and interactions among multiple factors (mixtures of contaminants; gene-contaminant interactions; pharmaceuticals; subpopulations varying in genetic susceptibility; nutrition, and lifestyle; complex dose-response relationships). Study designs must also be broadened to incorporate the possibility of multigenerational, epigenetic transmission of effects; consider a multiplicity of causal pathways and endpoints; and examine impacts on population-level endpoints such as sex ratio.

3: Research on wildlife populations and mechanistic studies in animals and cell cultures have proven invaluable in identifying new categories of risk and elucidating the biological mechanisms linking cause to effect. A vigorous research agenda using these approaches should be continued and expanded. These animal studies would ideally involve multidisciplinary approaches that develop biomarkers of exposure and disease in animal models and translate them for use in epidemiological and clinical studies. They should assess syndromes of impacts in addition to single effects. Human epidemiological data identifying fertility impairments can help guide the animal research.

4: Some human data are consistent with the reproductive effects observed in animals, but epidemiological studies confirming human impacts are rarely definitive, due in part to the multiplicity of variables in human studies. Therefore, a high priority should be placed on expanding relevant animal data and improving the sensitivity of animal test protocols, as well as developing better study protocols for testing hypotheses in humans.

5: Prospective studies of exposures, outcomes, and covariates, with high degrees of public participation and cooperation, are likely to be most helpful. For example, the National Children's Study plans to include the recruitment of couples prior to conception to explore fecundity-related impairments in relation to a host of environmental factors including chemicals. This landmark study could also include newly proposed developmental landmarks indicative of endocrine function in infants and be extended to evaluate fertility/fecundity in adulthood, as well as population level outcomes (such as changes in sex ratios, twinning, and birth rates).

6: Factors contributing to differential vulnerability to environmental exposures are diverse and include age, gender, genetic and epigenetic variation, nutritional status and obesity, infections, lifestyle behaviors, pharmaceutical use, occupation, socioeconomic and racial disparities, and physical proximity to certain industries or industrial accidents. All of these factors need to be evaluated to help identify biologically sensitive and otherwise vulnerable subgroups. More systematic attention to these subgroups is likely to improve sensitivity and accuracy of epidemiological research designed to assess risks associated with exposures.

7: Developing tools of toxicogenomics, proteomics, metabolomics, and the study of genetic variation (toxicogenetics) should be integrated with biomonitoring in epidemiological studies. These tools need to be developed to the point of defining specific biomarkers of susceptibility, exposure, and disease. Specific markers for ovarian and testicular responses need to be developed. Increased sensitivity, availability, and affordability of assays for measuring contamination levels in people would enhance research in epidemiology and clinical settings.

8: Testicular dysgenesis syndrome is emerging as a useful construct for organizing hypotheses about some aspects of male reproductive health, including infertility. Human patterns appear to be consistent with animal data, and information about impacts of contaminants on gene expression thought to be important for male reproductive development is providing insights into molecular mechanisms. We need a comprehensive national program, coordinated with efforts underway elsewhere in the world, in order to fully evaluate the TDS hypothesis—including TDS prevalence and etiology. This research program should combine epidemiological and clinical perspectives with in vivo and in vitro experimental research that targets mechanisms.

9: Research on both prevalence trends in and environmental causes of female infertility factors is of equally high priority and must be encouraged. Premature ovarian failure (POF), premature menopause, thyroid disruption, autoimmune disorders, menstrual cycle defects, PCOS, uterine fibroids, endometriosis, meiotic aneuploidy, and repeat pregnancy loss are examples of proximate explanations for female factor infertility that call for specific examination to develop understanding of potential environmental etiologic links.

10: A coherent environmental reproductive health research strategy should include a pointed emphasis on high priority compounds, i.e., those that are underinvestigated, those that are bioactive at low doses, and those for which potential for exposure is widespread due to persistence or continuous use.

High priority compounds include (but are not limited to):

- current-use pesticides;
- phthalates;
- bisphenol A;
- polybrominated flame retardants (PBDEs);

- perfluorinated compounds (PFCs);
- octyl/nonylphenols.

Conclusion

The scientific evidence we have reviewed indicates that while environmental contaminants are unlikely to be the sole etiologic factor underlying human infertility, some exposures cause adverse reproductive health outcomes that contribute to infertility. What proportion of infertility today is environmentally induced is a question of profound human, scientific, and public policy significance. Existing animal and human data suggest that a greater proportion is environmentally caused than has yet been generally realized or can be demonstrated with scientific certainty.

Nothing is more fundamental to the human prospect than the ability to reproduce. Uncertain as the science on environmental causes of infertility is, it is sufficient to raise troubling questions about the future of human reproductive health, and serious debate about how to communicate the information accumulated to date to physicians, patients, and the public. This amply justifies an accelerated research program built around interdisciplinary coordination and collaboration to resolve important uncertainties that currently prevail, particularly around issues involving low-level developmental exposures. A coherent, enhanced research agenda will help identify new strategies to prevent infertility, through actions that individuals can take as well as those that public health/regulatory agencies can pursue. As these investigations progress, it will be increasingly important to engage physicians, other health professionals, patients, and the public in formalized educational efforts that delineate and encourage opportunities for prevention that are elucidated by the research.

1. In the U.S., only 14 states have any form of mandate requiring health insurers to cover or offer coverage for infertility treatments, and more often than not such coverage is only partial at best.

Section 12.2

Fetal Exposures Can Lead to Adult Diseases

"Linking Early Environmental Exposures to Adult Diseases,"
National Institute of Environmental Health Sciences
(www.niehs.nih.gov), October 2008.

All complex diseases have been shown to have both a genetic and environmental component. A growing body of research is beginning to suggest that many chronic adult diseases and disorders, including asthma, diabetes, and obesity, may be traced back to exposures that occur during development. Research supported by the National Institute of Environmental Health Sciences (NIEHS) and others are finding that in utero or neonatal exposures to environmental, dietary, and behavioral changes may make people more susceptible to diseases later in life.

The Developmental Hypothesis

The reason people think that susceptibility to disease may be established during pre-birth is due to both human and developmental toxicology studies in animals. Researchers like David Barker, for example, put forward the "fetal programming or developmental basis of health and disease" hypothesis, after finding an association between low birth weight and coronary heart disease. Barker found that a malnourished fetus will adapt its metabolism in the womb to survive until birth, but these changes then increase a person's risk of disease later in life, such as heart disease, diabetes, and possibly cancer. This idea that the human fetus is vulnerable to outside influences, and that what women eat and perhaps even breathe during pregnancy can impact children into adulthood and possibly even future generations as well, is a growing area of research. Little is currently known about the mechanisms by which fetal insults lead to altered programming and to disease later in life.

Research Findings

It would be difficult to follow humans for 60 years to see if they develop diseases based on what they were exposed to before birth. For this reason, almost all data showing developmental exposures leading to increased susceptibility to disease later in life have been done in animal models. With the use of new technologies, however, researchers are able to examine gene expression changes in tissues during development and to link them to onset of disease later in life, providing a framework to understand the impact that environmental factors may be having on programming the body for future diseases. Some human studies have corroborated what we have seen in animals, including the long-term effects of DES, smoking, and some heavy metals like mercury.

DES, a medication used from the 1940s–1970s to prevent miscarriages in high risk pregnancies, is the best proof of principle supporting the developmental basis of adult disease hypothesis. DES has been shown to cause an increased risk of vaginal, uterine, and breast cancer in humans and animal models. It has also been shown to cause uterine fibroids in mouse models and DES-exposed women. NIEHS researchers also found that the adverse effects of DES in mice can be passed to subsequent generations, even though they were not directly exposed. Researchers have also linked developmental exposures to a variety of environmental chemicals to increased susceptibility to infertility, endometriosis, uterine fibroids, obesity, neurodegenerative diseases, and cardiovascular and lung diseases. There are also some data suggesting that infertility due to environmental exposures during development can be transmitted up to four generations after exposure. These studies indicate that a person's fertility may even be the result of what her great grandmother was exposed to while she was in utero, suggesting again that what a woman may be exposed to during her pregnancy can affect the fertility of her children, grandchildren, and great grandchildren. Mechanisms involved in the transmission of the altered programming due to exposures during development have been shown to involve epigenetic events or changes in gene function that occur without a change in the DNA sequence.

Timing and Duration of Exposure

From NIH [National Institutes of Health]–supported research we know that there are critical periods of vulnerability in the developmental process. This is when cell growth is occurring, tissues are forming, and the body is still without an immune system, blood brain barrier, DNA repair system, or any detoxification system to rid itself of chemicals or to protect itself, making the timing and duration of environmental exposures critical. The developmental period is also the most sensitive time for the development of the epigenetic system. This system controls gene expression in tissues and these changes can be transmitted across generations. Thus, changes in the epigenetic system provide a mechanism for environmental exposures to have effects long after the exposure.

The level of response to a given dose may change dramatically depending on the stage of development at which a fetus is exposed. All of this new research is indicating that a four-century-old paradigm, which states that "the dose makes the poison," needs to be expanded to emphasize that "the timing makes the poison" as well.

Even seemingly minor exposures during early development can lead to functional deficits and increased disease risks later in life.

Early Prevention Is Critical

If the "developmental basis of disease" hypothesis proves true, then there is an even greater need to change our focus from treating diseases after they are detected to prevention. Doctors have long hoped for ways to prevent or reverse health problems before they become chronic diseases. Given that many disorders arise during fetal development from disruptions in the dynamic but still poorly understood interplay of genes, environment, and nutrition, prevention may have to occur decades before a symptom even appears.

NIEHS Research Directions

NIEHS is committed to understanding the link between early environmental exposures and adult diseases. To accomplish this, NIEHS will do the following:

- Continue to lead a trans-NIH to determine the factors, such as the environment, that regulate or turn genes on and off (the Roadmap Epigenomic Program will produce a map of the epigenomes of normal human cells to serve as a reference for diseased cells, allowing us to understand how environmental factors can change patterns related to the link between exposures and disease)
- Encourage the development of more sensitive exposure assessments
- Encourage the use of stored human samples obtained at birth, to link developmental exposures to diseases in humans later in life
- Work with others to define biomarkers of exposure and effect in rodent models that can be translated to humans, to indicate potential increase in susceptibility to disease later in life

- Continue to play a leadership role in promoting partnerships between scientists and community members, to study environmental health concerns, and translate the results to the public, including encouraging more participation by members of the media and communication experts

Section 12.3

Endocrine Disruptors and Reproductive Disorders

"Endocrine Disruptors," National Institute of Environmental Health Sciences (www.niehs.nih.gov), February 2007.

Chemicals that disrupt the endocrine system are found in many of the everyday products we use including some plastic bottles, metal food cans, detergents, flame retardants, food, toys, cosmetics, and pesticides. Although limited scientific information is available on the potential adverse human health effects, concern arises because endocrine disrupting chemicals, while present in the environment at very low levels, have been shown to have adverse effects in wildlife species, as well as in laboratory animals, at these low levels.

The difficulty of assessing public health effects is increased by the fact that people are typically exposed to multiple endocrine disruptors simultaneously. NIEHS and the National Toxicology Program (NTP) support research to understand how these chemicals work and to understand the effects that they may have in various animal and human populations with the long-term goals of developing prevention and intervention strategies to reduce any adverse effects.

What Are Endocrine Disruptors?

Endocrine disruptors are naturally occurring compounds or man-made chemicals that may interfere with the production or activity of hormones of the endocrine system leading to adverse health effects. Many of these chemicals have been linked with developmental, reproductive, neural, immune, and other problems in wildlife and laboratory animals.

Some scientists think these chemicals also are adversely affecting human health in similar ways, resulting in declined fertility and increased incidences or progression of some diseases including endometriosis and cancers. These chemicals have also been referred to as endocrine modulators, environmental hormones, and endocrine active compounds. Environmental chemicals with estrogenic activity are probably the most well studied; however, chemicals with anti-estrogen, androgen, antiandrogen, progesterone, or thyroid-like activity have also been identified.

What Is the Endocrine System and Why Is It Important?

The endocrine system is one of the body's main communication networks and is responsible for controlling and coordinating numerous body functions. Hormones are first produced by the endocrine tissues, such as the ovaries, testes, pituitary, thyroid, and pancreas, and then secreted into the blood to act as the body's chemical messengers where they direct communication and coordination among other tissues throughout the body.

Over the past decade, a growing body of evidence suggests that numerous chemicals, both natural and man-made, may interfere with the endocrine system and produce adverse effects in humans, wildlife, fish, or birds. Scientists often refer to these chemicals as "endocrine disruptors."

For example, hormones work with the nervous system, reproductive system, kidneys, gut, liver, and fat to help maintain and control the following:

- Body energy levels
- Reproduction
- Growth and development
- Internal balance of body systems, called homeostasis
- Responses to surroundings, stress, and injury

Endocrine disrupting chemicals may interfere with the body's own hormone signals because of their structure and activity.

How Do Endocrine Disruptors Work?

From animal studies, researchers have learned much about the mechanisms through which endocrine disruptors influence the endocrine system and alter hormonal functions.

Endocrine disruptors can do the following:

- Mimic or partly mimic naturally occurring hormones in the body like estrogens (the female sex hormone) and androgens (the male sex hormone) and thyroid hormones, potentially producing overstimulation
- Bind to a receptor within a cell and block the endogenous hormone from binding—the normal signal then fails to occur and the body fails to respond properly (examples of chemicals that block or antagonize hormones are anti-estrogens or anti-androgens)
- Interfere or block the way natural hormones or their receptors are made or controlled, for example by blocking their metabolism in the liver

What Are Some Examples of Endocrine Disruptors?

A wide and varied range of substances are thought to cause endocrine disruption. Chemicals that are known endocrine disruptors include the drug DES, dioxin and dioxin-like compounds, PCBs, DDT [dichlorodiphenyltrichloroethane], and some other pesticides. Some chemicals, particularly pesticides and plasticizers, such as bisphenol A, are suspected endocrine disruptors based on animal studies.

Bisphenol A (BPA) is a chemical produced in large quantities for use primarily in the production of polycarbonate plastics and epoxy resins.

Some endocrine disruptors occur among a group of chemicals referred to as phthalates, a class of chemicals that soften and increase the flexibility of polyvinyl chloride plastics.

Di (2-ethylhexyl) phthalate (DEHP) is an example of a phthalate. DEHP is a high production volume chemical used in the manufacture of a wide variety of consumer food packaging, some children's products, and some polyvinyl chloride medical devices. Recently, an independent panel of experts assembled by the NTP found that DEHP may pose a risk to human development, especially critically ill male infants.

Phytoestrogens are naturally occurring substances in plants that have hormone-like activity. Examples of phytoestrogens are genistein and daidzein, which can be found in soy-derived products.

To specifically evaluate the effects that chemicals have on human reproduction, the NTP developed the Center for the Evaluation of Risks to Human Reproduction (CERHR). This center has evaluated the endocrine disruptor effects of seven phthalates and the phytoestrogen genistein found in soy infant formulas.

How Are People Exposed to Endocrine Disruptors?

People may be exposed to endocrine disruptors through the food and beverages they consume, medicine they take, and cosmetics they use. So, exposures may be through the diet, air, and skin. Some environmental endocrine disrupting chemicals, such as DDT, are highly persistent and slow to degrade in the environment, making them potentially hazardous over an extended period of time.

What Is NIEHS Research Telling Us about Endocrine Disruptors?

The NIEHS has been a pioneer in conducting research on the health effects of endocrine disruptors for more than three decades, starting with the endocrine disrupting effects of the pharmaceutical DES. From the 1940s–70s, DES was used to treat women with high risk pregnancies with the mistaken belief that it prevented miscarriage. In 1972, prenatal exposure to DES was linked with the development of a rare form of vaginal cancer in the DES-daughters, and with numerous noncancerous changes in both sons and daughters. NIEHS researchers developed animal models of DES exposure that successfully replicated and predicted human health problems and have been useful in studying the mechanisms involved in DES-toxic effects. NIEHS researchers also showed the effects of DES and other endocrine disruptors involved in the estrogen receptor protein mechanism. Researchers are playing a lead role in uncovering the mechanisms of action of endocrine disruptors.

Today, scientists are working on the following:

- Developing new models and tools to better understand how endocrine disruptors work
- Developing high throughput assays to determine which chemicals have endocrine disrupting activity
- Examining the long-term effects of exposure to various endocrine disrupting compounds during development, and on disease and dysfunction later in life
- Conducting epidemiological studies in human populations

- Developing new assessment and biomarkers to determine exposure and toxicity levels, especially how mixtures of chemicals impact individuals
- Developing intervention and prevention strategies

Some examples of findings in important research areas are provided below.

Developmental Exposures

Research shows that endocrine disruptors may pose the greatest risk during prenatal and early postnatal development when organ and neural systems are developing. In animals, adverse consequences, such as subfertility, premature reproductive senescence, and cancer, are linked to early exposure, but they may not be apparent until much later in life.

Researchers supported by NIEHS at the University of Cincinnati and the University of Illinois found that animals exposed to low doses of the natural human estrogen estradiol, or the environmental estrogen bisphenol A (BPA), during fetal development and estradiol as adults were more likely to develop a precursor of prostate cancer than those who were not exposed. This suggests that exposure to environmental and natural estrogens during fetal development could affect the way prostate genes behave, and may lead to higher rates of prostate disease during aging.

Exposures at Low Levels

In 2000, an independent panel of experts convened by the NIEHS and the NTP found that there was "credible evidence" that some hormone-like chemicals can affect test animals' bodily functions at very low levels—well below the "no effect" levels determined by traditional testing. Although there is little evidence to prove that low-dose exposures are causing adverse human health effects, there is a large body of research in experimental animals and wildlife suggesting that endocrine disruptors may cause the following:

- Reductions in male fertility and declines in the numbers of males born
- Abnormalities in male reproductive organs
- Female reproductive diseases including fertility problems, early puberty, and early reproductive senescence
- Increases in mammary, ovarian, and prostate cancers

There are data showing that exposure to bisphenol A as well as other endocrine disrupting chemicals with estrogenic activity may have effects on obesity and diabetes. These data, while preliminary and only in animals, indicate the potential for endocrine disrupting agents to have effects on other endocrine systems not yet fully examined.

Transgenerational Effects

There is some evidence that endocrine disruptors may not only impact the individual directly exposed, but also future generations.

Research from NIEHS investigators have shown that the adverse effects of DES in mice can be passed to subsequent generations even though they were not directly exposed. The increased susceptibility for tumors was seen in both the granddaughters and grandsons of mice who were developmentally exposed to DES. Mechanisms involved in the transmission of disease were shown to involve epigenetic events.

New research funded by the NIEHS also found that endocrine disruptors may affect not just the offspring of mothers exposed during pregnancy, but future offspring as well. The researchers found that two endocrine disrupting chemicals caused fertility defects in male rats that were passed down to nearly every male in subsequent generations. This study suggests that the two compounds may have caused changes in the developing male germ cells and that endocrine disruptors may be able to reprogram or change the expression of genes without mutating DNA.

The role of environmental endocrine disrupting chemicals in the transmission of disease from one generation to another is of great research interest to the NIEHS.

Chapter 13

The Link between Autism and the Environment

Chapter Contents

Section 13.1

Research on Potential Environmental Causes of Autism

"Epidemiologic Approaches to Autism and the Environment," by Craig J. Newschaffer. © 2006 Autism Society of America (www.autism-society.org). Reprinted with permission.

The science of epidemiology often is critical to discovering links between environmental exposures and particular diseases. Epidemiologists study how health outcomes are distributed across populations and, by making comparisons across population subgroups, they learn what factors are likely to increase risk of disease.

The two most common approaches used to establish that environmental factors play a role in causing a disease are to contrast disease rates in a single population at different points in time and to compare disease rates at the same point in time across different populations. If disease rates change markedly within a population over time, it is a strong sign that some environmental factors are at play since changes in disease risk due to genetic predisposition evolve over the course of generations, not decades. If rates at a single point in time are markedly different across distinct populations (e.g., in different countries), this also suggests environmental causes, especially if the rates correlate with factors influencing the nature of environmental exposures in the populations compared (for example, degree of industrialization, or dietary preferences).

These basic epidemiologic approaches work best for diseases that are diagnosed quickly, definitively, and inexpensively. When this is the case, epidemiologists are confidant that the variation in disease rates seen when they make comparisons are not by-products of differences in the manner in which the condition is diagnosed.

Autism by the Numbers

Because there is no medical test for autism, with diagnosis based on complex behavioral criteria, the diagnostic process is time-consuming, involves periods of uncertainty, and can be quite expensive. This is horribly frustrating to parents searching for help for their child and also is challenging for epidemiologists seeking to understand patterns of disease in groups.

Over the last two decades there has been a tremendous increase in the number of children in the United States diagnosed with autism spectrum disorders—that is unquestioned—and the numbers demonstrate conclusively that autism is a major public health problem. Being certain that these trends represent true changes in risk also would provide strong support for the notion that environmental factors are involved in causing autism. Unfortunately, there are considerable challenges to either proving that the trend represents real risk or to disproving that the trend is caused by shifting diagnostic practice over time.

It is nearly impossible to substantiate that a time trend in disease rates reflects real risk when the mechanisms or risk factors underlying that disease are unknown. Although recent strides have been made in understanding the biology underlying autism, we don't yet know what fundamental process or processes go awry in the brain leading to autism.

On the other hand, to disprove that a trend is due to diagnostic changes, good data must be available to show how diagnostic practice has or has not changed. Unfortunately, there is a dearth of real data on this for autism. We know that there have been considerable changes in the understanding and awareness of autism in the medical and educational communities, but when it comes to quantifying the extent of these changes and determining how they impact the prevalence of autism, there is a great deal of anecdote and speculation and very little data.

For a disease like melanoma, a deadly form of skin cancer where there also has been a large increase in rates over recent years, epidemiologists have good data available on relevant diagnostic practice, namely the rate at which screening biopsies are used. With these data, screening-biopsy rates in a community can correlate to that community's melanoma rates. If high rates of screening biopsy are associated with high rates of melanoma, this suggests that melanoma rate trends are related to diagnostic approach.

Further, melanoma rates by disease stage (early- vs. late-stage disease) can be examined separately. If communities with high biopsy rates tend to have higher rates of early- as opposed to late-stage melanoma, this adds evidence that the increasing rates are due to changes in the way the cancer is diagnosed, not real risk, because early-stage melanoma is much more likely to be detected through the screening biopsy approach.

For autism, shifts in diagnostic approach do not involve something easily trackable like biopsy rates. Even changes we can track, such as rephrasing the guidelines that describe behavior indicative of autism, likely capture only a small portion of the evolving understanding of this complex condition. The informal shifts in interpretation of criteria are more likely to have impact, and quantifying the magnitude of these changes and their impact on rates of diagnosis is extremely difficult.

Even though the most common approaches used to establish connections between environmental exposures and disease face fundamental challenges when applied to autism, epidemiology still offers support for continued research of a link between autism and the environment. Although much of this evidence is indirect, it is still compelling.

Genetics and the Environment

In the late 1970s, studies of twins indicated conclusively that genes strongly influence the risk of autism. These twin studies were landmark research with tremendous impact for families, establishing the biologic basis for autism and scuttling the long-standing conventional wisdom that it was parents' interactions with their children caused autism. So it is not surprising that the initial interpretation of this work emphasized the large influence genes appeared to play. In fact, based on these studies, it often is said that autism is "highly heritable."

However, these twin studies also indicated unequivocally that genetic influences did not completely explain autism risk. The numerous genetic epidemiology studies that followed have brought us closer to identifying specific genes that influence autism risk. But they also consistently have indicated that the genetic mechanisms underlying autism are extremely complicated.

Complexity in genetic inheritance can come from a number of different sources, one of which is interaction between genes and environmental exposures. Gene-environment interaction in autism means that genes passed on to a child may contribute to that child's autism, not because the genes directly influence the developing nervous system, but because they affect that child's biologic response to an environmental exposure that, in turn, dysregulates the developing brain.

We know that hundreds of chemicals have the potential to disturb basic brain development processes; for instance, the way growing brain cells move and connect. What we don't know is how harmful these chemicals can be at low levels of exposure, and which specific genes might make some children more vulnerable to low-dose exposure than others. However, if genetic susceptibility and environmental exposures interact, many of the epidemiologic studies done to date that have characterized only genes, but have not measured environmental exposures, have had little choice but to "count" autism caused by the interaction between genes and environmental exposures as being caused by genes.

So the argument that says, "because genetic epidemiology has shown autism to be highly heritable, there is little room for environmental influences" should be viewed with skepticism. Moreover, we are just now learning about entirely new sets of biologic mechanisms, referred to as "epigenetics," that influence the expression of genes—whether genes are "turned on" or "turned off." Early indications are that epigenetic processes are highly influenced by environmental exposures.

To date, there have been few epidemiologic studies completed that have directly linked environmental exposures and autism. Some studies have suggested that during pregnancy, both viral infection and the use of certain medications known to cause birth defects elevate autism risk. More recent research has reported associations of certain air pollutant exposures, most notably airborne mercury, cadmium, nickel, and chlorinated and diesel particulates, with autism. But caution should be used when interpreting this work due to limitations in the way air pollution exposure was measured and the way autism cases were counted.

There are other chemicals with direct neurotoxic effects or with the potential to alter neurodevelopment by acting on the endocrine or immune system that could warrant consideration in autism research. These include polychlorinated biphenyls (PCBs), complex mixtures of persistent contaminants stored in lipid; brominated fire retardants (BFRs), chemicals that are structurally similar to PCBs and found in increasing concentrations in people and the environment; and phthalates, substances used in making plastics and certain pesticides. Epidemiologic study of these chemicals as risk factors for autism is only the beginning.

The Challenges of Studying Autism and the Environment

As work continues in the area of environmental exposures and autism, it is critical to remember that, just as gene environment interaction creates complexity for genetic research, it also will complicate studies focused on environmental exposures. When the samples used in epidemiologic studies include mixes of children with differing degrees of genetic susceptibility to environmental exposures, the overall estimated effect on autism risk can appear very small, but may in fact be very large in a subgroup of children who are most highly genetically susceptible.

For example, mercury has well-known adverse neurotoxic effects, and for several years there has been mounting concern over thimerosal, a mercury-containing preservative used in multi-dose vials of vaccines. Childhood vaccine-related thimerosal exposure now has been investigated in several epidemiologic studies, and the findings have been quite consistent in indicating that thimerosal exposure is not responsible for the dramatic increases in autism cases witnessed over the past few decades.

However, although there is no discernible effect in the population overall, there still may be an effect in a subgroup of the population especially susceptible to mercury. There is a continuing need for research on susceptibility to low-dose mercury exposure via thimerosal, as well as via other routes. Autism epidemiologists wait for these findings, as well as for findings on markers of susceptibility to other neurotoxicants.

Although the debate continues over whether the increase in autism is attributable to changes in risk versus changes in diagnostic tendencies, resolution of this debate is not a precondition for moving forward with epidemiologic research on autism and the environment. The complex picture emerging from work on the genetic epidemiology of autism, coupled with what is known from animal and human research on the neurodevelopmental effects of a variety of environmental exposures and the limited existing epidemiologic data on environmental factors and autism, is sufficient to motivate more work in this area.

The next generation of autism epidemiology studies is moving ahead by capturing information on a range of different exposures while simultaneously collecting DNA samples to allow genetic characterization. This will allow investigation of select hypotheses right now and will ensure that these data can be returned to as findings on markers of susceptibility become available.

Section 13.2

Vaccinations, Thimerosal, and Autism

This section excerpted from "Thimerosal in Vaccines: Frequently Asked Questions," U.S. Food and Drug Administration (www.fda.gov), June 7, 2007.

What are preservatives and why are they added to vaccines?

Preservatives are compounds that kill or prevent the growth of microorganisms, such as bacteria or fungi. They are used in vaccines to prevent bacterial or fungal growth in the event that the vaccine is accidentally contaminated, as might occur with repeated puncture of multi-dose vials. Vaccines, both in the United States and throughout other parts of the world, are commonly packaged in multi-dose vials. In some cases, preservatives are added during manufacture to prevent microbial growth; with changes in manufacturing technology, however, the need to add preservatives during the manufacturing process has decreased markedly.

Preservatives have been used in vaccines for over 70 years. The requirement for a preservative in multi-dose, multi-entry vials was placed into the Code of Federal Regulations (21 CFR 610.15) in January 1968. There are exceptions to this requirement for preservative, primarily involving the live-attenuated viral vaccines.

The general need for preservatives in multi-dose vials has been underscored by cases in which multi-dose vials that did not contain preservatives become contaminated during use and caused fatal infections in vaccine recipients.

What is thimerosal?

Thimerosal is a preservative that has been used in some vaccines since the 1930s, when it was first introduced by Eli Lilly Company. It is 49.6% mercury by weight and is metabolized or degraded into ethylmercury and thiosalicylate. At concentrations found in vaccines, it meets the requirements for a preservative as set forth by the United States Pharmacopeia; that is, it kills the specified challenge organisms and is able to prevent the growth of the challenge fungi. Prior to its introduction in the 1930s, data were available in several animal species and humans providing evidence for its safety and effectiveness as a preservative. Since then, thimerosal has a long record of safe and effective use preventing bacterial and fungal contamination of vaccines, with no ill effects established other than minor local reactions at the site of injection.

As a vaccine preservative, thimerosal is used in concentrations of 0.003% to 0.01%. A vaccine containing 0.01% thimerosal as a preservative contains 50 micrograms of thimerosal per 0.5 mL dose, or approximately 25 micrograms of mercury per 0.5 mL dose. The use of mercury-containing preservatives in vaccines has declined markedly since 1999.

The Food and Drug Administration (FDA) is continuing its efforts toward reducing or removing thimerosal from all existing vaccines. Much progress has been made to date. FDA has been actively working with manufacturers, particularly those that manufacture childhood vaccines, to reach the goal of eliminating thimerosal from vaccines, and has been collaborating with other Public Health Service (PHS) agencies to further evaluate the potential health effects of thimerosal. In this regard, all vaccines routinely recommended for children six years of age or younger and marketed in the U.S. contain no thimerosal or only trace amounts (one microgram or less mercury per dose), with the exception of inactivated influenza vaccine, which was first recommended by the Advisory Committee on Immunization Practices in 2004 for routine use in children 6 to 23 months of age.

What has FDA done to address the issue of mercury-containing preservatives in vaccines?

Under the FDA Modernization Act (FDAMA) of 1997, FDA carried out a comprehensive review of the use of thimerosal in childhood vaccines. Conducted in 1999, this review found no evidence of harm from the use of thimerosal as a vaccine preservative, other than local hypersensitivity reactions.

As part of the FDAMA review, FDA evaluated the amount of mercury an infant might receive in the form of ethylmercury from vaccines under the U.S. recommended childhood immunization schedule and compared these levels with existing guidelines for exposure to methylmercury, as there are no existing guidelines for ethylmercury, the metabolite of thimerosal. At the time of this review in 1999, the maximum cumulative exposure to mercury from vaccines in the recommended childhood immunization schedule was within acceptable limits for the methylmercury exposure guidelines set by FDA, Agency for Toxic Substances and Disease Registry (ATSDR), and the World Health Organization (WHO). However, depending on the vaccine formulations used and the weight of the infant, some infants could have been exposed to cumulative levels of mercury during the first six months of life that exceeded Environmental Protection Agency (EPA) recommended guidelines for safe intake of methylmercury. As a precautionary measure, the Public Health Service (including FDA, National Institutes of Health [NIH], Centers for Disease Control and Prevention [CDC], and Health Resources and Services Administration [HRSA]) and the American Academy of Pediatrics issued a Joint Statement, urging vaccine manufacturers to reduce or eliminate thimerosal in vaccines as soon as possible. The U.S. Public Health Service agencies have collaborated with various investigators to initiate further studies to better understand any possible health effects from exposure to thimerosal in vaccines.

Available data has been reviewed in several public forums including the Workshop on Thimerosal, held in Bethesda in August 1999 and sponsored by the National Vaccine Advisory Committee, two meetings of the Advisory Committee on Immunization Practices of the CDC, held in October 1999 and June 2000, and by the Institute of Medicine's Immunization Safety Review Committee in July 2001 and February 2004. Data reviewed did not demonstrate convincing evidence of toxicity from doses of thimerosal used in vaccines. In case reports of accidental high-dose exposures in humans to thimerosal or ethylmercury toxicity was demonstrated only at exposures that were 100 or 1,000 times that found in vaccines.

In its report of October 1, 2001, the Institute of Medicine (IOM)'s Immunization Safety Review Committee concluded that the evidence is inadequate to either accept or reject a causal relationship between thimerosal exposure from childhood vaccines and the neurodevelopmental disorders of autism, attention deficit hyperactivity disorder (ADHD), and speech or language delay. At that time the committee's conclusion was based on the fact that there were no published epidemiological studies examining the potential association between thimerosal-containing vaccines and neurodevelopmental disorders. The committee did conclude that the hypothesis that exposure to thimerosal-containing vaccines could be associated with neurodevelopmental disorders was biologically plausible. However, additional studies were needed to establish or reject a causal relationship. The committee stated that the effort to remove thimerosal from vaccines was "a prudent measure in support of the public health goal to reduce mercury exposure of infants and children as much as possible."

In 2004, the IOM's Immunization Safety Review Committee again examined the hypothesis that vaccines, specifically the MMR vaccines and thimerosal-containing vaccines, are causally associated with autism. In this report, the committee incorporated new epidemiological evidence from the United States, Denmark, Sweden, and the United Kingdom and studies of biologic mechanisms related to vaccines and autism that had become available since its report in 2001. The committee concluded that this body of evidence favors rejection of a causal relationship between thimerosal-containing vaccines and autism, and that hypotheses generated to date concerning a biological mechanism for such causality are theoretical only. Further, the committee stated that the benefits of vaccination are proven and the hypothesis of susceptible populations is presently speculative, and that widespread rejection of vaccines would lead to increases in incidences of serious infectious diseases like measles, whooping cough, and Hib bacterial meningitis.

FDA is continuing its efforts toward reducing or removing thimerosal from all existing vaccines. Much progress has been made to date. FDA has been actively working with manufacturers, particularly those that manufacture childhood vaccines, to reach the goal of eliminating thimerosal from vaccines, and has been collaborating with other PHS agencies to further evaluate the potential health effects of thimerosal. Since 2001, all vaccines recommended for children six years of age and younger have contained either no thimerosal or only trace amounts, with the exception of inactivated influenza vaccines, which are marketed in both the preservative-free and thimerosal-preservative-containing formulations. Thimerosal-preservative-free influenza vaccine licensed for use in children 6 to 59 months of age is available in limited supply. Nevertheless, FDA is in discussions with manufacturers of influenza vaccine regarding their capacity to increase the supply of vaccine without thimerosal as a preservative. Additionally, new pediatric vaccines that have received licensure do not contain thimerosal.

What progress has been made towards the goal of eliminating thimerosal from vaccines?

Great progress has been made in removing thimerosal from vaccines. Manufacturers have been able to accomplish this goal through changing their manufacturing processes, including a switch from multi-dose vials, which generally require a preservative, to single-dose vials or syringes. Since 2001, all vaccines manufactured for the U.S. market and routinely recommended for children less than six years of age have contained no thimerosal or only trace amounts (≤ 1 microgram of mercury per dose remaining from the manufacturing process), with the exception of inactivated influenza vaccine. In addition, all of the routinely recommended vaccines that had been previously manufactured with thimerosal as a preservative (some formulations of DTaP [tetanus, diphtheria, and acellular pertussis], Hib [*Haemophilus influenzae* B conjugate], and hepatitis B vaccines) had reached the end of their shelf life by January 2003.

In the past, prior to the initiative to reduce or eliminate thimerosal from childhood vaccines, the maximum cumulative exposure to mercury via routine childhood vaccinations during the first six months of life was 187.5 micrograms. With the introduction of thimerosal-preservative-free formulations of DTaP, hepatitis B, and Hib, the maximum cumulative exposure from these vaccines decreased to less than three micrograms of mercury in the first six months of life. With the addition of influenza vaccine to the recommended vaccines, an infant could receive a thimerosal-containing influenza vaccine at six and seven months of age. This would result in a maximum exposure of 28 micrograms via routine childhood vaccinations. This level is well below the EPA-calculated exposure guideline for methylmercury of 65 micrograms for a child in the fifth percentile body weight during the first six months of life.

Currently, all hepatitis vaccines manufactured for the U.S. market contain either no thimerosal or only trace amounts. Also, DT [diphtheria and tetanus toxoids], Td [tetanus and diphtheria toxoids], and tetanus toxoid vaccines are now available in formulations that contain no thimerosal or only trace amounts.

Furthermore, all new vaccines licensed since 1999 are free of thimerosal as a preservative. Inactivated influenza vaccine was added to the routinely recommended vaccines for children 6 to 23 months of age in 2004. FDA has approved thimerosal-preservative-free formulations (containing either no or only trace amounts of thimerosal) for the inactivated influenza vaccines manufactured by Sanofi Pasteur and Chiron. These influenza vaccines continue to be marketed in both the preservative-free and thimerosal-preservative-containing formulations. In addition, in August 2005, FDA licensed GlaxoSmithKline's inactivated influenza vaccine, which contains 1.25 micrograms mercury per dose. Of the three licensed inactivated influenza vaccines, Sanofi Pasteur's Fluzone is the only one approved for use in children down to six months of age. Chiron's Fluvirin is approved for individuals four years of age and older, and GSK's Fluarix is approved for individuals 18 years of age and older. The live attenuated influenza vaccine (FluMist, manufactured by MedImmune), which contains no thimerosal, is approved for individuals 5 to 49 years of age. For the 2005–2006 season, Sanofi Pasteur was able to manufacture up to eight million doses of thimerosal-preservative-free influenza vaccine. Based on an estimated annual birth cohort in the United States of four million, there are six million infants and children between the ages of 6 and 23 months, most of whom would need two doses each. Thus, the amount of thimerosal-preservative-free vaccine that is available based on current manufacturing capacity is well below the number of doses needed to fully vaccinate this age group. FDA is in discussions with manufacturers of influenza vaccine regarding their capacity to further increase the supply of preservative-free formulations.

Why are some vaccines noted to be "thimerosal-free" while some are "thimerosal-reduced"? What is the difference between "thimerosal-free" and "preservative-free"?

Thimerosal may be added at the end of the manufacturing process to act as a preservative to prevent bacterial or fungal growth in the event that the vaccine is accidentally contaminated, as might occur with repeated puncture of multi-dose vials. When thimerosal is used as preservative in vaccines, it is present in concentrations up to 0.01% (50 micrograms thimerosal per 0.5 mL dose or 25 micrograms mercury per 0.5 mL dose). In some cases, thimerosal is used during the manufacturing process and is present in small amounts in the final vaccine (one microgram mercury or less per dose).

The term "preservative-free" indicates that no preservative (thimerosal or otherwise) is used in the vaccine; however, traces used during the manufacturing process may be present in the final formulation. For example, some vaccines may be preservative-free but may contain traces of thimerosal (one microgram mercury or less per dose); in such settings, this information is noted in the package insert. Similarly, the term "thimerosal-reduced" usually indicates that thimerosal is not added as a vaccine preservative, but trace amounts (one microgram mercury per dose or less) may remain from use in the manufacturing process. Such trace amounts are not felt to be clinically significant, nor would they result in exposure exceeding any federal guideline for mercury exposure. Vaccines may be termed "thimerosal-free" if no thimerosal can be measured; i.e., thimerosal content is below the limit of detection.

Why is exposure to mercury a concern?

Mercury is an element that is dispersed widely around the earth. Most of the mercury in the water, soil, plants, and animals is found as inorganic mercury salts. Mercury accumulates in the aquatic food chain, primarily in the form of the methylmercury, an organomercurial. Methylmercury is more easily absorbed and is less readily eliminated from the body than inorganic mercury. Exposure to one chemical with mercury, i.e., methylmercury, has been shown to pose a variety of health risks to humans. Extremely high levels, such as that observed in poisoning episodes in Japan and Iraq, has caused neurological damage and death. The fetus is considered more sensitive to health effects of methylmercury than adults. In recent years some studies have found adverse health effects of methylmercury at levels previously thought to be safe. Other studies, however, have shown conflicting results.

It is important to note that the preservative thimerosal contains ethylmercury, a related though distinct chemical from methylmercury. Moreover, recent studies in animal models exposed to thimerosal-containing vaccines or oral methylmercury suggest that methylmercury may not be a suitable reference to assess the risk from exposure to thimerosal. In addition, data from studies in human infants that were given routine immunizations with thimerosal-containing vaccines showed that mercury levels in blood and urine were uniformly below safety guidelines for methylmercury and that unlike methylmercury excretory profiles, infants excreted significant amounts of mercury in stool after thimerosal (ethylmercury) exposure, thus removing mercury from their bodies.

Is it safe for children to receive an influenza vaccine that contains thimerosal?

Yes. There is no convincing evidence of harm caused by the small doses of thimerosal preservative in influenza vaccines, except for minor effects like swelling and redness at the injection site.

Recent research suggests that healthy children under the age of two are more likely than older children and as likely as people over the age of 65 to be hospitalized with flu complications. Therefore, vaccination with thimerosal-preservative-containing influenza vaccine and thimerosal-reduced influenza vaccine is encouraged when feasible in children, including those that are 6–23 months of age.

Is it safe for pregnant women to receive an influenza vaccine that contains thimerosal?

Yes. A study of influenza vaccination examining over 2,000 pregnant women demonstrated no adverse fetal effects associated with influenza vaccine. Case reports and limited studies indicate that pregnancy can increase the risk for serious medical complications of influenza. One study found that out of every 10,000 women in their third trimester of pregnancy during an average flu season, 25 will be hospitalized for flu-related complications.

Additionally, influenza-associated excess deaths among pregnant women have been documented during influenza pandemics. Because pregnant women are at increased risk for influenza-related complications and because a substantial safety margin has been incorporated into the health guidance values for organic mercury exposure, the benefits of thimerosal–reduced influenza vaccine or thimerosal-preservative-containing influenza vaccine outweighs the theoretical risk, if any, of thimerosal.

You have said that thimerosal is no longer used as a preservative in vaccines routinely recommended for children six years or less of age, with the exception of influenza vaccine. What is being done about the thimerosal content of other vaccines and other biological products given to infants, children, and pregnant women?

FDA is continuing its efforts to reduce the exposure of infants, children, and pregnant women to mercury from vaccines. FDA is in discussions with manufacturers of influenza vaccine regarding their capacity to further increase the supply of preservative-free formulations. Of note, all hepatitis B vaccines for the U.S., including for adults, are now available only as thimerosal-free or thimerosal-reduced formulations.

Td, which is indicated for children seven years of age or older and adults, is now also available in thimerosal-free formulations. In addition, all vaccines licensed since 1999 with the exception of inactivated influenza vaccine have not contained thimerosal as a preservative. Also, all immune globulin preparations including hepatitis B immune globulin and Rho(D) immune globulin preparations are manufactured without thimerosal.

Part Three

Outdoor Environmental Hazards: Air, Water, and Soil

Chapter 14

Air Pollution

Chapter Contents

Section 14.1

Ozone (Smog)

"Air Quality Guide for Ozone," AIRNow: U.S. Office of Air Quality and Radiation (www.airnow.gov), March 2008.

You may have seen the Air Quality Index reported in your newspaper. This section provides you with more detailed information about what this index means to you. This section will help you determine ways to protect your family's health when ozone levels reach the unhealthy range and ways you can help reduce ozone air pollution.

Air pollution can affect your health and the environment. There are actions every one of us can take to reduce air pollution and keep the air cleaner, and precautionary measures you can take to protect your health.

What You Should Know about Ozone and Your Health

- Ozone in the air we breathe can harm our health—particularly on hot, sunny days when ozone can reach unhealthy levels.
- Even relatively low levels of ozone can cause health effects.
- People with lung disease, children, older adults, and people who are active outdoors may be particularly sensitive to ozone.
- Ozone exposure may also increase the risk of premature death from heart or lung disease.

What is ozone?

Ozone is a colorless gas found in the air we breathe. Ozone can be good or bad depending on where it occurs:

- Ozone occurs naturally in the Earth's upper atmosphere (the stratosphere), where it shields the Earth from the sun's ultraviolet rays.
- At ground level, ozone is an air pollutant that can harm human health.

Table 14.1. Air Quality Guide for Ozone

Air Quality Index	Protect Your Health
Good (0–50)	No health impacts are expected when air quality is in this range.
Moderate (51–100)	Unusually sensitive people should consider limiting prolonged outdoor exertion.
Unhealthy for Sensitive Groups (101–150)	The following groups should limit prolonged outdoor exertion: • People with lung disease, such as asthma • Children and older adults • People who are active outdoors
Unhealthy (151–200)	The following groups should avoid prolonged outdoor exertion: • People with lung disease, such as asthma • Children and older adults • People who are active outdoors Everyone else should limit prolonged outdoor exertion.
Very Unhealthy (201–300)	The following groups should avoid all outdoor exertion: • People with lung disease, such as asthma • Children and older adults • People who are active outdoors Everyone else should limit outdoor exertion.

Where does ground-level ozone come from?

Ground-level ozone is formed when two types of pollutants react in the presence of sunlight. These pollutants are known as volatile organic compounds (VOCs) and oxides of nitrogen. They are found in emissions from the following sources:

- Vehicles such as automobiles, trucks, buses, aircraft, and locomotives
- Construction equipment
- Lawn and garden equipment
- Sources that combust fuel, such as large industries and utilities
- Small industries such as gas stations and print shops
- Consumer products, including some paints and cleaners

Does my area have high ozone levels?

- Ozone is particularly likely to reach unhealthy levels on hot, sunny days in urban environments. It is a major part of urban smog.
- Ozone can also be transported long distances by wind. For this reason, even rural areas can experience high ozone levels.
- The AIRNow website at airnow.gov provides daily air quality reports for many areas. These reports use the Air Quality Index (or AQI) to tell you how clean or polluted the air is.
- Enviroflash, a free service, can alert you via e-mail when your local air quality is a concern. Sign up at www.enviroflash.info.

How does ozone affect health?

Ozone can affect health in the following ways:

- Make it more difficult to breathe deeply and vigorously
- Cause shortness of breath and pain when taking a deep breath
- Cause coughing and sore or scratchy throat
- Inflame and damage the lung lining
- Make the lungs more susceptible to infection
- Aggravate lung diseases such as asthma, emphysema, and chronic bronchitis
- Increase the frequency of asthma attacks
- Continue to damage the lungs even when the symptoms have disappeared

These effects may lead to increased school absences, visits to doctors and emergency rooms, and hospital admissions. Research also indicates that ozone exposure may increase the risk of premature death from heart or lung disease.

Who is sensitive to ozone?

Some people are more sensitive to ozone than others. Sensitive groups include children; people with lung disease, such as asthma, emphysema, or chronic bronchitis; and older adults. Even healthy adults who are active outdoors can experience ozone's harmful effects.

What is an Air Quality Action Day for Ozone?

Your state or local air quality agency may declare an Air Quality Action Day for Ozone when ozone levels are forecast to reach unhealthy levels. On ozone action days, you can take simple steps (see the following) to reduce the pollution that results in ground-level ozone.

Keep the Air Cleaner

- Conserve energy—at home, at work, everywhere. Turn off lights you are not using.
- Carpool or use public transportation.
- When air quality is healthy, bike or walk instead of driving.
- Combine errands to reduce vehicle trips.
- Limit engine idling.
- When refueling: Stop when the pump shuts off. Putting more fuel in is bad for the environment and can damage your vehicle. Avoid spilling fuel. Always tighten your gas cap securely.
- Keep your car, boat, and other engines tuned up.
- Inflate your car's tires to the recommended pressure.
- Use environmentally safe paints and cleaning products whenever possible.
- Follow manufacturers' recommendations to use and properly seal cleaners, paints, and other chemicals so smog-forming chemicals can't evaporate.

On Air Quality Action Days, you should also take the following precautions:

- Refuel cars and trucks after dusk, when emissions are less likely to produce ozone.
- Delay using gasoline-powered lawn and garden equipment until air quality is healthy again.
- Delay using household, workshop, and garden chemicals until air quality is healthy again.

Section 14.2

Particle Pollution

This section includes "Particulate Matter: Basic Information," and "Particulate Matter: Health and Environment," Environmental Protection Agency (www.epa.gov), May 9, 2008.

Particle pollution (also called particulate matter or PM) is the term for a mixture of solid particles and liquid droplets found in the air. Some particles, such as dust, dirt, soot, or smoke, are large or dark enough to be seen with the naked eye. Others are so small they can only be detected using an electron microscope.

Particle pollution includes "inhalable coarse particles," with diameters larger than 2.5 micrometers and smaller than 10 micrometers, and "fine particles," with diameters that are 2.5 micrometers and smaller. How small is 2.5 micrometers? Think about a single hair from your head. The average human hair is about 70 micrometers in diameter—making it 30 times larger than the largest fine particle.

These particles come in many sizes and shapes and can be made up of hundreds of different chemicals. Some particles, known as primary particles, are emitted directly from a source, such as construction sites, unpaved roads, fields, smokestacks, or fires. Others form in complicated reactions in the atmosphere of chemicals such as sulfur dioxides and nitrogen oxides that are emitted from power plants, industries, and automobiles. These particles, known as secondary particles, make up most of the fine particle pollution in the country.

The Environmental Protection Agency (EPA) regulates inhalable particles (fine and coarse). Particles larger than 10 micrometers (sand and large dust) are not regulated by EPA.

- **Health:** Particle pollution contains microscopic solids or liquid droplets that are so small that they can get deep into the lungs and cause serious health problems. The size of particles is directly linked to their potential for causing health problems. Small particles less than 10 micrometers in diameter pose the greatest problems, because they can get deep into your lungs, and some may even get into your bloodstream.

- **Visibility:** Fine particles (PM 2.5) are the major cause of reduced visibility (haze) in parts of the United States, including many of our treasured national parks and wilderness areas.
- **Reducing particle pollution:** EPA's national and regional rules to reduce emissions of pollutants that form particle pollution will help state and local governments meet the Agency's national air quality standards.

Health and Environment

The size of particles is directly linked to their potential for causing health problems. Small particles less than 10 micrometers in diameter pose the greatest problems, because they can get deep into your lungs, and some may even get into your bloodstream.

Exposure to such particles can affect both your lungs and your heart. Small particles of concern include "inhalable coarse particles" (such as those found near roadways and dusty industries), which are larger than 2.5 micrometers and smaller than 10 micrometers in diameter; and "fine particles" (such as those found in smoke and haze), which are 2.5 micrometers in diameter and smaller.

The Clean Air Act requires EPA to set air quality standards to protect both public health and the public welfare (e.g., crops and vegetation). Particle pollution affects both.

Particle pollution—especially fine particles—contains microscopic solids or liquid droplets that are so small that they can get deep into the lungs and cause serious health problems. Numerous scientific studies have linked particle pollution exposure to a variety of problems, including the following:

- Increased respiratory symptoms, such as irritation of the airways, coughing, or difficulty breathing, for example
- Decreased lung function
- Aggravated asthma
- Development of chronic bronchitis
- Irregular heartbeat
- Nonfatal heart attacks
- Premature death in people with heart or lung disease

People with heart or lung diseases, children, and older adults are the most likely to be affected by particle pollution exposure. However, even if you are healthy, you may experience temporary symptoms from exposure to elevated levels of particle pollution. For more information about asthma, visit www.epa.gov/asthma.

Section 14.3

Acid Rain

This section excerpted from "What is Acid Rain?" Environmental Protection Agency (www.epa.gov), June 8, 2007.

What Is Acid Rain?

"Acid rain" is a broad term referring to a mixture of wet and dry deposition (deposited material) from the atmosphere containing higher than normal amounts of nitric and sulfuric acids. The precursors, or chemical forerunners, of acid rain formation result from both natural sources, such as volcanoes and decaying vegetation, and man-made sources, primarily emissions of sulfur dioxide (SO_2) and nitrogen oxides (NO_x) resulting from fossil fuel combustion. In the United States, roughly 2/3 of all SO_2 and 1/4 of all NO_x come from electric power generation that relies on burning fossil fuels, like coal. Acid rain occurs when these gases react in the atmosphere with water, oxygen, and other chemicals to form various acidic compounds. The result is a mild solution of sulfuric acid and nitric acid. When sulfur dioxide and nitrogen oxides are released from power plants and other sources, prevailing winds blow these compounds across state and national borders, sometimes over hundreds of miles.

Wet Deposition

Wet deposition refers to acidic rain, fog, and snow. If the acid chemicals in the air are blown into areas where the weather is wet, the acids can fall to the ground in the form of rain, snow, fog, or mist. As this acidic water flows over and through the ground, it affects a variety of plants and animals. The strength of the effects depends on several factors, including how acidic the water is; the chemistry and buffering capacity of the soils involved; and the types of fish, trees, and other living things that rely on the water.

Dry Deposition

In areas where the weather is dry, the acid chemicals may become incorporated into dust or smoke and fall to the ground through dry deposition, sticking to the ground, buildings, homes, cars, and trees. Dry deposited gases and particles can be washed from these surfaces by rainstorms, leading to increased runoff. This runoff water makes the resulting mixture more acidic. About half of the acidity in the atmosphere falls back to earth through dry deposition.

Human Health

Acid rain looks, feels, and tastes just like clean rain. The harm to people from acid rain is not direct. Walking in acid rain, or even swimming in an acid lake, is no more dangerous than walking or swimming in clean water. However, the pollutants that cause acid rain—sulfur dioxide (SO_2) and nitrogen oxides (NO_x)—do damage human health. These gases interact in the atmosphere to form fine sulfate and nitrate particles that can be transported long distances by winds and inhaled deep into people's lungs. Fine particles can also penetrate indoors. Many scientific studies have identified a relationship between elevated levels of fine particles and increased illness and premature death from heart and lung disorders, such as asthma and bronchitis.

Based on health concerns, SO_2 and NO_x have historically been regulated under the Clean Air Act, including the Acid Rain Program. In the eastern United States, sulfate aerosols make up about 25% of fine particles. By lowering SO_2 and NO_x emissions from power generation, the Acid Rain Program will reduce the levels of fine sulfate and nitrate particles and so reduce the incidence and the severity of these health problems. When fully implemented by the year 2010, the public health benefits of the Acid Rain Program are estimated to be valued at $50 billion annually, due to decreased mortality, hospital admissions, and emergency room visits.

Decreases in NO_x emissions are also expected to have a beneficial impact on human health by reducing the nitrogen oxides available to react with volatile organic compounds and form ozone. Ozone impacts on human health include a number of morbidity and mortality risks associated with lung inflammation, including asthma and emphysema.

Reducing Acid Rain—Take Action as Individuals

It may seem like there is not much that one individual can do to stop acid deposition. However, like many environmental problems, acid deposition is caused by the cumulative actions of millions of individual people. Therefore, each individual can also reduce their contribution to the problem and become part of the solution. Individuals can contribute directly by conserving energy, since energy production causes the largest portion of the acid deposition problem. For example, you can follow these guidelines:

- Turn off lights, computers, and other appliances when you're not using them.
- Use energy-efficient appliances: lighting, air conditioners, heaters, refrigerators, washing machines, etc. For more information, see EPA's ENERGY STAR Program (www.energystar.gov/).
- Only use electric appliances when you need them.
- Keep your thermostat at 68° F in the winter and 72° F in the summer. You can turn it even lower in the winter and higher in the summer when you are away from home.
- Insulate your home as best you can.
- Carpool, use public transportation, or better yet, walk or bicycle whenever possible
- Buy vehicles with low NO_x emissions, and properly maintain your vehicle.
- Be well informed.

Chapter 15

Climate Change and Extreme Heat

Introduction

Extreme heat events, characterized by stagnant, warm air masses and consecutive nights with high minimum temperatures, are a significant public health problem in the U.S. that will be exacerbated by the synergistic effects of a warming climate, urbanization, and an aging population. In fact, extreme heat events (EHE), or heatwaves, are the most prominent cause of weather-related human mortality in the U.S., responsible for more deaths annually than hurricanes, lightning, tornadoes, floods, and earthquakes combined.

Although all heat-related deaths and illness are preventable, many people succumb to extreme heat every year. Over a five-year period, from 1999 to 2003, a total of 3,442 heat-related deaths were reported in the U.S. (an annual average of 688). Extreme heatwaves, such as that witnessed across Europe in 2003, can result in a significantly higher mortality.

Despite the high mortality associated with EHE and projections of a warming climate, there is a lack of public recognition of the hazard of extreme heat exposure, and U.S. metropolitan areas gen-

---

Excerpted from the *American Journal of Preventive Medicine*, Volume 35, Issue 35. George Luber, MA, PhD, and Michael McGeehin, PhD, MSPH. Climate Change and Extreme Heat Events, pages 429–435. To view the complete text of this article including references, visit http://www.ajpm-online.net or http://www.sciencedirect.com/science/journal/07493797.

erally lack preparedness measures such as heatwave-response plans. Part of the problem lies in the fact that heatwaves are silent killers—natural disasters that do not leave a trail of destruction in their wake. Like other natural disasters they are sporadic phenomena, but unlike hurricanes, which leave lasting reminders of the devastation, memories of the heatwave disappear once cooler weather arrives.

This chapter reviews the clinical and epidemiologic features of heat-related deaths in the U.S. and discusses the potential impacts of climate change, urbanization, and demographic trends on EHE-related mortality. It also discusses the application of new methodologies for identifying locations and populations at greatest risk of exposure to extreme heat stress and their contribution to efforts to bolster public health preparedness for heatwaves.

Heat-Related Illness: Clinical and Epidemiologic Aspects

Prolonged exposure to high temperatures can cause heat-related illnesses, including heat cramps, heat syncope, heat exhaustion, heat stroke, and death. Heat exhaustion is the most common heat-related illness. Signs and symptoms include intense thirst, heavy sweating, weakness, paleness, discomfort, anxiety, dizziness, fatigue, fainting, nausea or vomiting, and headache. Core body temperature can be normal, below normal, or slightly elevated, and the skin can be cool and moist. If unrecognized and untreated, these mild to moderate signs and symptoms may progress to heat stroke. Heat stroke is a severe illness clinically defined as core body temperature ≥40.6° C (≥105° F), accompanied by hot, dry skin and central nervous system abnormalities, such as delirium, convulsions, or coma.

Those at particularly high risk of adverse health effects from extreme heat exposure include the elderly, those living alone, and people without access to air conditioning. In addition, people with chronic mental disorders or pre-existing medical conditions (e.g., cardiovascular disease, obesity, neurologic or psychiatric disease), and those receiving medications that interfere with salt and water balance (e.g., diuretics, anticholinergic agents, and tranquilizers that impair sweating), are at greater risk for heat-related illness and death. Drinking alcoholic beverages, ingesting narcotics (e.g., cocaine or amphetamines), and participating in strenuous outdoor physical activities (e.g., sports or manual labor) in hot weather also are risk behaviors associated with heat-related illnesses.

U.S. Heat-Related Morbidity and Mortality

Several dramatic events, such as the 1995 Chicago and the 2003 European heatwaves, have demonstrated the stunning lethality of extreme heat exposure. Estimating the death toll of less extreme heatwaves is difficult in the U.S. because heat-related illnesses such as heat stroke and heat exhaustion are not notifiable conditions (i.e., conditions requiring reporting to public health agencies by hospitals and health care providers) and because heat-related deaths are often misclassified or unrecognized.

In the U.S., many causes of death also increase during heatwaves. In addition to classic heat stroke, deaths from cardiovascular and respiratory diseases have been shown to rise. Because heat-related illnesses can cause various symptoms and exacerbate a wide variety of existing medical conditions, the etiology can be difficult to establish when the illness onset or death is not witnessed by a physician.

Although many medical examiners accurately document heat-related deaths, the criteria used to determine heat-related causes of death vary among states and can lead to underreporting of heat-related deaths, or to the reporting of heat as a factor contributing to death rather than the underlying cause. Therefore, estimates of mortality from hyperthermia likely underdocument the true magnitude. Often, medical examiners attribute heat exposure as a primary or contributing cause of death only if they record a core body temperature >40.6° C (>105° F). In the National Association of Medical Examiners' revised criteria, a death also can be classified as heat-related if the person is "found in an enclosed environment with a high ambient temperature without adequate cooling devices and the individual had been known to be alive at the onset of the heatwave."

Few studies have attempted to assess the impact of EHEs on morbidity. Semenza and colleagues analyzed hospital admissions in Chicago during the July 1995 EHE and estimated that it was responsible for over 1,000 excess hospital admissions, particularly among people with pre-existing diabetes, respiratory illnesses, and nervous system disorders. Schwartz and others found an association between elevated temperatures and short-term increases in cardiovascular-related hospital admissions for 12 U.S. cities. Similarly, a recent analysis of emergency medical services dispatch data in Phoenix concluded that the greatest incidence of heat-related medical dispatches occurred during the times of peak solar irradiance, maximum diurnal temperature, and elevated heat indices (combined temperature and relative humidity). Analysis of short- and long-term outcomes of heat-stroke patients who survived the 2003 heatwaves in France demonstrated that heat-stroke victims suffered a dramatic reduction in functional status that restricted discharge to home and resulted in early mortality.

As a result of differences in climate and the prevalence of adaptations such as air conditioning, heat-related mortality rates can be expected to vary among cities. In fact, studies of mortality following EHEs in the U.S. show significant regional variation. Historically, EHEs have had the greatest impact in the Northeast and Midwest and the least impact in the South and Southwest. These findings may suggest that populations in vulnerable cities are less acclimated to high temperatures and have reduced prevalence of adaptations such as air-conditioning.

Extreme heat event–related mortality is characterized by temperatures and humidities substantially greater than the mean for a specific time of year. Relative humidity is a critical factor in the impact of heat on human health, because of its effect on the body's ability to cool by evaporation. When relative humidity is high, the rate of evaporative cooling of sweat on the skin is reduced, making thermoregulation more difficult. Because residents adapt to warmer temperatures over the summer, heatwaves occurring early in the summer pose an increased risk of adverse health outcomes. The duration of the EHE and the number of days of elevated minimum temperatures are additional meteorologic conditions associated with high mortality.

High ambient heat also affects human health through its effect on air pollution. A positive association has been found between temperatures >32° C (>90° F) and ground-level ozone production, and increasing evidence suggests that ozone and high temperature affect mortality synergistically. Similarly, heatwave mortality is greatest on days with high PM 10 (particulate matter with diameter under 10μ).

Future Drivers of Heat-Related Mortality

Climate Change

Mounting evidence that the earth's climate is changing has led the UN Intergovernmental Panel on Climate Change (IPCC) to conclude that "warming of the climate system is unequivocal, as is now evident from observations of increases in global average air and ocean temperatures, widespread melting of snow and ice, and rising of global average sea level." In fact, climate model simulations project that, for the first half of the twenty-first century, year-round temperatures across North America will warm approximately 1°–3° C (2°–5° F). Late in the twenty-first century, projected annual warming is likely to be 2°–3° C (3°–5° F) across the western, southern, and eastern continental edges, but more than 5° C (9° F) at high latitudes, where many U.S. urban areas that have been affected by lethal heatwaves are located.

The impact of climate change on U.S. heatwaves may have already begun, as observed by the significant upward trend in the frequency of heatwaves from 1949 to 1995 ($p<0.01$) for the eastern and western U.S., indicating approximately a 20% overall increase in the number of heatwaves during that period. For the twenty-first century, the IPCC projects with high confidence that extreme heat events will intensify in magnitude and duration over portions of the U.S. where they already occur. As a consequence, populations in Northeastern and Midwestern U.S. cities are likely to experience the greatest number of illnesses and deaths in response to changes in summer temperatures.

Analyses of U.S. climate change scenarios through General Circulation Models (GCMs) project that, for the period 2080 to 2099, Chicago will experience a 25% increase in the number of heatwaves, and the number of annual heatwave days in Los Angeles, for the 2070 to 2099 time period, will increase from 12 to 44–95. In a study on the impact of future climate scenarios on mortality in 44 cities, Kalkstein and Greene estimate that by 2020, under a business-as-usual emissions scenario, excess annual summer deaths will increase from 1,840 to 1,981–4,100 (depending on the GCM used), and by 2050 up to 3,190–4,748 excess deaths will occur each summer.

The Urban Heat Island Effect

Cities and climate are co-evolving in a manner that will certainly amplify both the health effects of heat and the vulnerability of urban populations to heat-related death. More than half the world's population now lives in cities, up from 30% only 50 years ago. This rapid urbanization has quickly transformed environments from native vegetation to an engineered infrastructure that increases thermal-storage capacity, resulting in significant change in the urban climate compared with adjacent rural regions, known as the urban heat island (UHI) effect.

The UHI effect can be a powerful force in local climate. The combined effect of the high thermal mass provided by concrete and blacktop roads, the low ventilation ability of the urban "canyons" created by tall buildings, and "point-source" heat emitted from vehicles and air conditioners, magnifies the temperature increases created by climate change. In real terms, relative to the surrounding rural and suburban areas, the UHI effect can add from 1° C to 6° C (2° to 10° F) to ambient air temperature. More importantly, the UHI effect serves to absorb heat during the daytime and radiate it out at night, raising the nighttime minimum temperatures, which have been linked epidemiologically with excess mortality.

Other features of the built environment and urban sociodemographics have been shown to increase the risk of heat-related death, including access to transportation, medical care, and cooling centers as well as crime, housing type, and neighborhood land use. In a study looking at the role of the urban form in mitigating exposure to extreme heat within the UHI, Harlan and colleagues compared eight neighborhoods within metro Phoenix and looked for differences in exposure to heat stress and availability of adaptive resources such as air conditioning. They found statistically significant differences in thermal stress among the study neighborhoods, which were amplified during a heatwave. High settlement density, typified by apartment buildings, sparse vegetation, and lack of green space in the neighborhood were significantly correlated with higher temperatures and thermal comfort index. Lower socioeconomic and ethnic minority groups were more likely to live in warmer neighborhoods and not only have greater exposure to heat stress but also lack resources to cope with it. In sum, people in warmer neighborhoods were more vulnerable to heat exposure because they had greater exposure to heat and fewer social and material resources.

Demographic Trends

Advanced age represents one of the most significant risk factors for heat-related death in the U.S. In addition to having diminished thermoregulatory and physiologic heat-adaptation ability, the elderly are more likely to live alone, have reduced social contacts, and experience poor health. The prevalence of these social and physiological vulnerabilities to extreme heat will increase as the elderly become an increasingly larger proportion of the U.S. population.

Analysis of demographic trends in the U.S. project that the number of adults aged ≥65 years will nearly triple from 35 million in 2000 to almost 90 million by 2060. Similarly, the proportion of the total U.S. population aged ≥65 years will increase from 12.4% in 2000 to over 20% in 2060. Another demographic trend affecting vulnerability to extreme heat is population movement toward urban areas, which are gaining an estimated 67 million people globally per year—about 1.3 million every week. By 2030, approximately 60% of the projected global population of 8.3 billion will live in cities. In addition to the impact the UHI effect has on electrical use, large cities' demands on power during heatwaves can severely tax the power grid infrastructure leading to rolling brown-outs or a large-scale power failure, as was observed in the 2006 heatwave in New York City.

Communicating Risk and Effecting Behavior Change

At a fundamental level, the success of public health efforts to prevent morbidity and mortality during heatwaves hinges on their ability to effect behavior change in individuals during these events. Despite the lethality of heat and heatwaves, public recognition of the hazard of extreme heat exposure is still lacking. Recent studies suggest that although extreme heat advisories are effective in alerting the public to the dangers of these events, many at-risk individuals are unaware, or unwilling, to take appropriate preventive measures. A survey of individuals aged ≥65 years in four North American cities found that, whereas community knowledge of heatwave advisories was high, knowledge about appropriate preventive actions was low.

Bridging the gap between EHE planning efforts and individual action requires serious attention to health communication activities, including audience segment analysis and message testing.

Heatwaves pose a unique challenge to health communicators for several reasons. First, as noted above, heatwaves are less dramatic and conspicuous than other natural disasters. Second, whereas most natural disasters pose a sudden and abrupt risk to human health, the danger of hyperthermia gradually increases with duration of exposure, as a person's ability to withstand excessive heat gradually diminishes over time; the epidemiologic evidence for this can be seen in the two- to three-day lag in mortality following the start of a heatwave. Additionally, although individuals might be willing to adjust their activities for the first day or two of an extreme heat advisory, an individual's perceived threat of the heatwaves diminishes the longer the event lasts.

Along with individual perceptions of the risk of heat stroke during hot weather, economic factors also play a role. The high costs of running air conditioners during a heatwave imposes a significant economic burden, especially on the elderly living on a fixed income, many of whom decide to endure the heat rather than incur large bills. Sheridan and colleagues report in their survey that more than a third of study respondents considered cost as a factor in deciding whether to run the air conditioning in their home. Reflecting the under-appreciation of heat exposure as a health hazard, many state-run energy assistance programs, including the Low Income Home Energy Assistance Program (LIHEAP), provide energy assistance only for heating costs, not cooling costs. In fact, in 2007, only 16 states offered cooling-related energy assistance programs under LIHEAP.

Vulnerability Mapping

One important finding of epidemiologic investigations of EHE-related morbidity and mortality is that poor and minority populations, located in urban neighborhoods, are disproportionately affected. Techniques to characterize the UHI and surface temperature, through the use of satellite remote sensing instruments, now have a degree of spatial resolution that allows for the characterization on a neighborhood scale. These high-resolution remote sensing technologies enable the mapping of vegetation, land use, and thermal profiles, and can be integrated, through GIS [geographic information systems], with indicators of social vulnerability such as demographic profiles, income, housing stock, prevalence of air-conditioning, and access to transportation infrastructure. The refinement of these mapping techniques ultimately will provide local emergency response personnel with novel tools to improve planning and preparation for heatwaves, by allowing for better resource allocation and tailoring of health communication messages to specific ethnic or demographic groups. Additionally, state and local energy policy managers can apply these mapping techniques to prioritize locations for suspension of electricity shut-offs, or for provisioning of LIHEAP cooling assistance during EHEs.

Conclusion

Heatwaves are a significant public health threat in the U.S. Although climate change, urbanization, and demographic trends will continue to contribute to risk, preventive approaches can help reduce the morbidity and mortality associated with these events. Public health practitioners can play an active role in developing adaptation measures such as city-specific heat response plans. The development and implementation of these plans should be guided by the best evidence, generated by epidemiologic studies and ecologic models, on the relationship between hazard and health outcomes.

Chapter 16

Noise Pollution

The hubbub of the city—the phrase conveys the excitement, the hustle and bustle of urban life, the throng of crowds and traffic, traders, shoppers, rowdy diversion, and entertainment. In ancient Rome the clatter of iron wheels of wagons on the stone pavements disturbed the sleep and so annoyed citizens that legislation was enacted to control movement. Some cities of medieval Europe prohibited horse and carriage traffic to protect the sleep of the inhabitants.

The noise problems of the past are incomparable with those plaguing modern society: the roar of aircraft, the thunder of heavily laden lorries, and the thumps and whines of industry provide a noisy background to our lives. But such noise can be not only annoying but also damaging to health, and is increasing with economic development.

Health Impact

The recognition of noise as a serious health hazard as opposed to a nuisance is a recent development and the health effects of hazardous noise exposure are now considered to be an increasingly important public health problem.

"Occupational and Community Noise," Fact Sheet Number 258, February 2001, http://www.who.int/mediacentre/factsheets/fs258/en/index.html. Reviewed by David A. Cooke, MD, FACP, June 2009.

- Globally, some 120 million people are estimated to have disabling hearing difficulties.
- More than half citizens of Europe live in noisy surroundings; a third experience levels of noise at night that disturb sleep.
- In the United States in 1990 about 30 million people were daily exposed to a daily occupational noise level above 85 dB [decibels], compared with more than nine million people in 1981; these people were mostly in the production and manufacturing industries.
- In Germany and other developed countries as many as four to five million, that is 12–15% of all employed people, are exposed to noise levels of 85 dB or more. In Germany, an acquired noise-related hearing impairment that results in 20% or more reduction in earning ability is compensatable; in 1993, nearly 12,500 new such cases were registered.
- Prolonged or excessive exposure to noise, whether in the community or at work, can cause permanent medical conditions, such as hypertension and ischemic heart disease.
- Noise can adversely affect performance, for example in reading, attentiveness, problem solving, and memory. Deficits in performance can lead to accidents.
- Noise above 80 dB may increase aggressive behavior.
- A link between community noise and mental health problems is suggested by the demand for tranquilizers and sleeping pills, the incidence of psychiatric symptoms, and the number of admissions to mental hospitals.

Noise can cause hearing impairment, interfere with communication, disturb sleep, cause cardiovascular and psycho-physiological effects, reduce performance, and provoke annoyance responses and changes in social behavior. The main social consequence of hearing impairment is the inability to understand speech in normal conditions, which is considered a severe social handicap.

Whereas in the developed world hearing impairment is mostly restricted to the work setting, in cities in the developing world the problems are worse, with increasing hearing impairment due to community noise.

Sound and the Ear

At birth the inner ear is fully developed and has its full complement of hair cells, supporting cells, and nerve fibers. Unlike most other tissues in the body, mammalian hair cells and nerve fibers do not regenerate when damaged.

The response of the human ear to sound depends both on the sound frequency (measured in Hertz, Hz) and the sound pressure, measured in decibels (dB). A normal ear in a healthy young person can detect sounds with frequencies from 20 Hz to 20,000 Hz. Speech frequency ranges from 100 to 6,000 Hz.

Community Noise

Noise-induced hearing impairment is by no means restricted to occupational situations—noise levels associated with impairment are experienced at open-air concerts, discotheques, motor sports events, etc.

Such nonindustrial noise is referred to as community noise, also known as environmental, residential, or domestic noise. The main indoor sources are ventilation systems, office machines, home appliances, and neighbors. Other typical sources of neighborhood noise include the catering trade (restaurants, cafeterias, etc.), live or recorded music, sports, playgrounds, car parks, barking dogs.

For most people, lifetime's continuous exposure to an environmental average noise level of 70 dB will not cause hearing impairment. An adult person's ear can tolerate an occasional noise level of up to 140 dB, but for children such an exposure should never exceed 120 dB.

Continued growth in transport systems—highways, airports, and railways—generate more noise. Many countries have regulations on community noise from rail, road, construction, and industrial plants based on emission standards, but few have any regulations on neighborhood community noise, probably owing to difficulties with its definition, measurement, and control. This and the insufficient knowledge of the effects of noise on people handicap attempts to prevent and control the problem.

Occupational Noise

Occupational Sources of Noise

The many and varied sources of noise in industrial machinery and processes include: rotors, gears, turbulent fluid flow, impact processes, electrical machines, internal combustion engines, pneumatic equipment, drilling, crushing, blasting, pumps, and compressors. Furthermore, the emitted sounds are reflected from floors, ceiling, and equipment. Noise is a common occupational hazard in many workplaces.

The major sources of noise that damages hearing are impact processes, material handling, and industrial jets.

- Air jets—widely used, for example, for cleaning, drying, power tools, and steam valves—can generate sound levels of 105 dB.
- Workers in a cigarette factory in Brazil involved in compressed air cleaning were exposed to sound levels equivalent to 92 dB for eight hours.
- In the woodworking industry the sound levels of saws can be as high as 106 dB.
- Average sound levels range between 92 and 96 dB in industries such as foundries, shipyards, breweries, weaving factories, paper and saw mills. The recorded peak values were between 117 and 136 dB.
- In most developing countries, industrial noise levels are higher than those in developed countries.
- Noise-induced hearing impairment is the most common irreversible (and preventable) occupational hazards worldwide.

Cheaper, more cost-effective production is a driving force in economic development. However, new processes introduced on grounds of cost-effectiveness are often noisier than previous ones. The associated rise in noise levels is often overlooked. Thus, even though noise-reducing measures may have been incorporated in the design of machinery, greater output may generate higher noise levels. For example, for every doubling of the speed of rotary machines the noise emission rises by about 7 dB, of warp knitting looms—12 dB, of diesel engines—9 dB, of petrol engines—15 dB, and of fans—between 18 to 24 dB.

- Exposure for more than eight hours a day to sound in excess of 85 dB is potentially hazardous.

After exposure to a typical hazardous industrial sound around 90 dB for an eight-hour work day, the ear tires and hearing is temporarily impaired.

- Industrial workers exposed to noise often turn the volume of their car radios up when they leave work, but turn it down in the morning, because it is too loud. After a time, hearing recovery becomes less complete and impairment becomes permanent. This can be noticeable within 6–12 months of starting a job where levels of sound are hazardous.

- Transient tinnitus (ringing in the ear) is a common occupational hearing condition, especially in people exposed to impact noise. It should be considered as a warning of excessive exposure to sound and a trigger for appropriate preventive action.

Warning sounds: One sound can sometimes interfere with the perception of another. Because lower frequency sounds can mask higher sounds, warning sounds should be pitched at lower frequencies than the dominant industrial background noise.

Occupational Exposure Limits

Occupational exposure limits specify the maximum sound pressure levels and exposure times to which nearly all workers may be repeatedly exposed without adverse effect on their ability to hear and understand normal speech. An occupational exposure limit of 85 dB for eight hours should protect most people against a permanent hearing impairment induced by noise after 40 years of occupational exposure.

Noise Reduction

Noise-induced hearing impairment is preventable.

- Protection against hazardous noise exposure should be included into overall hazard prevention and control programs in workplaces. The dangers of noise should be recognized before workers start complaining of hearing difficulties.

Machine Safety

A European Union directive requires that machines are so designed and constructed that hazards from noise emissions are minimized. Declarations of the noise emissions of machines are required, to allow potential buyers not only to select the least hazardous equipment but also to calculate the noise impact at workplaces and to help with noise-control planning.

- It is 10 times less expensive (unit cost per decibel reduction) to make noise-generating processes quieter than to make a barrier to screen the noise.

Noise levels can be lowered by the use of noise-control enclosures, absorbers, silencers, and baffles and by the use of personal protective equipment, such as earmuffs. Where technical methods are insufficient, noise exposure may be reduced by use of hearing protection and by administrative controls—such as limiting the time spent in noisy environment and scheduling noisy operations outside normal shifts or at distant locations.

Essential elements of noise-control programs are education and training of the workers as well as regular hearing tests.

WHO [World Health Organization] Response

WHO has responded in two main ways: by developing and promoting the concept of noise management, and by drawing up community noise guidelines. The field is marked by a scarcity of literature, especially for developing countries. Some 20 years after its last publication on noise, WHO has issued "Guidelines for Community Noise." This publication, the outcome of a WHO expert task force meeting in London in March 1999, includes guideline values for community noise (listing also critical health effects ranging from annoyance to hearing impairment), for example [see the levels in Table 16.1]:

Table 16.1. Guideline Values for Community Noise

Environment	Critical health effect	Sound level dB(A)*	Time hours
Outdoor living areas	Annoyance	50–55	16
Indoor dwellings	Speech intelligibility	35	16
Bedrooms	Sleep disturbance	30	8
School classrooms	Disturbance of communication	35	During class
Industrial, commercial, and traffic areas	Hearing impairment	70	24
Music through earphones	Hearing impairment	85	1
Ceremonies and entertainment	Hearing impairment	100	4

*The ear has different sensitivities to different frequencies, being least sensitive to extremely high and extremely low frequencies. Because of this varied sensitivity, the term "A weighting" is used: All the different frequencies that make up the sound are assessed to give a sound pressure level. The sound pressure level measured in dB is referred to as "A-weighted" and expressed as dB(A).

The guidelines also offer recommendations to governments for implementation, such as extending (and enforcing) existing legislation and including community noise in environmental impact assessments. The role of WHO is to provide leadership and technical support.

Chapter 17

Ultraviolet (UV) Light

Too Much Sun Is Dangerous

Sunlight, an essential prerequisite for life, may be extremely dangerous to human health. Excessive exposure to the sun is known to be associated with increased risks of various skin cancers, cataracts and other eye diseases, as well as accelerated skin aging. It may also adversely affect people's ability to resist infectious diseases and compromise the effectiveness of vaccination programs.

Sunlight is electromagnetic energy, which is propagated by electromagnetic waves. Health wise, the most important parts of the sunlight electromagnetic spectrum are: ultraviolet radiation (UV), invisible to the eye; visible light that allows us to see; and infrared radiation, which is our main source of heat but is also invisible. Excessive exposures to them pose particular risks to health.

Skin

Excessive UV exposure results in a number of chronic skin changes. These include various skin cancers of which melanoma is the most life threatening, an increased number of moles (benign abnormalities of melanocytes), and a range of other alterations arising from UV

"Ultraviolet Radiation: Solar Radiation and Human Health," Fact Sheet Number 227, August 1999, http://www.who.int/mediacentre/factsheets/fs227/en/index.html. Reviewed by David A. Cooke, MD, FACP, June 2009.

damage to keratinocytes and blood vessels. UV damage to fibrous tissue is often described as "photoaging." Photoaging makes people look older because their skin loses its tightness and so sags or wrinkles.

- United Nations Environment Programme (UNEP) has estimated that more than two million nonmelanoma skin cancers and 200,000 malignant melanomas occur globally each year.
- In the event of a 10% decrease in stratospheric ozone, an additional 300,000 nonmelanoma and 4,500 melanoma skin cancers could be expected worldwide.
- Caucasians have a higher risk of skin cancer because of the relative lack of skin pigmentation.
- The worldwide incidence of malignant melanoma continues to increase and is strongly related to frequency of recreational exposure to the sun and to history of sunburn.
- There is evidence that risk of melanoma is also related to intermittent exposure to UV, especially in childhood, and to exposure to sunlamps. However, the latter results are still preliminary.

Eye

UV exposure of the eye depends on many factors: ground reflection, the degree of brightness in the sky leading to activation of the squint reflex, the amount of atmospheric refection, and the use of eyewear.

- The acute effects of UV on the eye include the development of photokeratitis and photoconjunctivitis, which are like sunburn of the delicate skin-like tissue on the surface of the eyeball (cornea) and eyelids. While painful, they are reversible, easily prevented by protective eyewear, and have not been associated with any long-term damage.
- Chronic effects include the possible development of pterygium (a white or cream-colored opaque growth attached to the cornea), squamous cell cancer of the conjunctiva (scaly or plate-like malignancy), and cataracts.
- Some 20 million people worldwide are currently blind as a result of cataracts. Of these, WHO [World Health Organization] estimates that as many as 20% may be due to UV exposure. Experts believe that each 1% sustained decrease in stratospheric ozone would result in an increase of 0.5% in the number of cataracts caused by solar UV.

- Direct viewing of the sun and other extremely bright objects can also seriously damage the very sensitive part of the retina called the yellow spot, fovea, or macula lutea. When cells of the fovea are destroyed, people can no longer view fine detail. This is a serious visual impairment making it impossible to read, sew, watch TV, recognize faces, drive a vehicle, or do any task which requires recognition of fine details.

Immune System

UV also appears to alter immune response by changing the activity and distribution of the cells responsible for triggering these responses. A number of studies indicate that UV exposures at environmental levels suppress immune responses in both rodents and humans. In rodents, this immune suppression results in enhanced susceptibility to certain infectious diseases with skin involvement and some systemic infections. Mechanisms associated with UV-induced immunosuppression and host defense that protect against infectious agents are similar in rodents and humans. It is therefore reasonable to assume that UV exposure may enhance the risk of infection and decrease the effectiveness of vaccines in humans. Additional research is necessary to substantiate this.

Thermal Effects

Heating of tissues in the human body is the principal effect of infrared radiation. Excessive infrared radiation can result in heat strokes and other similar reactions particularly in elderly, infirm, or very young individuals. At moderate levels of exposure, the warmth experienced from being in the sun is relaxing and restorative.

Protective Measures

Methods for personal protection from solar UV exposure include adequate clothing, hats, and the proper use of sunscreens to protect UV-exposed skin. For eye protection, UV-absorbing sunglasses are needed.

Changes in behavior could minimize solar UV exposure. These include staying out of the sun, either indoors or in shaded areas, during the four-hour period around solar noon when UV levels are at their highest. During summer, when daylight saving time is in effect, solar noon in most of Europe is at 14.00 hours (2 p.m.); in the U.K. and countries with a similar longitude, it is at 13.00 hours (1 p.m.).

Broad-spectrum sunscreens should be used when other means of protection are not feasible, and then to reduce exposure rather than lengthen the period of exposure. While topical applications of sunscreen are preferred for absorbing UVB, some preparations do not absorb the longer wavelength UVA effectively. Moreover, some preparations have been found to contain ingredients that are mutagenic in sunlight. People using sunscreens should use those with a high sun protection factor (SPF) and be aware that they are to protect from the sun and not for tanning purposes.

The reflective properties of the ground have an influence on UV exposure. Most natural surfaces such as grass, soil, and water reflect less than 10% of incident UV. However, fresh snow reflects nearly 80% while sand reflects 10–25%, significantly increasing UV exposure for skiers and bathers.

Chapter 18

Drinking Water

Chapter Contents

Section 18.1

Drinking Water Hazards

This section excerpted from "Water on Tap," Environmental Protection Agency (www.epa.gov), October 2003. Revised by David A. Cooke, MD, FACP, June 2009.

The Nation's Drinking Water

The United States enjoys one of the best supplies of drinking water in the world. Nevertheless, many of us who once gave little or no thought to the water that comes from our taps are now asking the question: "Is my water safe to drink?" While tap water that meets federal and state standards is generally safe to drink, threats to drinking water are increasing. Short-term disease outbreaks and water restrictions during droughts have demonstrated that we can no longer take our drinking water for granted.

Consumers have many questions about their drinking water. How safe is my drinking water? What is being done to improve security of public water systems? Where does my drinking water come from, and how is it treated? Do private wells receive the same protection as public water systems? What can I do to help protect my drinking water?

This section provides the answers to these and other frequently asked questions. Additionally, the Safe Drinking Water Hotline (800-426-4791) is available to answer your questions.

Are some populations more vulnerable to water-supply issues?

Some people may be more vulnerable to contaminants in drinking water than the general population. People undergoing chemotherapy or living with HIV/AIDS, transplant patients, children and infants, the frail elderly, and pregnant women and their fetuses can be particularly at risk for infections.

If you have special health care needs, consider taking additional precautions with your drinking water, and seek advice from your health care provider. For more information, see www.epa.gov/safewater/healthcare/special.html.

Drinking Water Safety

What law keeps my drinking water safe?

Congress passed the Safe Drinking Water Act (SDWA) in 1974 to protect public health by regulating the nation's public drinking water supply and protecting sources of drinking water. SDWA is administered by the U.S. Environmental Protection Agency (EPA) and its state partners.

The following items summarize highlights of the Safe Drinking Water Act:

- Authorizes EPA to set enforceable health standards for contaminants in drinking water.
- Requires public notification of water systems violations and annual reports (Consumer Confidence Reports) to customers on contaminants found in their drinking water (www.epa.gov/safewater/ccr).
- Establishes a federal-state partnership for regulation enforcement.
- Includes provisions specifically designed to protect underground sources of drinking water (www.epa.gov/safewater/uic).
- Requires disinfection of surface water supplies, except those with pristine, protected sources.
- Establishes a multi-billion-dollar state revolving loan fund for water system upgrades (www.epa.gov/safewater/dwsrf).
- Requires an assessment of the vulnerability of all drinking water sources to contamination (www.epa.gov/safewater/protect).

What is a public water system?

The Safe Drinking Water Act defines a public water system (PWS) as one that serves piped water to at least 25 persons or 15 service connections for at least 60 days each year. There are approximately 161,000 public water systems in the United States. Such systems may be publicly or privately owned. Community water systems (CWSs) are public water systems that serve people year-round in their homes. Most people in the U.S. (268 million) get their water from a community water system. EPA also regulates other kinds of public water systems, such as those at schools, campgrounds, factories, and restaurants. Private water supplies, such as household wells that serve one or a few homes, are not regulated by EPA.

Will water systems have adequate funding in the future?

Nationwide, drinking water systems have spent hundreds of billions of dollars to build drinking water treatment and distribution systems. From 1995 to 2000, more than $50 billion was spent on capital investments to fund water quality improvements.

With the aging of the nation's infrastructure, the clean water and drinking water industries face a significant challenge to sustain and advance their achievements in protecting public health. EPA's Clean Water & Drinking Water Infrastructure Gap Analysis has found that if present levels of spending do not increase, there will be a significant funding gap by the year 2019.

Where can I find information about my local water system?

Since 1999, water suppliers have been required to provide annual Consumer Confidence Reports to their customers. These reports are due by July 1 each year, and contain information on contaminants found in the drinking water, possible health effects, and the water's source. Some Consumer Confidence Reports are available at www.epa.gov/safewater/dwinfo.htm.

Water suppliers must promptly inform you if your water has become contaminated by something that can cause immediate illness. Water suppliers have 24 hours to inform their customers of violations of EPA standards "that have the potential to have serious adverse effects on human health as a result of short-term exposure." If such a violation occurs, the water system will announce it through the media, and must provide information about the potential adverse effects on human health, steps the system is taking to correct the violation, and the need to use alternative water supplies (such as boiled or bottled water) until the problem is corrected.

Systems will inform customers about violations of less immediate concern in the first water bill sent after the violation, in a Consumer Confidence Report, or by mail within a year. In 1998, states began compiling information on individual systems, so you can evaluate the overall quality of drinking water in your state. Additionally, EPA must compile and summarize the state reports into an annual report on the condition of the nation's drinking water. To view the most recent annual report, see www.epa.gov/safewater/annual.

How often is my water supply tested?

EPA has established pollutant-specific minimum testing schedules for public water systems. To find out how frequently your drinking water is tested, contact your water system or the agency in your state in charge of drinking water.

If a problem is detected, immediate retesting requirements go into effect along with strict instructions about how the system informs the public. Until the system can reliably demonstrate that it is free of problems, the retesting is continued.

In 2001, one out of every four community water systems did not conduct testing or report the results for all of the monitoring required to verify the safety of their drinking water. Although failure to monitor does not necessarily suggest safety problems, conducting the required reporting is crucial to ensure that problems will be detected. Consumers can help make sure certain monitoring and reporting requirements are met by first contacting their state drinking water agency to determine if their water supplier is in compliance. If the water system is not meeting the requirements, consumers can work with local and state officials and the water supplier to make sure the required monitoring and reporting occurs.

A network of government agencies monitor tap water suppliers and enforce drinking water standards to ensure the safety of public water supplies. These agencies include EPA, state departments of health and environment, and local public health departments. Nevertheless, problems with local drinking water can, and do, occur.

What problems can occur?

Actual events of drinking water contamination are rare, and typically do not occur at levels likely to pose health concerns. However, as development in our modern society increases, there are growing numbers of activities that can contaminate our drinking water. Improperly disposed-of chemicals, animal and human wastes, wastes injected underground, and naturally occurring substances have the potential to contaminate drinking water. Likewise, drinking water that is not properly treated or disinfected, or that travels through an improperly maintained distribution system, may also pose a health risk. Greater vigilance by you, your water supplier, and your government can help prevent such events in your water supply.

Contaminants can enter water supplies either as a result of human and animal activities, or because they occur naturally in the environment. Threats to your drinking water may exist in your neighborhood, or may occur many miles away. For more information on drinking water threats, see www.epa.gov/safewater/publicoutreach/landscapeposter.html. Some typical examples are microbial contamination, chemical contamination from fertilizers, and lead contamination.

Common sources of pollution include the following:

- *Naturally Occurring:* Microorganisms (wildlife and soils), radionuclides (underlying rock), nitrates and nitrites (nitrogen compounds in the soil), heavy metals (underground rocks containing arsenic, cadmium, chromium, lead, and selenium), fluoride.
- *Human Activities:* Bacteria and nitrates (human and animal wastes—septic tanks and large farms), heavy metals (mining construction, older fruit orchards), fertilizers and pesticides (used by you and others, anywhere crops or lawns are maintained), industrial products and wastes (local factories, industrial plants, gas stations, dry cleaners, leaking underground storage tanks, landfills, and waste dumps), household wastes (cleaning solvents, used motor oil, paint, paint thinner), lead and copper (household plumbing materials), water treatment chemicals (wastewater treatment plants), prescription medications (improperly disposed medications).

Microbial Contamination: The potential for health problems from microbial-contaminated drinking water is demonstrated by localized outbreaks of waterborne disease. Many of these outbreaks have been linked to contamination by bacteria or viruses, probably from human or animal wastes. For example, in 1999 and 2000, there were 39 reported disease outbreaks associated with drinking water, some of which were linked to public drinking water supplies.

Certain pathogens (disease-causing microorganisms), such as *Cryptosporidium*, may occasionally pass through water filtration and disinfection processes in numbers high enough to cause health problems, particularly in vulnerable members of the population. *Cryptosporidium* causes the gastrointestinal disease cryptosporidiosis and can cause serious, sometimes fatal, symptoms, especially among sensitive members of the population. A serious outbreak of cryptosporidiosis occurred in 1993 in Milwaukee, Wisconsin, causing more than 400,000 persons to be infected with the disease, and resulting in at least 50 deaths. This was the largest recorded outbreak of waterborne disease in United States history.

When microorganisms such as those that indicate fecal contamination are found in drinking water, water suppliers are required to issue "Boil Water Notices." Boiling water for one minute kills the microorganisms that cause disease. Therefore, these notices serve as a precaution to the public (see www.epa.gov/safewater/faq/emerg.html).

Chemical Contamination from Fertilizers: Nitrate, a chemical most commonly used as a fertilizer, poses an immediate threat to infants when it is found in drinking water at levels above the national standard. Nitrates are converted to nitrites in the intestines. Once absorbed into the bloodstream, nitrites prevent hemoglobin from transporting oxygen. (Older children have an enzyme that restores hemoglobin.) Excessive levels can cause "blue baby syndrome," which can be fatal without immediate medical attention. Infants most at risk for blue baby syndrome are those who are already sick, and while they are sick, consume food that is high in nitrates or drink water or formula mixed with water that is high in nitrates. Avoid using water with high nitrate levels for drinking. This is especially important for infants and young children, nursing mothers, pregnant women, and certain elderly people.

Do NOT boil water to attempt to reduce nitrates. Boiling water contaminated with nitrates increases its concentration and potential risk. If you are concerned about nitrates, talk to your health care provider about alternatives to boiling water for baby formula.

Lead Contamination: Lead, a metal found in natural deposits, is commonly used in household plumbing materials and water service lines. The greatest exposure to lead is swallowing lead paint chips or breathing in lead dust. But lead in drinking water can also cause a variety of adverse health effects. In babies and children, exposure to lead in drinking water above the action level of lead (0.015 milligram per liter) can result in delays in physical and mental development, along with slight deficits in attention span and learning abilities. Adults who drink this water over many years could develop kidney problems or high blood pressure. Lead is rarely found in source water, but enters tap water through corrosion of plumbing materials. Very old and poorly maintained homes may be more likely to have lead pipes, joints, and solder. However, new homes are also at risk: pipes legally considered to be "lead-free" may contain up to 8% lead. These pipes can leach significant amounts of lead in the water for the first several months after their installation. For more information on lead contamination, see www.epa.gov/safewater/contaminants/dw_contamfs/lead.html.

Do NOT boil water to attempt to reduce lead. Boiling water increases lead concentration. Always use water from the cold tap for preparing baby formula, cooking, and drinking. Flush pipes first by running the water before using it. Allow the water to run until it's cold. If you have high lead levels in your tap water, talk to your health care provider about alternatives to using boiled water in baby formula.

Where can I find more information about my drinking water?

Drinking water varies from place to place, depending on the water's source and the treatment it receives. If your drinking water comes from a community water system, the system will deliver to its customers annual drinking water quality reports (or Consumer Confidence Reports). These reports will tell consumers what contaminants have been detected in their drinking water, how these detection levels compare to drinking water standards, and where their water comes from. The reports must be provided annually before July 1, and, in most cases, are mailed directly to customers' homes. Contact your water supplier to get a copy of your report, or see if your report is posted online at www.epa.gov/safewater/dwinfo.htm. Your state's department of health or environment can also be a valuable source of information. For help in locating these agencies, call the Safe Drinking Water Hotline (800-426-4791).

For more information on drinking water contaminants that are regulated by EPA visit www.epa.gov/safewater/mcl.html.

Where Drinking Water Comes from and How It Is Treated

Your drinking water comes from surface water or ground water. The water that systems pump and treat from sources open to the atmosphere, such as rivers, lakes, and reservoirs, is known as surface water. Water pumped from wells drilled into underground aquifers, geologic formations containing water, is called ground water. The quantity of water produced by a well depends on the nature of the rock, sand, or soil in the aquifer from which the water is drawn. Drinking water wells may be shallow (50 feet or less) or deep (more than 1,000 feet). More water systems have ground water than surface water as a source (approx. 147,000 v. 14,500), but more people drink from a surface water system (195 million v. 101,400). Large-scale water supply systems tend to rely on surface water resources, while smaller water systems tend to use ground water. Your water utility or public works department can tell you the source of your public water supply.

How does water get to my faucet?

An underground network of pipes typically delivers drinking water to the homes and businesses served by the water system. Small systems serving just a handful of households may be relatively simple, while large metropolitan systems can be extremely complex—sometimes consisting of thousands of miles of pipes serving millions of people. Drinking water must meet required health standards when it leaves the treatment plant. After treated water leaves the plant, it is monitored within the distribution system to identify and remedy any problems such as water main breaks, pressure variations, or growth of microorganisms.

How is my water treated to make it safe?

Water utilities treat nearly 34 billion gallons of water every day. The amount and type of treatment applied varies with the source and quality of the water. Generally, surface water systems require more treatment than ground water systems because they are directly exposed to the atmosphere and runoff from rain and melting snow.

Water suppliers use a variety of treatment processes to remove contaminants from drinking water. These individual processes can be arranged in a "treatment train" (a series of processes applied in a sequence). The most commonly used processes include coagulation (flocculation and sedimentation), filtration, and disinfection. Some water systems also use ion exchange and adsorption. Water utilities select the treatment combination most appropriate to treat the contaminants found in the source water of that particular system.

Flocculation: This step removes dirt and other particles suspended in the water. Alum and iron salts or synthetic organic polymers are added to the water to form tiny sticky particles called "floc," which attract the dirt particles.

Sedimentation: The flocculated particles then settle naturally out of the water.

Filtration: Many water treatment facilities use filtration to remove all particles from the water. Those particles include clays and silts, natural organic matter, precipitates from other treatment processes in the facility, iron and manganese, and microorganisms. Filtration clarifies the water and enhances the effectiveness of disinfection.

Disinfection: Disinfection of drinking water is considered to be one of the major public health advances of the twentieth century. Water is often disinfected before it enters the distribution system to ensure that dangerous microbial contaminants are killed. Chlorine, chlorinates, or chlorine dioxides are most often used because they are very effective disinfectants, and residual concentrations can be maintained in the water system. Some systems may also expose the water to intense ultraviolet light, which kills microorganisms.

Disinfection of drinking water is one of the major public health advances of the twentieth century. However, sometimes the disinfectants themselves can react with naturally occurring materials in the water to form unintended byproducts, which may pose health risks. EPA recognizes the importance of removing microbial contaminants while simultaneously protecting the public from disinfection byproducts, and has developed regulations to limit the presence of these byproducts. For more information, see www.epa.gov/safewater/mdbp.html.

Water Security

What security measures are in place to protect water systems?

Drinking water utilities today find themselves facing new responsibilities due to concerns over water system security and counterterrorism. EPA is committed to the safety of public drinking water supplies and has taken numerous steps to work with utilities, other government agencies, and law enforcement to minimize threats.

The Public Health Security and Bioterrorism Preparedness and Response Act of 2002 requires that all community water systems serving more than 3,300 people evaluate their susceptibility to potential threats and identify corrective actions. EPA has provided assistance to help utilities with these Vulnerability Assessments by giving direct grants to large systems, supporting self-assessment tools, and providing technical help and training to small and medium utilities. For more information on water system security, see www.epa.gov/safewater/security.

How can I help protect my drinking water?

Local drinking water and wastewater systems may be targets for terrorists and other would-be criminals wishing to disrupt and cause harm to your community water supplies or wastewater facilities.

Because utilities are often located in isolated areas, drinking water sources and wastewater collection systems may cover large areas that are difficult to secure and patrol. Residents can be educated to notice and report any suspicious activity in and around local water utilities. Any residents interested in protecting their water resources and community as a whole can join together with law enforcement, neighborhood watch groups, water suppliers, wastewater operators, and other local public health officials. If you witness suspicious activities, report them to your local law enforcement authorities.

Examples of suspicious activities might include the following:

- People climbing or cutting a utility fence
- People dumping or discharging material to a water reservoir
- Unidentified truck or car parked or loitering near waterway or facilities for no apparent reason
- Suspicious opening or tampering with manhole covers, fire hydrants, buildings, or equipment
- People climbing or on top of water tanks
- People photographing or videotaping utility facilities, structures, or equipment
- Strangers hanging around locks or gates

Do not confront strangers. Instead report suspicious activities to local authorities.

When reporting an incident, follow these steps:

- State the nature of the incident.
- Identify yourself and your location.
- Identify location of activity.
- Describe any vehicle involved (color, make, model, plate number).
- Describe the participants (how many, sex, race, color of hair, height, weight, clothing).

What can I do if there is a problem with my drinking water?

Local incidents, such as spills and treatment problems, can lead to short-term needs for alternative water supplies or in-home water treatment. In isolated cases, individuals may need to rely on alternative sources for the long-term, due to their individual health needs or problems with obtaining new drinking water supplies.

What alternative sources of water are available?

Bottled water is sold in supermarkets and convenience stores. Some companies lease or sell water dispensers or bubblers and regularly deliver large bottles of water to homes and businesses. It is expensive compared to water from a public water system. The bottled water quality varies among brands, because of the variations in the source water used, costs, and company practices. Analyses of various bottled water brands have shown many of them to be no different than tap water, and in some cases to have elevated levels of contaminants.

The U.S. Food and Drug Administration (FDA) regulates bottled water used for drinking. While most consumers assume that bottled water is at least as safe as tap water, there are still potential risks. Although required to meet the same safety standards as public water supplies, bottled water does not undergo the same testing and reporting as water from a treatment facility. Water that is bottled and sold in the same state may not be subject to any federal standards at all. Those with compromised immune systems may want to read bottled water labels to make sure more stringent treatments have been used, such as reverse osmosis, distillation, UV radiation, or filtration by an absolute one micron filter.

Check with NSF International to see if your bottled water adheres to FDA and international drinking water standards. The International Bottled Water Association can also provide information on which brands adhere to even more stringent requirements.

Can I do anything in my house to improve the safety of my drinking water?

Most people do not need to treat drinking water in their home to make it safe. However, a home water treatment unit can improve water's taste, or provide a factor of safety for those people more vulnerable to waterborne disease. There are different options for home treatment systems. Point-of-use (POU) systems treat water at a single tap. Point-of-entry (POE) systems treat water used throughout the house. POU systems can be installed in various places in the home, including the counter top, the faucet itself, or under the sink. POE systems are installed where the water line enters the house.

POU and POE devices are based on various contaminant removal technologies. Filtration, ion exchange, reverse osmosis, and distillation are some of the treatment methods used. All types of units are generally available from retailers, or by mail order. Prices can reach well into the hundreds and sometimes thousands of dollars, and depending on the method and location of installation, plumbing can also add to the cost.

Activated carbon filters absorb organic contaminants that cause taste and odor problems. Depending on their design, some units can remove chlorination byproducts, some cleaning solvents, and pesticides. To maintain the effectiveness of these units, the carbon canisters must be replaced periodically. Activated carbon filters are efficient in removing metals such as lead and copper if they are designed to absorb or remove lead.

Because ion exchange units can be used to remove minerals from your water, particularly calcium and magnesium, they are sold for water softening. Some ion exchange softening units remove radium and barium from water. Ion exchange systems that employ activated alumina are used to remove fluoride and arsenate from water. These units must be regenerated periodically with salt.

Reverse osmosis treatment units generally remove a more diverse list of contaminants than other systems. They can remove nitrates, sodium, other dissolved inorganics, and organic compounds.

Distillation units boil water and condense the resulting steam to create distilled water. Depending on their design, some of these units may allow vaporized organic contaminants to condense back into the product water, thus minimizing the removal of organics.

You may choose to boil your water to remove microbial contaminants. Keep in mind that boiling reduces the volume of water by about 20%, thus concentrating those contaminants not affected by the temperature of boiling water, such as nitrates and pesticides.

No one unit can remove everything. Have your water tested by a certified laboratory prior to purchasing any device. Do not rely on the tests conducted by salespeople that want to sell you their product.

Maintaining Treatment Devices: All POU and POE treatment units need maintenance to operate effectively. If they are not maintained properly, contaminants may accumulate in the units and actually make your water worse. In addition, some vendors may make claims about their effectiveness that have no merit. Units are tested for their safety and effectiveness by two organizations, NSF International and Underwriters Laboratory. In addition, the Water Quality Association represents the household, commercial, industrial, and small community treatment industry and can help you locate a professional that meets their code of ethics. EPA does not test or certify these treatment units.

Protect Your Drinking Water

Stormwater runoff threatens our sources of drinking water. As this water washes over roofs, pavement, farms, and grassy areas, it picks up fertilizers, pesticides, and litter and deposits them in surface water and ground water. Here are some other threats to our drinking water:

Every year the following occur:

- We apply 67 million pounds of pesticides that contain toxic and harmful chemicals to our lawns.
- We produce more than 230 million tons of municipal solid water—approximately five pounds of trash or garbage per person per day—that contain bacteria, nitrates, viruses, synthetic detergents, and household chemicals.
- Our more than 12 million recreational and houseboats and 10,000 boat marinas release solvents, gasoline, detergents, and raw sewage directly into our rivers, lakes, and streams.
- Prescription medications are increasingly being recognized as significant water contaminants. Some are present in water supplies in sufficient levels that they might have effects on wildlife, and possibly humans as well. While some drugs are being released from the urine and stool of patients taking medications, most of the contamination is from people dumping unused medication down sinks and toilets.

Drinking water protection is a shared responsibility. Many actions are underway to protect our nation's drinking water, and there are many opportunities for citizens to become involved.

How can I be involved in protecting my water?

EPA activities to protect drinking water include setting drinking water standards and overseeing the work of states that enforce federal standards—or stricter ones set by the individual state. EPA holds many public meetings on issues ranging from proposed drinking water standards to the development of databases. You can also comment on proposed drafts of other upcoming EPA documents. A list of public meetings and regulations open for comment can be found at www.epa.gov/safewater/pubinput/html.

How can I be informed about water safety?

- Read the annual Consumer Confidence Report provided by your water supplier. Some Consumer Confidence Reports are available at www.epa.gov/safewater/dwinfo.htm.
- Use information from your state's Source Water Assessment to learn about potential threats to your water source.
- If you are one of the 15% of Americans who uses a private source of drinking water—such as a well, cistern, or spring—find out what activities are taking place in your watershed that may impact your drinking water, talk to local experts, test your water periodically, and maintain your well properly.
- Find out if the Clean Water Act standards for your drinking water source are intended to protect water for drinking, in addition to fishing and swimming.

What should I look for regarding water safety?

- Look around your watershed and look for announcements in the local media about activities that may pollute your drinking water.
- Form and operate a citizens watch network within your community to communicate regularly with law enforcement, your public water supplier, and wastewater operator. Communication is key to a safer community.
- Be alert. Get to know your water/wastewater utilities, their vehicles, routines, and their personnel.
- Become aware of your surroundings. This will help you to recognize suspicious activity as opposed to normal daily activities.

What other ways are there to get involved?

- Attend public hearings on new construction, storm water permitting, and town planning.
- Keep your public officials accountable by asking to see their environmental impact statements.
- Ask questions about any issue that may affect your water source.
- Participate with your government and your water system as they make funding decisions.

- Volunteer or help recruit volunteers to participate in your community's contaminant monitoring activities.
- Help ensure that local utilities that protect your water have adequate resources to do their job.
- If you see any suspicious activities in or around your water supply, please notify local authorities or call 911 immediately to report the incident.

What can help reduce water contamination?

- Reduce paved areas: Use permeable surfaces that allow rain to soak through, not run off.
- Reduce or eliminate pesticide application: Test your soil before applying chemicals, and use plants that require little or no water, pesticides, or fertilizers.
- Reduce the amount of trash you create: Reuse and recycle.
- Recycle used oil: One quart of oil can contaminate two million gallons of drinking water—take your used oil and antifreeze to a service station or recycling center.
- Take the bus instead of your car one day a week: You could prevent 33 pounds of carbon dioxide emissions each day.
- Keep pollutants away from boat marinas and waterways: Keep boat motors well-tuned to prevent leaks, select nontoxic cleaning products and use a drop cloth, and clean and maintain boats away from the water.
- If you are prescribed medications, be sure to finish them if instructed to do so by your physician. If you need to dispose of old or unused medications, do not dump them down the sink or toilet. Instead, close bottles tightly and seal the caps with duct tape. Double-bag the medications in plastic bags and tightly tie or tape shut, and then dispose in the trash. A few communities and pharmacies offer medication "take back" programs; use them if they are available.

For more information on how you can help protect your local drinking water source, call the Safe Drinking Water Hotline, or check www.epa.gov/safewater/publicoutreach.

Section 18.2

Lead in Drinking Water

"Lead in Drinking Water: Basic Information," Environmental Protection Agency (www.epa.gov), August 24, 2006.

What is lead?

Lead is a toxic metal that was used for many years in products found in and around homes. Even at low levels, lead may cause a range of health effects including behavioral problems and learning disabilities. Children six years old and under are most at risk because this is when the brain is developing. The primary source of lead exposure for most children is lead-based paint in older homes. Lead in drinking water can add to that exposure.

How does lead get into tap water?

Typically, lead gets into your water after the water leaves your local treatment plant or your well. That is, the source of lead in your home's water is most likely from pipes or solder in your home's own plumbing. The most common cause is corrosion, a reaction between the water and the lead pipes or solder. Dissolved oxygen, low pH (acidity), and low mineral content in water are common causes of corrosion. All kinds of water, however, may have high levels of lead.

What are the health effects of lead?

The health effects of lead are most severe for infants and children. For infants and children, exposure to high levels of lead in drinking water can result in delays in physical or mental development. For adults, it can result in kidney problems or high blood pressure. Although the main sources of exposure to lead are ingesting paint chips and inhaling dust, EPA estimates that 10 to 20% of human exposure to lead may come from lead in drinking water. Infants who consume mostly mixed formula can receive 40 to 60% of their exposure to lead from drinking water.

How can I reduce lead in drinking water at home?

Flush your pipes before drinking, and only use cold water for consumption. The more time water has been sitting in your home's pipes, the more lead it may contain. Anytime the water in a particular faucet has not been used for six hours or longer, "flush" your cold-water pipes by running the water until it becomes as cold as it will get. This could take as little as 5 to 30 seconds if there has been recent heavy water use such as showering or toilet flushing. Otherwise, it could take two minutes or longer. Your water utility will inform you if longer flushing times are needed to respond to local conditions.

Use only water from the cold-water tap for drinking, cooking, and especially for making baby formula. Hot water is likely to contain higher levels of lead. The two actions recommended above are very important to the health of your family. They will probably be effective in reducing lead levels because most of the lead in household water usually comes from the plumbing in your house, not from the local water supply.

How can I tell if my water contains too much lead?

You should have your water tested for lead by a certified laboratory. (Lists are available from your state or local drinking water authority.) Testing costs between $20 and $100. Since you cannot see, taste, or smell lead dissolved in water, testing is the only sure way of telling whether there are harmful quantities of lead in your drinking water. You should be particularly suspicious if your home has lead pipes (lead is a dull gray metal that is soft enough to be easily scratched with a house key), if you see signs of corrosion (frequent leaks, rust-colored water, stained dishes or laundry), or if your non-plastic plumbing is less than five years old. Your water supplier may have useful information, including whether the service connector used in your home or area is made of lead. Testing is especially important in high-rise buildings where flushing might not work.

Should I be concerned about lead in drinking water in my child's school or child care facility?

Children spend a significant part of their days at school or in a child care facility. The faucets that provide water used for consumption, including drinking, cooking lunch, and preparing juice and infant formula, should be tested.

What are the legal limits regarding lead and drinking water?

Section 1417 of the Safe Drinking Water Act prohibits any person from introducing into commerce any pipe, or plumbing fitting or fixture, that is not lead free after August 6, 1998, except for a pipe that is used in manufacturing or industrial processing. The law also required development of a voluntary standard to limit the leaching of lead into the drinking water for devices that are intended by the manufacturer to dispense water for human ingestion.

Lead and copper in drinking water are regulated by a treatment technique that requires systems to control the corrosiveness of their water. If more than 10% of tap water samples exceed the action level of 15 parts per billion, water systems must take additional steps to reduce corrosivity.

Section 18.3

Household Wells

"How Safe Is the Drinking Water in My Household Well?" excerpted from "Water on Tap," Environmental Protection Agency (www.epa.gov), October 2003.

EPA regulates public water systems; it does not have the authority to regulate private wells. Approximately 15% of Americans rely on their own private drinking water supplies, and these supplies are not subject to EPA standards. Unlike public drinking water systems serving many people, they do not have experts regularly checking the water's source and its quality before it is sent to the tap. These households must take special precautions to ensure the protection and maintenance of their drinking water supplies.

How much risk can I expect?

The risk of having problems depends on how good your well is—how well it was built and located, and how well you maintain it. It also depends on your local environment. That includes the quality of the aquifer from which your water is drawn and the human activities going on in your area that can affect your well.

Several sources of pollution are easy to spot by sight, taste, or smell. However, many serious problems can be found only by testing your water. Knowing the possible threats in your area will help you decide the kind of tests you may need.

What should I do?

There are six basic steps you can take to help protect your private drinking water supply:

1. Identify potential problem sources.
2. Talk with local experts.
3. Have your water tested periodically.
4. Have the test results interpreted and explained clearly.
5. Set and follow a regular maintenance schedule for your well, and keep up-to-date records.
6. Immediately remedy any problems.

Identify Potential Problem Sources: Understanding and spotting possible pollution sources is the first step to safeguarding your drinking water. If your drinking water comes from a well, you may also have a septic system. Septic systems and other onsite wastewater disposal systems are major potential sources of contamination of private water supplies if they are poorly maintained or located improperly, or if they are used for disposal of toxic chemicals. Information on septic systems is available from local health departments, state agencies, and the National Small Flows Clearinghouse (www.epa.gov/owm/mab/smcomm/nsfc.htm) at 800-624-8301. A septic system design manual and guidance on system maintenance are available from EPA (www.epa.gov/OW-OWM.html/mtb/decent/homeowner.htm).

Talk with Local Experts: Ground water conditions vary greatly from place to place, and local experts can give you the best information about your drinking water supply. Some examples are your health department's "sanitarian," local water-well contractors, public water system officials, county extension agents of the Natural Resources Conservation Service (NRCS), local or county planning commissions, and your local library.

Have Your Water Tested Periodically: Test your water every year for total coliform bacteria, nitrates, total dissolved solids, and pH levels. If you suspect other contaminants, test for these as well. As the tests can be expensive, limit them to possible problems specific to your situation. Local experts can help you identify these contaminants. You should also test your water after replacing or repairing any part of the system, or if you notice any change in your water's look, taste, or smell.

Often, county health departments perform tests for bacteria and nitrates. For other substances, health departments, environmental offices, or county governments should have a list of state-certified laboratories. Your State Laboratory Certification Officer can also provide you with this list. Call the Safe Drinking Water Hotline (800-426-4791) for the name and number of your state's certification officer. Any laboratory you use should be certified to do drinking water testing.

Have Your Test Results Interpreted and Explained Clearly: Compare your well's test results to federal and state drinking water standards (visit www.epa.gov/safewater/mcl.html or call the Safe Drinking Water Hotline). You may need to consult experts to aid you in understanding your results, such as the state agency that licenses water-well contractors, your local health department, or your state's drinking water program.

Set a Regular Maintenance Schedule for Your Well and Your Septic System: Proper well and septic system construction and continued maintenance are keys to the safety of your water supply. Your state water well and septic system contractor licensing agency, local health department, or local public water system professional can provide information on well construction. Make certain your contractors are licensed by the state, if required, or certified by the National Ground Water Association.

Maintain your well, fixing problems before they reach crisis levels, and keep up-to-date records of well installation and repairs, as well as plumbing and water costs. Protect your own well area from contamination.

Immediately Remedy Any Problems: If you find that your well water is contaminated, fix the problem as soon as possible. Consider connecting into a nearby community water system, if one is available. You may want to install a water treatment device to remove impurities. If you connect to a public water system, remember to close your well properly.

How can I protect my ground water supply?

- Periodically inspect exposed parts of the well for problems such as the following:
  - Cracked, corroded, or damaged well casing
  - Broken or missing well cap
  - Settling and cracking of surface seals
- Slope the area around the well to drain surface runoff away from the well.
- Install a well cap or sanitary seal to prevent unauthorized use of, or entry into, the well.
- Disinfect drinking water wells at least once per year with bleach or hypochlorite granules, according to the manufacturer's directions.
- Have the well tested once a year for coliform bacteria, nitrates, and other constituents of concern.
- Keep accurate records of any well maintenance, such as disinfection or sediment removal, that may require the use of chemicals in the well.
- Hire a certified well driller for any new well construction, modification, or abandonment and closure.
- Avoid mixing or using pesticides, fertilizers, herbicides, degreasers, fuels, and other pollutants near the well.
- Do not dispose of wastes in dry wells or in abandoned wells.
- Do not cut off the well casing below the land surface.
- Pump and inspect septic systems as often as recommended by your local health department.
- Never dispose of hazardous materials in a septic system.

Section 18.4

Fluoride

Keeping kids' teeth healthy requires more than just daily brushing. During a routine well-child exam, you may be surprised to find the doctor examining your child's teeth and asking you about your water supply. That's because fluoride, a substance that's found naturally in water, plays an important role in healthy tooth development and cavity prevention.

What Is Fluoride?

Fluoride exists naturally in water sources and is derived from fluorine, the thirteenth most common element in the Earth's crust. It is well known that fluoride helps prevent and even reverse the early stages of tooth decay.

Tooth decay occurs when plaque—that sticky film of bacteria that accumulates on your teeth—breaks down sugars in food. The bacteria produce damaging acids that dissolve the hard enamel surfaces of teeth. If the damage is not stopped or treated, the bacteria can penetrate through the enamel causing tooth decay (also called cavities or caries). Cavities weaken teeth and can lead to pain, tooth loss, or even widespread infection in the most severe cases.

Fluoride combats tooth decay in two ways. It is incorporated into the structure of developing teeth when it is ingested and also works when it comes in contact with the surface of the teeth. Fluoride prevents the acid produced by the bacteria in plaque from dissolving, or demineralizing, tooth enamel, the hard and shiny substance that protects the teeth. Fluoride also allows teeth damaged by acid to repair, or remineralize, themselves. Fluoride cannot repair cavities, but it can reverse low levels of tooth decay and thus prevent new cavities from forming.

Despite the good news about dental health, tooth decay remains one of the most common diseases of childhood. According to the Centers for Disease Control and Prevention (CDC), more than one quarter of two- to five-year-olds and half of kids 12 to 15 years old have one or more cavities, and tooth decay has affected two thirds of 16- to 19-year-olds.

Fluoride and the Water Supply

For over 60 years, water fluoridation has proved to be a safe and cost-effective way to reduce dental caries. Today, water fluoridation is estimated to reduce tooth decay by 20–40%. As of 2002, the CDC statistics show that almost 60% of the U.S. population receives fluoridated water through the taps in their homes. Some communities have naturally occurring fluoride in their water; others add it at water-processing plants.

Your child's doctor or dentist may know whether local water supplies contain optimal levels of fluoride, between 0.7 and 1.2 ppm (parts fluoride per million parts of water). If your water comes from a public system, you could also call your local water authority or public health department, or check online at the EPA's database of local water safety reports. If you use well water or water from a private source, fluoride levels should be checked by a laboratory or public health department.

Some parents purchase bottled water for their children to drink instead of tap water. Most bottled waters lack fluoride, but fluoridated bottled water is now available. If fluoride is added, the manufacturer is required to list the amount. If fluoride concentration is greater than 0.6 ppm up to 1.0 ppm, you might see the health claim "Drinking fluoridated water may reduce the risk of tooth decay" on the label.

The Controversy over Fluoride

Opponents of water fluoridation have questioned its safety and effectiveness; however, there has been little evidence to support these claims.

Scientific research continues to support the benefits of fluoride when it comes to prevention of tooth decay and its safety at current recommended levels of 0.7 to 1.2 ppm. Dramatic reductions in tooth decay in the past 30 years is attributed to fluoridation of the water supply, and parents and health professionals should continue to ensure that kids receive enough fluoride to prevent cavities.

The American Dental Association (ADA), the United States Public Health Service (USPHS), the American Academy of Pediatric (AAP), and the World Health Organization (WHO), among many other national and international organizations, endorse community water fluoridation. The CDC recognized fluoridation of water as one of the 10 greatest public health achievements of the twentieth century.

Kids' Fluoride Needs

So how much fluoride do kids need? In general, kids under the age of six months do not need fluoride supplements. Your child's six-month checkup offers a great chance to discuss fluoride supplementation with a health professional. If you live in a nonfluoridated area, your doctor or dentist may prescribe fluoride drops, tablets, or vitamins after your baby is six months old.

The AAP recommends that these fluoride supplements be given daily to kids between the ages of six months and 16 years. The dosage depends on how much fluoride naturally occurs in the water and the child's age. Only kids living in nonfluoridated areas or those who drink only nonfluoridated bottled water should receive supplements.

What about toothpastes, mouth rinses, and other products that contain fluoride? Here are a few tips:

- Kids under two years old should not use fluoride toothpaste unless instructed by a dentist or health professional.
- Kids younger than six may swallow too much toothpaste while brushing, so should be supervised when brushing and taught to spit, not swallow, toothpaste.
- Kids over age two should use a fluoride-containing toothpaste that carries the ADA's seal of acceptance.
- Kids should use only a pea-sized amount of toothpaste.
- Kids under age six should never use fluoride-containing mouth rinses. However, older kids at high risk for tooth decay may benefit from using them. Your dentist can talk with you about risk factors such as a family history of dental disease, recent periodontal surgery or disease, or a physical impediment to brushing regularly and thoroughly.

Your family dentist or pediatric dentist (one who specializes in the care of children's teeth) is a great resource for information about dental care and fluoride needs. A dentist can help you understand more about how fluoride affects the teeth, and once all of your child's primary teeth have come in, may recommend regular topical fluoride during routine dental visits.

Overexposure to Fluoride

If some fluoride is good, why isn't more fluoride better? As with most medications, including vitamins and mineral supplements, too much can be harmful. Most kids get the right amount of fluoride through a combination of fluoridated toothpaste and fluoridated water or supplements.

Too much fluoride before eight years of age, a time when teeth are developing, can cause enamel fluorosis, a discoloration or mottling of the permanent teeth. For most, the changes are subtle. In one study, 94% of identified fluorosis cases were very mild to mild. Most cases are due to inappropriate use of fluoride-containing dental products, including toothpaste and mouth rinses. Sometimes kids take daily fluoride supplements but may be getting adequate fluoride from other sources, which also puts them at risk.

Recently, the National Research Council found naturally occurring fluoride levels exceeded the optimal levels used in community fluoridation programs (0.7 to 1.2 ppm), putting kids under eight years old at risk for severe enamel fluorosis. The CDC recommends that in communities where fluoride levels are greater than 2 ppm, parents should provide kids with water from other sources.

The ADA also recognizes that infants need less fluoride than older kids and adults. Some infants may be getting too much fluoride in the water used to reconstitute infant formula. If you're concerned that your infant may be getting too much fluoride, talk with your doctor or dentist, who may recommend ready-to-feed formula or formula reconstituted with fluoride-free or low-fluoride water.

Very rarely, fluoride toxicity can occur when large amounts of fluoride are ingested during a short period of time. Kids under age six account for more than 80% of reports of suspected overingestion. Although outcomes are generally not serious, fluoride toxicity sends several hundred children to emergency rooms each year.

Symptoms of fluoride toxicity may include nausea, diarrhea, vomiting, abdominal pain, increased salivation, or increased thirst. Symptoms begin 30 minutes after ingestion and can last up to 24 hours. If you suspect your child may have eaten a substantial amount of a fluoridated product or supplement, call the poison control center or 911.

Be sure to keep toothpaste, supplements, mouth rinses, and other fluoride-containing products out of children's reach or in a locked cabinet. You should also supervise your young child's toothbrushing sessions to prevent swallowing of toothpaste or other fluoridated products.

If you have any questions about your water's fluoride content, the fluoridated products your child uses, or whether your child is receiving too much or too little fluoride, talk to your doctor or dentist.

Section 18.5

Chlorination and Water Disinfection Byproducts

This section includes "Chlorination of Drinking Water" and "Disinfection Byproducts: Chlorination of Drinking Water," © 2004 Washington State Department of Health (http://www.doh.wa.gov). Reprinted with permission. Reviewed by David A. Cooke, MD, FACP, June 2009.

Chlorination of Drinking Water

Note: This section deals with the practice of continuously adding chlorine to water, not the occasional use of chlorine to disinfect wells, pipes, and other water system equipment.

Why Water Systems Continuously Add Chlorine to Their Water

Many public water systems add chlorine (a process known as "chlorination") to their water supply for the purpose of disinfection. Disinfection kills or inactivates harmful microorganisms which can cause illnesses such as typhoid, cholera, hepatitis, and giardiasis. Sometimes, water systems use chlorination for taste and odor control, iron and manganese removal, and to stop nuisance growths in wells, water pipes, storage facilities, and conduits.

Chlorine is also added for its "residual" properties. Chlorine remaining in the water supply, or added after disinfection is first accomplished, is available to fight against potential contamination in water distribution and storage systems that might enter through leaks and pipe breakages. This is called "secondary disinfection."

Chlorine can be added to water as a gas or in the form of hypochlorite either as liquid or solid. Gas chlorination requires more sophisticated equipment and more training to apply safely. Adding chlorine as a hypochlorite is much simpler, requires less training, and is safer. If large amounts of chlorine are required, the overall cost of gas chlorination may be lower.

History of Chlorination

Techniques for chlorination of water supplies were developed in the late 19th and early 20th centuries. In 1908, Jersey City Water Works became the first system in the United States to practice large-scale chlorination on a permanent basis.

As more water systems adopted the practice of chlorination, there was a corresponding decrease in the number of waterborne disease outbreaks. Health professionals regard the chlorination of water as one of the most important advances in the field of public health. Waterborne diseases, such as typhoid, caused thousands of deaths annually in the United States in the early 1900s and are now considered rare.

Does Chlorination Result in Harmful Compounds?

When chlorine is added to water, it reacts with organic substances that occur naturally in the water. The compounds formed are called "disinfection byproducts (DBPs)." The amount formed depends on the amount of chlorine used and contact time between the organic substances and the chlorine.

Some studies of human health effects from exposure to chlorinated water show increased risk to cancer and reproductive and developmental effects. Other studies show no additional risk. Since there may be potential health effects, the EPA adopted the Stage 1 Disinfectants and Disinfection Byproducts Rule (DBPR), which specifies maximum allowable levels and monitoring requirements for disinfectants and DBPs.

Other Disinfectants or Methods of Disinfection

There are other disinfectants used for treatment of water. These include:

- **Chloramines:** These are formed by a combination of chlorine (from gas or hypochlorite) and ammonia.

- **Chlorine Dioxide (ClO_2):** This compound is always produced on-site using sodium chlorite and either chlorine or hydrochloric acid.
- **Ozone (O_3):** This compound is produced by an electrical discharge through air or oxygen.
- **Ultraviolet Radiation (UV):** This is a nonchemical method of disinfection by using ultraviolet radiation at certain wavelengths.

All disinfectants have advantages and disadvantages in their effectiveness, residual qualities, and byproduct formation, depending on the application circumstances and water quality. For a more thorough discussion of other disinfectants, request or download Washington State Department of Health publication "Alternate Disinfectants" (www.doh.wa.gov/ehp/dw/Publications/alternate_disinfectants.htm).

Is Chlorination Right for Your Water System?

The reason your water system chlorinates depends upon the needs of the water system. Most public water systems in the state of Washington use groundwater exclusively. Disinfection alone is sufficient treatment against bacteria and viruses. Since most groundwaters have low levels of dissolved organic substances, the formation of DBPs is not a serious health concern. All factors considered—cost, simplicity of operation, and residual qualities—the use of chlorine (as gas or hypochlorite) is a good choice of disinfectant for most water systems.

Future Challenges

Disinfection of drinking water, especially when the supply originates from a surface source, is needed to maintain water quality and protect public health. The challenge is to maintain the level of microbial protection while minimizing the exposure of the consumers to DBPs. Research still continues, especially in the field of health effects of disinfectants other than chlorine.

Disinfection Byproducts

What Are Disinfection Byproducts and How Are They Formed?

Chlorine is added to drinking water to kill or inactivate harmful organisms that cause various diseases. This process is called disinfection. However, chlorine is a very active substance and it reacts with naturally occurring substances to form compounds known as disinfection byproducts. The most common DBPs formed when chlorine is used are trihalomethanes (THMs) and haloacetic acids (HAAs).

What Types of Water Systems Are Most Likely to Have DBPs?

Water systems using sources with higher amounts of organic substances will form more DBPs when disinfected than those that do not. Sources with higher organics levels include:

- surface waters, such as lakes, rivers, and streams;
- springs and wells that are shallow and/or located near surface waters.

Groundwater, especially those from deep wells, tends to contain little organic substances. Even if they chlorinate the water, lesser amounts of DBPs are typically found.

Do DBPs Have Harmful Health Effects?

Scientists have conducted studies on health effects of exposure to high levels of DBPs on laboratory animals. These studies have shown that several DBPs cause cancer in laboratory animals. In addition, some DBPs cause undesirable effects in the animals' growth and reproduction. It is, however, difficult to estimate how the results of these high-dosage studies on laboratory animals can be applied to low-dosage, long-term exposure for humans.

Scientists have also studied the relationship between drinking chlorinated water and cancer rates. Some of these studies suggest an increased cancer risk to those using chlorinated drinking water, while others found no increased risk. Other studies that investigate whether chlorinated drinking water has an effect on reproduction and development also show inconsistent results. At the present time, the EPA does not believe there is enough evidence to state conclusively that DBPs cause these types of health effects. Research on the health effects of DBPs is not complete and the federal government continues funding research on this topic.

Are There Regulations Regarding DBPs?

Although, at present, there is no conclusive evidence showing DBPs in water is associated with cancer or other health effects, there are some concerns, given the research information and the large number of people drinking chlorinated water.

In 1979, EPA established total trihalomethane (TTHM) levels for certain types of water systems. In 1998, EPA finalized the Stage 1 Disinfectants and Disinfection Byproducts Rule. These new rules replace the original TTHM Rule. The Washington State Department of Health incorporated these rules into the State's Drinking Water Regulations in April 2003, and these rules became effective January 1, 2004.

Why Can't One Simply Remove the DBPs Formed during Treatment?

DBP formation is not instantaneous. The amount formed depends upon factors such as chlorine concentration, temperature, and length of contact time between the chlorine and water. The rules specify that some or all the samples must be collected at the end of the distribution system from locations that represent maximum residence time.

What Can Be Done to Reduce the Amount of DBPs Formed?

Sometimes, it is possible to reduce the amount of DBPs formed by one or more of the following methods:

- Removing the organic substances that react with the chlorine to produce DBPs
- Avoid maintaining residuals that are higher than necessary for public health protection
- Changing the location where the chlorine is added
- Using a different type of disinfectant

Disinfectants other than chlorine have certain advantages and disadvantages and some form other types of DBPs. For a more thorough discussion of alternative disinfectants, request or download the fact sheet "Alternative Disinfectants" (www.doh.wa.gov/ehp/dw/Publications/alternate_disinfectants.htm).

Should Chlorination Be Discontinued in Order to Avoid DBPs?

The primary reason for adding chlorine to water is to make it safe to drink by killing or inactivating harmful microorganisms that cause diseases such as typhoid, cholera, dysentery, and giardiasis. Health professionals regard the chlorination of water as one of the most important advances in the field of public health protection. Chlorinating drinking water has saved millions of lives.

Research is still continuing on the health effects of DBPs and improvements in water treatment technology. Because of the immense benefits in reduction of infectious diseases, and the simplicity and low cost of water treatment using chlorine, chlorination is the most appropriate choice as a method of ensuring safe drinking water for most water systems.

Section 18.6

Bottled Water

"Bottled Water Quality Investigation: 10 Major Brands, 38 Pollutants," © 2008 Environmental Working Group. Reprinted with permission. The complete text of this document including references is available at http://www.ewg.org/reports/bottledwater.

The bottled water industry promotes an image of purity, but comprehensive testing by the Environmental Working Group (EWG) reveals a surprising array of chemical contaminants in every bottled water brand analyzed, including toxic byproducts of chlorination in Walmart's Sam's Choice and Giant Supermarket's Acadia brands, at levels no different than routinely found in tap water. Several Sam's Choice samples purchased in California exceeded legal limits for bottled water contaminants in that state. Cancer-causing contaminants in bottled water purchased in five states (North Carolina, California, Virginia, Delaware, and Maryland) and the District of Columbia substantially exceeded the voluntary standards established by the bottled water industry.

Unlike tap water, where consumers are provided with test results every year, the bottled water industry does not disclose the results of any contaminant testing that it conducts. Instead, the industry hides behind the claim that bottled water is held to the same safety standards as tap water. But with promotional campaigns saturated with images of mountain springs, and prices 1,900 times the price of tap water, consumers are clearly led to believe that they are buying a product that has been purified to a level beyond the water that comes out of the garden hose.

To the contrary, our tests strongly indicate that the purity of bottled water cannot be trusted. Given the industry's refusal to make available data to support their claims of superiority, consumer confidence in the purity of bottled water is simply not justified.

Laboratory tests conducted for EWG at one of the country's leading water quality laboratories found that 10 popular brands of bottled water, purchased from grocery stores and other retailers in nine states and the District of Columbia, contained 38 chemical pollutants altogether, with an average of 8 contaminants in each brand. More than one-third of the chemicals found are not regulated in bottled water. In the Sam's Choice and Acadia brands levels of some chemicals exceeded legal limits in California as well as industry-sponsored voluntary safety standards. Four brands were also contaminated with bacteria.

Walmart and Giant Brands No Different than Tap Water

Two of 10 brands tested, Walmart's and Giant's store brands, bore the chemical signature of standard municipal water treatment—a cocktail of chlorine disinfection byproducts, and for Giant water, even fluoride. In other words, this bottled water was chemically indistinguishable from tap water. The only striking difference: the price tag.

In both brands levels of disinfection byproducts exceeded safety standards established by the state of California and the bottled water industry:

- Walmart's Sam's Choice bottled water purchased at several locations in the San Francisco bay area was polluted with disinfection byproducts called trihalomethanes at levels that exceed the state's legal limit for bottled water. These byproducts are linked to cancer and reproductive problems and form when disinfectants react with residual pollution in the water. Las Vegas tap water was the source for these bottles, according to Walmart representatives.
- Also in Walmart's Sam's Choice brand, lab tests found a cancer-causing chemical called bromodichloromethanes at levels that exceed safety standards for cancer-causing chemicals under California's Safe Drinking Water and Toxic Enforcement Act of 1986. EWG is filing suit under this act to ensure that Walmart posts a warning on bottles as required by law: "WARNING: This product contains a chemical known to the State of California to cause cancer."

- These same chemicals also polluted Giant's Acadia brand at levels in excess of California's safety standards, but this brand is sold only in Mid-Atlantic states where California's health-based limits do not apply. Nevertheless, disinfection byproducts in both Acadia and Sam's Choice bottled water exceeded the industry trade association's voluntary safety standards for samples purchased in Washington, DC, and five states (Delaware, Maryland, Virginia, North Carolina, and California). The bottled water industry boasts that its internal regulations are stricter than the FDA bottled water regulations, but voluntary standards that companies are failing to meet are of little use in protecting public health.

Broad Range of Pollutants Found in 10 Brands

Altogether, the analyses conducted by the University of Iowa Hygienic Laboratory of these 10 brands of bottled water revealed a wide range of pollutants, including not only disinfection byproducts, but also common urban wastewater pollutants like caffeine and pharmaceuticals (Tylenol); heavy metals and minerals including arsenic and radioactive isotopes; fertilizer residue (nitrate and ammonia); and a broad range of other, tentatively identified industrial chemicals used as solvents, plasticizers, viscosity decreasing agents, and propellants.

The identity of most brands in this study are anonymous. This is typical scientific practice for market-basket style testing programs. We consider these results to represent a snapshot of the market during the window of time in which we purchased samples. While our study findings show that consumers can't trust that bottled water is pure or cleaner than tap water, it was not designed to indicate pollutant profiles typical over time for particular brands. Walmart and Giant bottled water brands are named in this study because our first tests and numerous follow-up tests confirmed that these brands contained contaminants at levels that exceeded state standards or voluntary industry guidelines.

The study also included assays for breast cancer cell proliferation, conducted at the University of Missouri. One bottled water brand spurred a 78% increase in the growth of the breast cancer cells compared to the control sample, with 1,200 initial breast cancer cells multiplying to 32,000 in four days, versus only 18,000 for the control sample, indicating that chemical contaminants in the bottled water sample stimulated accelerated division of cancer cells. When estrogen-blocking chemicals were added, the effect was inhibited, showing that the cancer-spurring chemicals mimic estrogen, a hormone linked to breast cancer. Though this result is considered a modest effect relative to the potency of some other industrial chemicals in spurring breast cancer cell growth, the sheer volume of bottled water people consume elevates the health significance of the finding. While the specific chemical(s) responsible for this cancer cell proliferation were not identified in this pilot study, ingestion of endocrine-disrupting and cancer-promoting chemicals from plastics is considered to be a potentially important health concern.

With Bottled Water, You Don't Know What You're Getting

Americans drink twice as much bottled water today as they did 10 years ago, for an annual total of over 9 billion gallons with producer revenues nearing 12 billions. Purity should be included in a price that, at a typical cost of $3.79 per gallon, is 1,900 times the cost of public tap water. But EWG's tests indicate that in some cases the industry may be delivering a beverage little cleaner than tap water, sold at a premium price. The health consequences of exposures to these complex mixtures of contaminants like those found in bottled water have never been studied.

Unlike public water utilities, bottled water companies are not required to notify their customers of the occurrence of contaminants in the water, or, in most states, to tell their customers where the water comes from, how and if it is purified, and if it is merely bottled tap water. Information provided on the U.S. EPA website clearly describes the lack of quality assurance for bottled water: "Bottled water is not necessarily safer than your tap water." The agency further adds following consumer information: "Some bottled water is treated more than tap water, while some is treated less or not treated at all. Bottled water costs much more than tap water on a per gallon basis... Consumers who choose to purchase bottled water should carefully read its label to understand what they are buying, whether it is a better taste, or a certain method of treatment."

In conjunction with this testing program, EWG conducted a survey of 228 brands of bottled water, compiling information from websites, labels, and other marketing materials. We found that fewer than half describe the water source (i.e., municipal or natural) or provide any information on whether or how the water is treated. In the absence of complete disclosure on the label, consumers are left in the dark, making it difficult for shoppers to know if they are getting what they expect for the price.

This study did not focus on the environmental impacts of bottled water, but they are striking and have been well publicized. Of the 36 billion bottles sold in 2006, only a fifth were recycled. The rest ended up in landfills, incinerators, and as trash on land and in streams, rivers, and oceans. Water bottle production in the U.S. uses 1.5 million barrels of oil per every year, according to a U.S. Conference of Mayors' resolution passed in 2007, enough energy to power 250,000 homes or fuel 100,000 cars for a year. As oil prices are continuing to skyrocket, the direct and indirect costs of making and shipping and landfilling the water bottles continue to rise as well.

Extracting water for bottling places a strain on rivers, streams, and community drinking water supplies as well. When the water is not bottled from a municipal supply, companies instead draw it from groundwater supplies, rivers, springs, or streams. This "water mining," as it is called, can remove substantial amounts of water that otherwise would have contributed to community water supplies or to the natural flow of streams and rivers.

Recommendations

Currently there is a double standard where tap water suppliers provide information to consumers on contaminants, filtration techniques, and source water; bottled water companies do not. This double standard must be eliminated immediately; bottled water should conform to the same right-to-know standards as tap water.

To bring bottled water up to the standards of tap water we recommend:

- full disclosure of all test results for all contaminants (this must be done in a way that is readily available to the public);
- disclosure of all treatment techniques used to purify the water; and
- clear and specific disclosure of the name and location of the source water.

To ensure that public health and the environment are protected, we recommend:

- Federal, state, and local policymakers must strengthen protections for rivers, streams, and groundwater that serve as America's drinking water sources. Even though it is not necessarily any healthier, some Americans turn to bottled water in part because they distrust the quality of their tap water. And sometimes this is for good reason. Some drinking water (tap and bottled) is grossly polluted at its source—in rivers, streams, and underground aquifers fouled by decades of wastes that generations of political and business leaders have dismissed, ignored, and left for others to solve. A 2005 EWG study found nearly 300 contaminants in drinking water all across the country. Source water protection programs must be improved, implemented, and enforced nationwide. The environmental impacts associated with bottled water production and distribution aggravate the nation's water quality problems rather than contributing to their solution.

- Consumers should drink filtered tap water instead of bottled water. Americans pay an average of two-tenths of a cent per gallon to drink water from the tap. A carbon filter at the tap or in a pitcher costs a manageable $0.31 per gallon (12 times lower than the typical cost of bottled water) and removes many of the contaminants found in public tap water supplies. A whole-house carbon filter strips out chemicals not only from drinking water, but also from water used in the shower, clothes washer, and dishwasher where they can volatilize into the air for families to breathe in. For an average four-person household, the cost for this system is about $0.25 per person per day. A single gallon of bottled water costs 15 times this amount.

EWG's study has revealed that bottled water can contain complex mixtures of industrial chemicals never tested for safety, and may be no cleaner than tap water. Given some bottled water companies' failure to adhere to the industry's own purity standards, Americans cannot take the quality of bottled water for granted. Indeed, test results like those presented in this study may give many Americans reason enough to reconsider their habit of purchasing bottled water and turn back to the tap.

Editor's Note: The information in this section represents the opinion of the copyright holder and is presented as one viewpoint on a complex subject.

Chapter 19

Swimming Water

What are recreational water illnesses (RWIs)?

RWIs are illnesses that are spread by swallowing, breathing, or having contact with contaminated water from swimming pools, spas, lakes, rivers, or oceans. Recreational water illnesses can cause a wide variety of symptoms, including gastrointestinal, skin, ear, respiratory, eye, neurologic, and wound infections. The most commonly reported RWI is diarrhea. Diarrheal illnesses can be caused by germs such as Crypto, short for *Cryptosporidium*, *Giardia*, *Shigella*, norovirus, and *E. coli* O157:H7.

Where are RWIs found?

RWIs can be spread through use of swimming pools, hot tubs, decorative water fountains, oceans, lakes, and rivers.

Swimming Pools, Waterparks, Spray Features: The most common illness spread through use of swimming pools is diarrhea. If swimmers are ill with diarrhea, the germs that they carry can contaminate the water if they have an "accident" in the pool. On average, people have about 0.14 grams of feces on their bottoms that,

---

This section includes "Answers to Your Questions about Recreational Water Illnesses (RWIs)," May 2, 2007, and "Six 'PLEAs' for Healthy Swimming: Protection against Recreational Water Illnesses (RWIs)," February 12, 2008, Centers for Disease Control and Prevention (www.cdc.gov).

when rinsed off, can contaminate recreational water. When people are ill with diarrhea, their stool can contain millions of germs. Therefore, swimming when ill with diarrhea can easily contaminate large pools or waterparks. As a result, if someone swallows water that has been contaminated with feces, he/she may become sick. Many of these diarrhea-causing germs do not have to be swallowed in large amounts to cause illness. Remember that standing water is not necessary for RWIs to spread so even spray decks can become contaminated (the water is just in a collection tank underground) and spread illness. To ensure that most germs are killed, chlorine or other disinfectant levels and pH should be checked regularly as part of good pool operation.

Hot Tubs: Skin infections like "hot tub rash" are the most common RWIs spread through hot tubs and spas. Chlorine and other disinfectant levels evaporate more quickly because of the higher temperature of the water in the tubs. Respiratory illnesses are also associated with hot tub use if the hot tub is not well maintained. Because of this it is important to check disinfectant levels even more regularly than in swimming pools. "Hot tub rash" can also be spread in pools and at the lake or beach.

Decorative Water Fountains: Not all decorative or interactive fountains are chlorinated or filtered. Therefore, when people, especially diaper-aged children, play in the water, they can contaminate the water with fecal matter. Swallowing this contaminated water can then cause diarrheal illness.

Lakes, Rivers, and Oceans: Lakes, rivers, and oceans can become contaminated with germs from sewage, animal waste, water runoff following rainfall, fecal accidents, and germs rinsed off the bottoms of swimmers. It is important to avoid swallowing the water because natural recreational water is not disinfected. Avoid swimming after rainfalls or in areas identified as unsafe by health departments. Contact your state or local health department for results of water testing in your area or go to EPA [Environmental Protection Agency]'s beach site or their National Health Protection Survey of Beaches.

How are RWIs spread?

Keep in mind that you share the water with everyone else in the pool, lake, or ocean.

Diarrheal Illnesses: If swimmers are ill with diarrhea, the germs that they carry can contaminate the water if they have an "accident" in the pool. Swimming when ill with diarrhea can easily contaminate large pools or waterparks. In addition, lakes, rivers, and the ocean can be contaminated by sewage spills, animal waste, and water runoff following rainfall. Some common germs can also live for long periods of time in salt water.

So, if someone swallows water that has been contaminated with feces, he/she may become sick. Many of these diarrhea-causing germs do not have to be swallowed in large amounts to cause illness.

Other RWIs: Many other RWIs (skin, ear, eye, respiratory, neurologic, wound, and other infections) are caused by germs that live naturally in the environment (water, soil). In the pool or hot tub, if disinfectant is not maintained at the appropriate levels, these germs can increase to the point where they can cause illness when swimmers breathe or have contact with water containing these germs.

Why doesn't chlorine kill these RWI germs?

Chlorine in swimming pools does kill the germs that may make people sick, but it takes time. Chlorine in properly disinfected pools kills most germs that can cause RWIs in less than an hour. Chlorine takes longer to kill some germs such as Crypto, which can survive for days in even a properly disinfected pool. This means that without your help, illness can spread even in well-maintained pools.

Healthy swimming behaviors are needed to protect you and your family from RWIs and will help stop germs from getting in the pool.

Who is most likely to get ill from an RWI?

Children, pregnant women, and people with compromised immune systems (such as those living with AIDS, those who have received an organ transplant, or those receiving certain types of chemotherapy) can suffer from more severe illness if infected. People with compromised immune systems should be aware that recreational water might be contaminated with human or animal waste that contains *Cryptosporidium* (or Crypto), which can be life threatening in persons with weakened immune systems. People with a compromised immune system should consult their health care provider before participating in behaviors that place them at risk for illness.

How can we prevent RWIs?

Healthy swimming behaviors are needed to protect you and your kids from RWIs and will help stop germs from getting in the pool in the first place.

Here are six "PLEAs" that promote healthy swimming:

Three "PLEAs" for All Swimmers: Practice these three "PLEAs" to stop germs from causing illness at the pool.

- **Please** don't swim when you have diarrhea. You can spread germs in the water and make other people sick. This is especially important for kids in diapers.
- **Please** don't swallow the pool water. In fact, avoid getting water in your mouth.
- **Please** practice good hygiene. Take a shower before swimming and wash your hands after using the toilet or changing diapers. Germs on your body end up in the water.

Three "PLEAs" for Parents of Young Kids: Follow these three "PLEAs" to keep germs out of the pool and your community.

- **Please** take your kids on bathroom breaks or check diapers often. Waiting to hear "I have to go" may mean that it's too late.
- **Please** change diapers in a bathroom or a diaper-changing area and not at poolside. Germs can spread to surfaces and objects in and around the pool and cause illness.
- **Please** wash your child thoroughly (especially the rear end) with soap and water before swimming. Everyone has invisible amounts of fecal matter on their bottoms that end up in the pool.

Chapter 20

Harmful Algae Blooms (Red Tides)

Algae are vitally important to marine and fresh-water ecosystems, and most species of algae are not harmful. However, a harmful algal bloom (HAB) can occur when certain types of microscopic algae grow quickly in water, forming visible patches that may harm the health of the environment, plants, or animals. HABs can deplete the oxygen and block the sunlight that other organisms need to live, and some HAB-causing algae release toxins that are dangerous to animals and humans. HABs can occur in marine, estuarine, and fresh waters, and HABs appear to be increasing along the coastlines and in the surface waters of the United States, according to the National Oceanic and Atmospheric Administration (NOAA).

Responding to this suspected increase, the U.S. Congress in 1998 passed a law that required NOAA to lead an Inter-Agency Task Force on Harmful Algal Blooms and Hypoxia, and funded research into the origins, types, and possible human health effects of HABs.

Although scientists do not yet understand fully how HABs affect human health, authorities in the United States and abroad are monitoring HABs and developing guidelines for HAB-related public health action. The U.S. Environmental Protection Agency (EPA) has added certain algae associated with HABs to its Drinking Water Contaminant

---

This section excerpted from "Harmful Algae Blooms (HABs)," Centers for Disease Control and Prevention, March 2004. Reviewed by David A. Cooke, MD, FACP, June 2009.

Candidate List. This list identifies organisms and toxins that EPA believes are priorities for investigation.

The Centers for Disease Control and Prevention (CDC) works with public health agencies, universities, and federal partners to investigate how the following algae, which can cause HABs, may affect public health:

Ciguatera

Ciguatera fish poisoning (or ciguatera) is an illness humans can get by eating fish that contain toxins produced by the microscopic marine algae *Gambierdiscus toxicus*. People who have ciguatera may experience nausea, vomiting, and neurologic symptoms such as tingling fingers or toes. They also may find that cold things feel hot and hot things feel cold. Ciguatera has no cure. Symptoms usually go away in days or weeks but can last for years. People who have ciguatera can receive treatment for their symptoms.

Cyanobacteria

Cyanobacteria are single-celled organisms that live in fresh, brackish, and marine water. They use sunlight to make their own food. In warm, nutrient-rich environments, microscopic cyanobacteria can grow quickly, creating blooms that spread across the water's surface and may become visible. Because of the color, texture, and location of these blooms, the common name for cyanobacteria is blue-green algae. However, cyanobacteria are related more closely to bacteria than to algae. Cyanobacteria are found worldwide, from Brazil to China, Australia to the United States. In warmer climates, these organisms can grow year-round.

Scientists have called cyanobacteria the origin of plants, and have credited cyanobacteria with providing nitrogen fertilizer for rice and beans. But blooms of cyanobacteria are not always helpful. When these blooms become harmful to the environment, animals, and humans, scientists call them cyanobacterial harmful algal blooms (CyanoHABs).

Freshwater CyanoHABs can use up the oxygen and block the sunlight that other organisms need to live. They also can produce powerful toxins that affect the brain and liver of animals and humans. Because of concerns about CyanoHABs, which can grow in drinking water and recreational water, the EPA has added cyanobacteria to its Drinking Water Contaminant Candidate List.

Assessing the Impact on Public Health: Reports of poisonings associated with CyanoHABs date back to the late 1800s. Anecdotal evidence and data from laboratory animal research suggest that cyanobacterial toxins can cause a range of adverse human health effects, yet few studies have explored the links between CyanoHABs and human health.

Humans can be exposed to cyanobacterial toxins by drinking water that contains the toxins, swimming in water that contains high concentrations of cyanobacterial cells, or breathing air that contains cyanobacterial cells or toxins (while watering a lawn with contaminated water, for example).

Health effects associated with exposure to high concentrations of cyanobacterial toxins include the following symptoms:

- Stomach and intestinal illness
- Trouble breathing
- Allergic responses
- Skin irritation
- Liver damage
- Neurotoxic reactions, such as tingling fingers and toes

Scientists are exploring the human health effects associated with long-term exposure to low levels of cyanobacterial toxins. Some studies have suggested that such exposure could be associated with chronic illnesses, such as liver cancer and digestive-system cancer.

In Australia, where cyanobacteria are prevalent and CyanoHAB-related poisonings are well-documented, health officials have set up intensive monitoring systems and have written guidelines for public-health response to CyanoHABs. Similar, less-intensive monitoring systems exist in the Lake Champlain Basin area of North America, and in states such as Maryland and Florida.

Pfiesteria

Pfiesteria piscicida (*P. piscicida*) is a microscopic alga that lives in estuaries—where freshwater streams or rivers mix with and salt water—along the Atlantic and Gulf coasts. Researchers at North Carolina State University first identified *P. piscicida* in 1988 in fish cultures. Since then, scientists have advanced many theories about the organism's life cycle and its possible effects on the health of fish and humans.

P. piscicida is a dinoflagellate, a free-swimming, single-celled organism that uses other organisms to create food from sunlight. Dinoflagellates are a natural part of the marine environment, and most dinoflagellates are not toxic. Some researchers have suggested that *P. piscicida* produces toxins that might be dangerous to humans, but so far researchers have not identified any such toxins.

In 1998, Congress appropriated funds to the CDC to address concerns about human health effects possibly associated with exposure to *P. piscicida*.

Assessing the Impact on Public Health: *P. piscicida* has been found near large groups of dead fish, prompting researchers to explore whether *P. piscicida* caused the fish to die. Scientists do not yet know if *P. piscicida* affects human health. However, anecdotal reports of symptoms such as headache, confusion, skin rash, and eye irritation in laboratory workers exposed to water containing high concentrations of *P. piscicida*—along with reports of similar symptoms in people living near waters where *P. piscicida* has been found—have caused concerns among the public.

Responding to these concerns, CDC continues to support research to identify toxins associated with *P. piscicida* and to evaluate the potential health effects of exposure to this organism.

- Beginning in 1998, CDC worked with six East Coast states to develop a surveillance system to collect information about exposure to estuarine water (where *P. piscicida* is found) and subsequent health effects.
- In 2003, CDC awarded Florida, Maryland, North Carolina, South Carolina, and Virginia an average of $900,000 each to expand their existing surveillance systems to include monitoring of human illnesses possibly associated with exposure to other harmful algal blooms.
- CDC has assisted state health agencies in creating appropriate public health messages regarding the presence of *P. piscicida* in coastal waters.
- CDC has supported Maryland, North Carolina, and Virginia in the study of potential acute and chronic health effects that might result from occupational exposure to *P. piscicida* or any toxins that *P. piscicida* might produce. The data generated by these studies currently is being analyzed.

Red Tide

Algae are vitally important to marine ecosystems, and most species of algae are not harmful. However, under certain environmental conditions, microscopic marine algae called *Karenia brevis* (*K. brevis*) grow quickly, creating blooms that can make the ocean appear red or brown. People often call these blooms "red tide."

K. brevis produces powerful toxins called brevetoxins, which have killed millions of fish and other marine organisms. Red tides have damaged the fishing industry, shoreline quality, and local economies in states such as Texas and Florida. Because *K. brevis* blooms move based on winds and tides, pinpointing a red tide at any given moment is difficult.

Red tides occur throughout the world, affecting marine ecosystems in Scandinavia, Japan, the Caribbean, and the South Pacific. Scientists first documented a red tide along Florida's Gulf Coast in fall 1947, when residents of Venice, Florida, reported thousands of dead fish and a "stinging gas" in the air, according to Mote Marine Laboratory. However, Florida residents have reported similar events since the mid-1800s.

Assessing the Impact on Public Health: In addition to killing fish, brevetoxins can become concentrated in the tissues of shellfish that feed on *K. brevis*. People who eat these shellfish may suffer from neurotoxic shellfish poisoning, a food poisoning that can cause severe gastrointestinal and neurologic symptoms, such as tingling fingers or toes.

The human health effects associated with eating brevetoxin-tainted shellfish are well documented. However, scientists know little about how other types of environmental exposures to brevetoxin—such as breathing the air near red tides or swimming in red tides—may affect humans. Anecdotal evidence suggests that people who swim among brevetoxins or inhale brevetoxins dispersed in the air may experience irritation of the eyes, nose, and throat, as well as coughing, wheezing, and shortness of breath. Additional evidence suggests that people with existing respiratory illness, such as asthma, may experience these symptoms more severely.

Chapter 21

Soil Contamination

Chapter Contents

Section 21.1

Pesticides

This section excerpted from "Chemical Trespass: Pesticides in Our Bodies and Corporate Accountability," by Kristin S. Schafer, Margaret Reeves, Skip Spitzer, and Susan E. Kegley. © 2004 Pesticide Action Network North America (www.panna.org). Reprinted with permission. The complete text of this report including references is available at http://www.panna.org/docsTrespass/chemicalTrespass2004.dv.html. *Health Reference Series* Medical Advisor's note added by David A. Cooke, MD, FACP, June 2009.

The human body is not designed to cope with synthetic pesticides. Yet we all carry a cocktail of chemicals designed to kill insects, weeds, and other agricultural and household pests.

Some of these pesticides are coursing through our systems at levels that can barely be detected with the most sophisticated monitoring equipment. Others occur in concentrations reflecting exposure levels known to be unsafe.

Many of the pesticides we carry in our bodies can cause cancer, disrupt our hormone systems, decrease fertility, cause birth defects, or weaken our immune systems. These are just some of the known detrimental effects of particular pesticides at very low levels of exposure. Almost nothing is known about the long-term impacts of multiple chemicals in the body over long periods.

For decades, pesticide manufacturers have argued that applying pesticides in our homes and introducing them into our environment is necessary and safe. When used correctly, they argue, pesticides harm pests, not people. But the claim that pesticides are necessary is rapidly eroding in light of the growing success of sustainable and organic agricultural production and alternative controls for household pests. And the safety argument is directly challenged by the data analyzed in this section documenting the presence of pesticides in the bodies of men, women, and children throughout the U.S.

Government Data Reveal Pesticide Body Burden

The U.S. Centers for Disease Control and Prevention (CDC) released its "Second National Report on Human Exposure to Environmental

Chemicals" in January 2003. The report reflects the results of testing 9,282 people for the presence in their bodies of 116 chemicals, including 34 pesticides.

This section takes a closer look at what the CDC data tell us about the pesticides we all carry, or our "pesticide body burden." Analysis of these data tell us which groups of people carry the most of which pesticides, and whether the levels we're exposed to are considered "safe" by U.S. authorities. We also review what is known (and what is not known) about the long-term health effects of daily exposure to this mix of synthetic chemicals, who is responsible for the pesticides in our bodies, and what can and must be done to prevent and eliminate pesticide body burdens. Key findings of our analysis are outlined in the following.

Many in the U.S. Are Exposed to Pesticides at Harmful Levels

Body burden data provide direct evidence of an individual's exposure to pesticides. In many cases, pesticide exposure levels indicated by CDC's body burden data were well above officially permitted thresholds established by government health and environmental agencies. Of the 13 pesticides in the evaluated set for which such "acceptable" exposure levels have been established, two—chlorpyrifos and methyl parathion—exceeded the thresholds dramatically. Chronic exposure to chlorpyrifos, an insecticide more commonly known by its commercial name Dursban, was furthest above the government safety threshold, with average levels for the different age groups 3 to 4.6 times what agencies consider "acceptable" for chronic exposure of vulnerable populations. This means that women, children, and elderly people in the sample population—reflecting many millions of people in the U.S.—exceed the officially established "acceptable" dose for chronic exposure.

Children Carry Heaviest Body Burden of Many Harmful Pesticides

CDC data show that the most vulnerable members of the population—our children—are exposed to the highest levels of the organophosphorus family of pesticides, which damage the nervous system. As CDC noted in the 2003 release of these data, young children carry particularly high body burdens—nearly twice that of adults—of a breakdown product (or "metabolite") specific to the insecticide chlorpyrifos.

Mexican Americans Carry Higher Body Burden of Many Agricultural Pesticides

A comparison of pesticide exposure levels among ethnic groups showed Mexican Americans had significantly higher concentrations of 5 of 17 pesticide metabolites measured in urine. Mexican Americans also had significantly higher body burdens than other ethnic groups of the waste and breakdown products of the insecticides lindane and DDT [dichlorodiphenyltrichloroethane] (*beta*-HCH [beta-hexachlorocyclohexane] and *p,p*-DDE [dichlorodiphenyl dichloroethylene], respectively).

Most People in the U.S. Carry Many Pesticides in Their Bodies

CDC found pesticides and their breakdown products in all of the people they tested. All but 5 of the 23 pesticides and pesticide metabolites evaluated in this report were found in at least half of the study subjects. Among those tested for pesticide residues in both blood and urine, the average person had 13 pesticides in his or her body. Two chemicals found in nearly all the test subjects were TCP [trichloropropane], a metabolite of the insecticide chlorpyrifos (found in 93% of those tested), and *p,p*-DDE, a breakdown product of DDT (found in 99% of those tested). Based on these data—which present results from testing for only a fraction of the pesticides that individuals are actually exposed to—it is clear that most people in the U.S. carry a significant body burden of pesticides and pesticide metabolites.

Future Generations Are at Risk

Adult women—including women of childbearing age—had the highest measured body burden levels of three of the six organochlorine pesticides evaluated. This is cause for serious concern, as many of these pesticides are known to have multiple harmful effects when crossing the placenta during fetal development. Potential negative impacts of fetal exposure include reduced infant birth weight; reproductive problems including low sperm counts and other fertility problems later in life; and disruption of neurological development during infancy, potentially leading to learning disabilities and other neurobehavioral problems. Elevated levels of *p,p*-DDE in mothers, for example, have been associated with both lower infant birth weight and reduced lactation, shortening the length of time mothers are able to breastfeed.

Pesticide Companies Must Be Held Accountable

Where did these harmful pesticides in our bodies come from? Who is responsible for this chemical trespass?

Primary responsibility must rest with pesticide manufacturers. Over the last 50 years, agrochemical companies have largely defined the range of pest control technologies available to farmers and nonagricultural users alike. They also use their political influence to promote and protect their interests by limiting health and safety regulations. Pesticide manufacturers have the greatest capacity to prevent pesticide body burdens, and the general public expects manufacturers to be responsible for the impacts of their products.

In an effort to begin quantifying the responsibilities of individual manufacturers for pesticide body burdens, PANNA [Pesticide Action Network North America] has developed a Pesticide Trespass Index (PTI). The PTI is a quantitative measure (a number between 0 and 1) of the fraction of chemical trespass attributable to a specific manufacturer for a pesticide, or group of pesticides, found in a population.

A test case using the pesticide chlorpyrifos as an example illustrates how the PTI works. Dow AgroSciences, a wholly owned subsidiary of Dow Chemical Corporation, is the primary manufacturer of chlorpyrifos. Using conservative market share estimates, Dow's PTI for chlorpyrifos can be calculated to be 0.8. This suggests that at least 80% of the population's chlorpyrifos body burden is the responsibility of Dow Chemical Corporation.

It would be difficult to make a case that anyone could be more responsible for the chlorpyrifos in our bodies than Dow Chemical Company. Dow developed and was the first to commercialize the pesticide for a wide range of agricultural, residential, and nonresidential uses, and remains the predominant producer of technical-grade chlorpyrifos to this day. The company continues to produce and promote the pesticide in the U.S. and internationally, despite strong evidence of significant public health impacts.

Real changes are needed to reduce pesticide body burdens. The fact that we all carry a mixture of toxic pesticides in our bodies reflects a dramatic failure of government efforts to protect public health and safety. Rather than focusing on preventing harm, current pesticide policies are designed to weigh health and environmental concerns against the powerful economic interests of pesticide manufacturers, users, and their allies. Systemic changes are needed to reduce our pesticide body burden, safeguard public health and safety, hold pesticide manufacturers accountable, and prevent further harm.

Health Reference Series Medical Advisor's Note: The effects of pesticides on human health are an active area of research, and some of the findings so far have been disturbing. However, the majority of research to date has been done on animals. It is not yet known whether all of the harmful effects observed in animals also occur in humans.

Editor's Note: The information in this section represents the opinion of the copyright holder and is presented as one viewpoint on a complex subject.

Section 21.2

Pharmaceuticals and Personal Care Products (PPCPs) as Pollutants

This section excerpted from "Pharmaceuticals and Personal Care Products (PPCPs) as Pollutants," Environmental Protection Agency (www.epa.gov), March 25, 2009.

What are PPCPs?

The acronym "PPCPs" was coined in the 1999 critical review published in *Environmental Health Perspectives* (www.epa.gov/ppcp/pdf/errata.pdf) to refer to pharmaceuticals and personal care products. PPCPs comprise a very broad, diverse collection of thousands of chemical substances, including prescription, veterinary, and over-the-counter (OTC) therapeutic drugs; fragrances; cosmetics; sunscreen agents; diagnostic agents; nutraceuticals (vitamins); biopharmaceuticals; growth-enhancing chemicals used in livestock operations; and many others. This broad collection of substances refers, in general, to any product used by individuals for personal health or cosmetic reasons.

What are the major sources of PPCPs in the environment?

- Human activity (e.g., bathing, shaving, swimming)
- Illicit drugs
- Veterinary drug use, especially antibiotics and steroids
- Agribusiness

- Residues from pharmaceutical manufacturing (well defined and controlled)
- Residues from hospitals

The importance of individuals adding chemicals to the environment has been largely overlooked. The discovery of PPCPs in water and soil shows even simple activities like shaving, using lotion, or taking medication affect the environment in which you live.

People contribute PPCPs to the environment when the following occur:

- Medication residues pass out of the body and into sewer lines
- Externally applied drugs and personal care products they use wash down the shower drain
- Unused or expired medications are placed in the trash

Personal use and manufacturing of illicit drugs are a less visible source of PPCPs entering the environment.

Many of the issues pertaining to the introduction of drugs to the environment from human usage also pertain to veterinary use, especially for antibiotics and steroids.

The discharge of pharmaceuticals and synthesis materials and by-products from manufacturing are already well defined and controlled.

What is the overall scientific concern?

Studies have shown that pharmaceuticals are present in our nation's water bodies. Further research suggests that certain drugs may cause ecological harm. More research is needed to determine the extent of ecological harm and any role it may have in potential human health effects. To date, scientists have found no evidence of adverse human health effects from PPCPs in the environment.

Reasons for concern are the following:

- Large quantities of PPCPs can enter the environment after use by individuals or domestic animals.
- Sewage systems are not equipped for PPCP removal. Currently, there are no municipal sewage treatment plants that are engineered specifically for PPCP removal or for other unregulated contaminants. Effective removal of PPCPs from treatment

plants varies based on the type of chemical and on the individual sewage treatment facilities.

- The risks are uncertain. The risks posed to aquatic organisms and to humans are unknown, largely because the concentrations are so low. While the major concerns have been the resistance to antibiotics and disruption of aquatic endocrine systems (the system of glands that produce hormones that help control the body's metabolic activity) by natural and synthetic sex steroids, many other PPCPs have unknown consequences. There are no known human health effects from such low-level exposures in drinking water, but special scenarios (one example being fetal exposure to low levels of medications that a mother would ordinarily be avoiding) require more investigation.
- The number of PPCPs are growing. In addition to antibiotics and steroids, over 100 individual PPCPs have been identified (as of 2007) in environmental samples and drinking water.

Where are PPCPs found in the environment?

PPCPs are found where people or animals are treated with drugs and people use personal care products. PPCPs are found in any water body influenced by raw or treated sewage, including rivers, streams, ground water, coastal marine environments, and many drinking water sources. PPCPs have been identified in most places sampled.

The U.S. Geological Survey (USGS) implemented a national reconnaissance to provide baseline information on the environmental occurrence of PPCPs in water resources. You can find more information about this project from the USGS's What's in Our Wastewaters and Where Does it Go? site (toxics.usgs.gov/highlights/whatsin.html).

PPCPs in the environment are frequently found in aquatic environments because PPCPs dissolve easily and don't evaporate at normal temperature and pressures. Practices such as the use of sewage sludge ("biosolids") and reclaimed water for irrigation brings PPCPs into contact with the soil.

How is the disposal of unused pharmaceuticals regulated by the U.S. EPA [Environmental Protection Agency]?

The Resource Conservation and Recovery Act (RCRA) is a federal law controlling the management and disposal of solid and hazardous wastes produced by a wide variety of industries and sources. The

RCRA program regulates the management and disposal of hazardous pharmaceutical wastes produced by pharmaceutical manufacturers and the health care industry. Under RCRA, a waste is a hazardous waste if it is specifically listed by the EPA or if it exhibits one or more of the following four characteristics: ignitability, corrosivity, reactivity, and toxicity.

How do I properly dispose of unwanted pharmaceuticals?

In February 2007, the White House Office of National Drug Control Policy issued the first consumer guidance for the "Proper Disposal of Prescription Drugs" (www.whitehousedrugpolicy.gov/publications/pdf/prescrip_disposal.pdf). Proper disposal of drugs is a straightforward way for individuals to prevent pollution.

RCRA does not regulate any household waste, which includes medications/pharmaceutical waste generated in a household. While discarded pharmaceuticals under the control of consumers are not regulated by RCRA, EPA encourages the public to take these steps:

- Take advantage of pharmaceutical take-back programs or household hazardous waste collection programs that accept pharmaceuticals.
- If there are no take-back programs near you, follow these guidelines:
    - Contact your state and local waste management authorities (the disposal of household waste is primarily regulated on the state and local levels) with questions about discarding unused pharmaceuticals, whether or not these materials meet the definition of hazardous waste.
    - Follow any specific disposal instructions that may be printed on the label or accompanying patient information.

In what quantities are PPCPs used or introduced to the environment?

As a whole, PPCPs are produced and used in large quantities. Personal care products tend to be made in extremely large quantities—thousands of tons per year. But quantities of production or consumption do not correspond with the quantities of PPCPs introduced to the environment. PPCPs manufactured in large quantities may not be found in the environment if they are easily broken down and processed by the human body or degrade quickly. PPCPs made in small quantities could be over represented in the environment if they are not easily broken down and processed by the human body and make their way into domestic sewers.

What are some major issues with respect to effects?

- The effects of PPCPs are different from conventional pollutants. Drugs are purposefully designed to interact with cellular receptors at low concentrations and to elicit specific biological effects. Unintended adverse effects can also occur from interaction with nontarget receptors.
- Environmental toxicology focuses on acute effects of exposure rather than chronic effects.
- Effects on aquatic life are a major concern. Exposure risks for aquatic organisms are much larger than those for humans. Aquatic organisms have the following exposures:
  - Continual exposures
  - Multigenerational exposures
  - Exposure to higher concentrations of PPCPs in untreated water
  - Possible low dose effects
- Effects may be subtle because PPCPs in the environment occur at low concentrations. There's a need to develop tests that detect more subtle end-points. Neurobehavioral effects and inhibition of efflux pumps are two examples. Subtle effects that accumulate may be significant.
- There are little aquatic/terrestrial toxicology data for PPCPs. There is substantially more data available for pesticides. For example, brief exposure of salmon to one ppb of the insecticide diazinon is known to affect signaling pathways (via olfactory disruption), leading to alteration in homing behavior (with obvious implications for predation, feeding, and mating). There's concern that low doses of PPCPs may also have effects.
- There are many drug classes of concern:
  - Antibiotics that are actively being researched
  - Antimicrobials

- Estrogenic steroids
- Antidepressants: Profound effects on spawning and other behaviors in shellfish can occur with antidepressant selective serotonin reuptake inhibitors (SSRIs)
- Calcium-channel blockers: Dramatic inhibition of sperm activity in certain aquatic organisms can be effected by calcium-channel blockers
- Antiepileptic drugs (e.g., phenytoin, valproate, carbamazepine): Potential as human neuroteratogens, triggering extensive apoptosis in the developing brain, leading to neurodegeneration
- Multidrug transporters (efflux pumps): Possible significance of efflux pump inhibitors (EPIs) in compromising aquatic health
- Musk fragrances are bioaccumulative and persistent
- Genotoxic drugs (primarily used at hospitals)

Section 21.3

Effects of Industrial Agriculture

"Concentrated Animal Feeding Operations (CAFOs)," Centers for Disease Control and Prevention (www.cdc.gov), March 2004. Reviewed by David A. Cooke, MD, FACP, June 2009.

During the past three decades, animal production in the United States has become increasingly specialized. Many farms function as links in the chain of animal production, housing and feeding cattle and poultry. In 2003, the nation's 238,000 feeding operations produced 500 million tons of manure. The EPA estimates that a small percentage of those facilities—called concentrated animal feeding operations (CAFOs)—accounted for more than half of the manure.

CAFOs are agricultural facilities that house and feed a large number of animals in a confined area for 45 days or more during any 12-month period. Federal regulations require CAFOs to carry a permit and to develop nutrient-management plans designed to keep animal waste from contaminating surface water and groundwater. The number and type(s) of animal(s) the operation houses, and the extent to which waste from the operation could pollute surface water and groundwater, determine whether EPA considers a feeding operation to be a CAFO.

EPA began regulating CAFOs during the 1970s. The latest EPA regulations, guidance, and other information on CAFOs are available at cfpub.epa.gov/npdes/afo/info.cfm?program_id=7.

Public Health Concerns

People who work with livestock may develop adverse health effects, including chronic and acute respiratory illnesses and musculoskeletal injuries, and may be exposed to infections that travel from animals to humans. Residents in areas surrounding CAFOs report nuisances, such as odor and flies. In studies of CAFOs, CDC has shown that chemical and infectious compounds from swine and poultry waste are able to migrate into soil and water near CAFOs. Scientists do not yet know whether or how the migration of these compounds affects human health.

Pollutants possibly associated with manure-related discharges at CAFOs include the following:

- Antibiotics, which may contribute to the development of antibiotic-resistant pathogens
- Pathogens, such as parasites, bacteria, and viruses, which can cause disease in animals and humans
- Nutrients, such as ammonia, nitrogen, and phosphorus, which can reduce oxygen in surface waters, encourage the growth of harmful algal blooms, and contaminate drinking-water sources
- Pesticides and hormones, which researchers have associated with hormone-related changes in fish
- Solids, such as feed and feathers, which can limit the growth of desirable aquatic plants in surface waters and protect disease-causing microorganisms
- Trace elements, such as arsenic and copper, which can contaminate surface waters and possibly harm human health

Researchers do not yet know whether or how these or other substances from CAFOs may affect human health. Therefore, CDC supports efforts to address these questions.

Section 21.4

Landfills

This section excerpted from "Frequently Asked Questions about Landfill Gas and How It Affects Public Health, Safety, and the Environment," Environmental Protection Agency (www.epa.gov), June 2008.

Approximately 64% of all municipal solid waste (MSW) generated in the United States is currently being disposed of in roughly 1,800 operational MSW landfills, as referenced in "EPA's Inventory of U.S. Greenhouse Gas Emissions and Sinks: 1990–2006." Landfills are the second-largest single human source of methane emissions in the United States, accounting for nearly 23% of all methane sources. Uncontrolled MSW landfills also emit nonmethane organic compounds (NMOC), which include volatile organic compounds (VOC) that contribute to ozone formation and hazardous air pollutants (HAP) that can affect human health when exposed. However, combustion of landfill gas significantly reduces emissions of methane and NMOC. More than 400 MSW landfills in the United States recover and combust landfill gas to generate heat or electricity, and more than 450 other MSW landfills flare the gas. EPA's air quality requirements and advances in landfill gas energy technologies have encouraged the combustion of landfill gas to benefit human health, safety, and the environment, as well as provide economic opportunities.

What are the public health, safety, and environmental concerns associated with landfill gas?

The public health, safety, and environmental concerns fall into three categories: subsurface migration, surface emissions/air pollution, and odor nuisance.

Subsurface Migration: Subsurface migration is the underground movement of landfill gas from landfills to other areas within the landfill property or outside the landfill property. (Note: Most subsurface migration occurs at older, unlined landfills because there is minimal barrier for lateral migration. The Resource Conservation and Recovery

Act began requiring all new or expanded landfills to be lined as of October 9, 1993. This requirement decreases the likelihood of subsurface migration.) Since landfill gas contains approximately 50% methane (a potentially explosive gas), it is possible for landfill gas to travel underground, accumulate in enclosed structures, and ignite. There have been incidences of subsurface migration causing fires and explosions on both landfill property and private property.

Surface Emissions: Possibly the biggest health and environmental concerns are related to the uncontrolled surface emissions of landfill gas into the air. As previously mentioned, landfill gas contains carbon dioxide, methane, VOC, HAP, and odorous compounds that can adversely affect public health and the environment. For example, carbon dioxide and methane are greenhouse gases that contribute to global climate change. Methane is of particular concern because it is 21 times more effective at trapping heat in the atmosphere than carbon dioxide. Emissions of VOC contribute to ground-level ozone formation (smog). Ozone is capable of reducing or damaging vegetation growth as well as causing respiratory problems in humans. Finally, exposure to HAP can cause a variety of health problems, such as cancerous illnesses, respiratory irritation, and central nervous system damage. Thermal treatment of NMOC (including HAP and VOC) and methane through flaring or combustion in an engine, turbine, boiler, or other device greatly reduces the emission of these compounds.

Odors: The final concern related to uncontrolled landfill gas emissions is their unpleasant odor. Compounds found in landfill gas are associated with strong, pungent odors. These smells can be transmitted off-site to nearby homes and business. Unpleasant odors can lower the quality of life for individuals that live near landfills and potentially reduce local property values.

What is EPA doing to protect public health, safety, and the environment?

EPA promulgated Criteria for Municipal Solid Waste Landfills (40 CFR Part 258) under the Resource Conservation and Recovery Act (RCRA) on October 9, 1991. The criteria contain location restrictions, design and operating standards, groundwater monitoring requirements, corrective actions, financial assurance requirements, landfill gas migration control, closure requirements, and post closure requirements. Under the design standards new landfills and lateral expansions that occur on or after October 9, 1993, are required to line the bottom and sides of the landfill prior to waste deposition. In addition, all landfills operating after October 9, 1991, must place a final cap over the landfill surface. The placement of liners and caps reduces the potential for subsurface and surface landfill gas migration and groundwater contamination. Recovery and combustion of landfill gas will reduce emissions of organic compounds that would otherwise be released from the landfill. Because of the benefits of collecting and controlling landfill gas, the 1996 EPA Standards of Performance for New Stationary Sources (NSPS) and Guidelines for Control of Existing Sources, and the 2003 National Emission Standards for Hazardous Air Pollutants (NESHAP), require "large" MSW landfills to collect landfill gas and combust it to reduce NMOC by 98% (or to an outlet concentration of 20 ppmv [parts per million by volume]). A "large" landfill is defined as having a design capacity of at least 2.5 million metric tons and 2.5 million cubic meters and a calculated or measured uncontrolled NMOC emission rate of at least 50 metric tons (megagrams) per year. Landfills are meeting these gas destruction standards using flares or energy recovery devices, including reciprocating engines, gas turbines, and boilers. In addition to gas destruction requirements, the NSPS and NESHAP require that gas collection systems be well designed and well operated. They require gas collection from all areas of the landfill, monthly monitoring at each collection well, and monitoring of surface methane emissions to ensure that the collection system is operating properly and to reduce fugitive emissions. Smaller MSW landfills are not required to control emissions by the NSPS or NESHAP but can still greatly reduce emissions of NMOC by collecting and combusting landfill gas for energy recovery or in a flare.

EPA's Landfill Methane Outreach Program (LMOP) is a voluntary assistance and partnership program that promotes the use of landfill gas as a renewable energy resource. By preventing emissions of methane through the development of landfill gas energy projects, LMOP helps businesses, states, and communities protect the environment and build a sustainable future. LMOP helps communities and landfill owner/operators learn more about the benefits of using landfill gas as an alternative energy source and helps them develop or participate in landfill gas energy projects. In addition, LMOP provides information, software tools, and marketing assistance, and access to technical experts to facilitate development of landfill gas energy projects. For more information about LMOP, please visit the LMOP website at www.epa.gov/lmop.

What are dioxins and furans and are they released from landfill gas combustion?

Dioxins and furans are a group of toxic chemical compounds, known as persistent organic pollutants, that share certain similar chemical structures and biological characteristics. Dioxins/furans are released into the air as by-products of many combustion processes, such as incinerating municipal waste, burning fuels (e.g., wood, coal, or oil), and some industrial processes such as the bleaching of pulp and paper. Some of the conditions that are conducive to dioxin/furan formation are the combustion of organic material in the presence of chlorine and particulate matter under certain thermodynamic conditions such as low combustion temperatures and brief combustion times. Sources of dioxin/furan include but are not limited to: MSW combustors (incinerators), residential and commercial coal combustion, residential and commercial oil combustion, backyard trash burning, residential fireplaces, cars, cigarettes, forest and brush fires, and the combustion of landfill gas. However, relative to many of these combustion sources, the characteristics of landfill gas combustion are less conducive to dioxin/furan formation.

EPA's review of the available data indicates that dioxins/furans can be released in small amounts when landfill gas is combusted by flare or for recovering energy. Based on national and international source tests, the concentration of dioxins from landfill gas combustion ranges from nondetectable to 0.1 nanograms (10^{-9} grams) of toxic equivalents (TEQ) per dry standard cubic meter of exhaust, at 7% oxygen. Because of the health threat from uncontrolled emissions of other organic compounds in landfill gas, EPA found, in developing emissions standards, that landfill gas destruction in a proper control device (e.g., flare or energy recovery unit) with minimal by-product generation of dioxins/furans is preferable to the release of uncontrolled landfill gas. In summary, EPA believes that the potential for dioxin emissions from the combustion of landfill gas is small.

How does landfill gas combustion affect mercury emissions?

Mercury, although present throughout the environment, is a health concern because it can bioaccumulate through the food chain as methylated mercury, an organic, more toxic form of mercury. Sources of mercury in MSW landfills can include batteries, fluorescent light bulbs, electrical switches, thermometers, and paints. Once mercury enters the waste stream, it will ultimately be released from the landfill and is contained in uncontrolled landfill gas. However, combustion of landfill gas reduces the toxicity of landfill gas emissions by converting the organic mercury compounds, including methylated mercury, to less toxic, less hazardous, inorganic mercury compounds. According to EPA's 1997 "Mercury Study Report to Congress," MSW landfills contributed less than 0.1% of the total mercury released from all man-made sources in the United States in 1994. When compared on an annual basis, mercury emissions from landfill gas are significantly less than mercury emissions generated by small oil-fired boilers used in homes and apartments.

Chapter 22

Bioterrorism and Chemical Emergencies

Biological Threats

Biological agents are organisms or toxins that can kill or incapacitate people, livestock, and crops. The three basic groups of biological agents that would likely be used as weapons are bacteria, viruses, and toxins. Most biological agents are difficult to grow and maintain. Many break down quickly when exposed to sunlight and other environmental factors, while others, such as anthrax spores, are very long lived. Biological agents can be dispersed by spraying them into the air, by infecting animals that carry the disease to humans, and by contaminating food and water. Delivery methods include the following:

- **Aerosols:** Biological agents are dispersed into the air, forming a fine mist that may drift for miles. Inhaling the agent may cause disease in people or animals.
- **Animals:** Some diseases are spread by insects and animals, such as fleas, mice, flies, mosquitoes, and livestock.
- **Food and Water Contamination**: Some pathogenic organisms and toxins may persist in food and water supplies. Most microbes can be killed, and toxins deactivated, by cooking food

---

This section includes "Terrorism: Biological Threats" and "Terrorism: Chemical Threats," Federal Emergency Management Agency (www.fema.gov), March 21, 2006.

and boiling water. Most microbes are killed by boiling water for one minute, but some require longer. Follow official instructions.

- **Person-to-Person:** Spread of a few infectious agents is also possible. Humans have been the source of infection for smallpox, plague, and the Lassa viruses.

Specific information on biological agents is available at the Centers for Disease Control and Prevention's website (www.bt.cdc.gov).

Before a Biological Attack

What You Should Do to Prepare: Check with your doctor to ensure all required or suggested immunizations are up to date. Children and older adults are particularly vulnerable to biological agents.

Consider installing a High Efficiency Particulate Air (HEPA) filter in your furnace return duct. These filters remove particles in the 0.3 to 10 micron range and will filter out most biological agents that may enter your house. If you do not have a central heating or cooling system, a stand-alone portable HEPA filter can be used.

Filtration in Buildings: Building owners and managers should determine the type and level of filtration in their structures and the level of protection it provides against biological agents. The National Institute of Occupational Safety and Health (NIOSH) provides technical guidance on this topic in their publication "Guidance for Filtration and Air-Cleaning Systems to Protect Building Environments from Airborne Chemical, Biological, or Radiological Attacks." To obtain a copy, call 800-35NIOSH or visit the NIOSH website (www.cdc.gov/niosh/pubs.html) and request or download NIOSH Publication 2003-136.

During a Biological Attack

In the event of a biological attack, public health officials may not immediately be able to provide information on what you should do. It will take time to determine what the illness is, how it should be treated, and who is in danger. Watch television, listen to radio, or check the Internet for official news and information including signs and symptoms of the disease, areas in danger, if medications or vaccinations are being distributed, and where you should seek medical attention if you become ill.

The first evidence of an attack may be when you notice symptoms of the disease caused by exposure to an agent. Be suspicious of any symptoms you notice, but do not assume that any illness is a result of the attack. Use common sense and practice good hygiene.

If you become aware of an unusual and suspicious substance nearby, take the following precautions:

- Move away quickly.
- Wash with soap and water.
- Contact authorities.
- Listen to the media for official instructions.
- Seek medical attention if you become sick.

If you are exposed to a biological agent, follow these steps:

- Remove and bag your clothes and personal items. Follow official instructions for disposal of contaminated items.
- Wash yourself with soap and water and put on clean clothes.
- Seek medical assistance. You may be advised to stay away from others or even quarantined.

Using HEPA Filters: HEPA filters are useful in biological attacks. If you have a central heating and cooling system in your home with a HEPA filter, leave it on if it is running or turn the fan on if it is not running. Moving the air in the house through the filter will help remove the agents from the air. If you have a portable HEPA filter, take it with you to the internal room where you are seeking shelter and turn it on.

If you are in an apartment or office building that has a modern, central heating and cooling system, the system's filtration should provide a relatively safe level of protection from outside biological contaminants.

HEPA filters will not filter chemical agents.

After a Biological Attack

In some situations, such as the case of the anthrax letters sent in 2001, people may be alerted to potential exposure. If this is the case, pay close attention to all official warnings and instructions on how to proceed. The delivery of medical services for a biological event may be handled differently to respond to increased demand. The basic public health procedures and medical protocols for handling exposure to biological agents are the same as for any infectious disease. It is important for you to pay attention to official instructions via radio, television, and emergency alert systems.

Chemical Threats

Chemical agents are poisonous vapors, aerosols, liquids, and solids that have toxic effects on people, animals, or plants. They can be released by bombs or sprayed from aircraft, boats, and vehicles. They can be used as a liquid to create a hazard to people and the environment. Some chemical agents may be odorless and tasteless. They can have an immediate effect (a few seconds to a few minutes) or a delayed effect (2 to 48 hours). While potentially lethal, chemical agents are difficult to deliver in lethal concentrations. Outdoors, the agents often dissipate rapidly. Chemical agents also are difficult to produce.

A chemical attack could come without warning. Signs of a chemical release include people having difficulty breathing; experiencing eye irritation; losing coordination; becoming nauseated; or having a burning sensation in the nose, throat, and lungs. Also, the presence of many dead insects or birds may indicate a chemical agent release.

Before a Chemical Attack

Take the following precautions to prepare for a chemical threat:

- Check your disaster supplies kit to make sure it includes these supplies:
    - A roll of duct tape and scissors
    - Plastic for doors, windows, and vents for the room in which you will shelter in place (to save critical time during an emergency, pre-measure and cut the plastic sheeting for each opening)
- Choose an internal room to shelter, preferably one without windows and on the highest level.

During a Chemical Attack

If you are instructed to remain in your home or office building, you should do the following:

- Close doors and windows and turn off all ventilation, including furnaces, air conditioners, vents, and fans.
- Seek shelter in an internal room and take your disaster supplies kit.
- Seal the room with duct tape and plastic sheeting.
- Listen to your radio for instructions from authorities.

If you are caught in or near a contaminated area, you should follow these steps:

- Move away immediately in a direction upwind of the source.
- Find shelter as quickly as possible.

After a Chemical Attack

Decontamination is needed within minutes of exposure to minimize health consequences. Do not leave the safety of a shelter to go outdoors to help others until authorities announce it is safe to do so.

A person affected by a chemical agent requires immediate medical attention from a professional. If medical help is not immediately available, decontaminate yourself and assist in decontaminating others.

Decontamination guidelines are as follows:

- Use extreme caution when helping others who have been exposed to chemical agents.
- Remove all clothing and other items in contact with the body. Contaminated clothing normally removed over the head should be cut off to avoid contact with the eyes, nose, and mouth. Put contaminated clothing and items into a plastic bag and seal it. Decontaminate hands using soap and water. Remove eyeglasses or contact lenses. Put glasses in a pan of household bleach to decontaminate them, and then rinse and dry.
- Flush eyes with water.
- Gently wash face and hair with soap and water before thoroughly rinsing with water.
- Decontaminate other body areas likely to have been contaminated. Blot (do not swab or scrape) with a cloth soaked in soapy water and rinse with clear water.

- Change into uncontaminated clothes. Clothing stored in drawers or closets is likely to be uncontaminated.
- Proceed to a medical facility for screening and professional treatment.

Part Four

Household and Indoor Hazards

Chapter 23

The Importance of Indoor Air Quality

Indoor Air Quality in Your Home

All of us face a variety of risks to our health as we go about our day-to-day lives. Driving in cars, flying in planes, engaging in recreational activities, and being exposed to environmental pollutants all pose varying degrees of risk. Some risks are simply unavoidable. Some we choose to accept because to do otherwise would restrict our ability to lead our lives the way we want. And some are risks we might decide to avoid if we had the opportunity to make informed choices. Indoor air pollution is one risk that you can do something about.

In the last several years, a growing body of scientific evidence has indicated that the air within homes and other buildings can be more seriously polluted than the outdoor air in even the largest and most industrialized cities. Other research indicates that people spend approximately 90% of their time indoors. Thus, for many people, the risks to health may be greater due to exposure to air pollution indoors than outdoors.

In addition, people who may be exposed to indoor air pollutants for the longest periods of time are often those most susceptible to the effects of indoor air pollution. Such groups include the young, the elderly, and the chronically ill, especially those suffering from respiratory or cardiovascular disease.

This section excerpted from "The Inside Story: A Guide to Indoor Air Quality," Consumer Product Safety Commission (www.cpsc.gov), April 2009.

While pollutant levels from individual sources may not pose a significant health risk by themselves, most homes have more than one source that contributes to indoor air pollution. There can be a serious risk from the cumulative effects of these sources. Fortunately, there are steps that most people can take both to reduce the risk from existing sources and to prevent new problems from occurring.

What Causes Indoor Air Problems?

Indoor pollution sources that release gases or particles into the air are the primary cause of indoor air quality problems in homes. Inadequate ventilation can increase indoor pollutant levels by not bringing in enough outdoor air to dilute emissions from indoor sources and by not carrying indoor air pollutants out of the home. High temperature and humidity levels can also increase concentrations of some pollutants.

Pollutant Sources: There are many sources of indoor air pollution in any home. These include combustion sources such as oil, gas, kerosene, coal, wood, and tobacco products; building materials and furnishings as diverse as deteriorated, asbestos-containing insulation, wet or damp carpet, and cabinetry or furniture made of certain pressed wood products; products for household cleaning and maintenance, personal care, or hobbies; central heating and cooling systems and humidification devices; and outdoor sources such as radon, pesticides, and outdoor air pollution.

The relative importance of any single source depends on how much of a given pollutant it emits and how hazardous those emissions are. In some cases, factors such as how old the source is and whether it is properly maintained are significant. For example, an improperly adjusted gas stove can emit significantly more carbon monoxide than one that is properly adjusted.

Some sources, such as building materials, furnishings, and household products like air fresheners, release pollutants more or less continuously. Other sources, related to activities carried out in the home, release pollutants intermittently. These include smoking; the use of unvented or malfunctioning stoves, furnaces, or space heaters; the use of solvents in cleaning and hobby activities; the use of paint strippers in redecorating activities; and the use of cleaning products and pesticides in housekeeping. High pollutant concentrations can remain in the air for long periods after some of these activities.

Amount of Ventilation: If too little outdoor air enters a home, pollutants can accumulate to levels that can pose health and comfort problems. Unless they are built with special mechanical means of ventilation, homes that are designed and constructed to minimize the amount of outdoor air that can "leak" into and out of the home may have higher pollutant levels than other homes. However, because some weather conditions can drastically reduce the amount of outdoor air that enters a home, pollutants can build up even in homes that are normally considered "leaky."

How Does Outdoor Air Enter a House?

Outdoor air enters and leaves a house by: infiltration, natural ventilation, and mechanical ventilation. In a process known as infiltration, outdoor air flows into the house through openings, joints, and cracks in walls, floors, and ceilings, and around windows and doors. In natural ventilation, air moves through opened windows and doors. Air movement associated with infiltration and natural ventilation is caused by air temperature differences between indoors and outdoors and by wind. Finally, there are a number of mechanical ventilation devices, from outdoor-vented fans that intermittently remove air from a single room, such as bathrooms and kitchen, to air handling systems that use fans and duct work to continuously remove indoor air and distribute filtered and conditioned outdoor air to strategic points throughout the house. The rate at which outdoor air replaces indoor air is described as the air exchange rate. When there is little infiltration, natural ventilation, or mechanical ventilation, the air exchange rate is low and pollutant levels can increase.

What If You Live in an Apartment?

Apartments can have the same indoor air problems as single-family homes because many of the pollution sources, such as the interior building materials, furnishings, and household products, are similar. Indoor air problems similar to those in offices are caused by such sources as contaminated ventilation systems, improperly placed outdoor air intakes, or maintenance activities.

Solutions to air quality problems in apartments, as in homes and offices, involve such actions as: eliminating or controlling the sources of pollution, increasing ventilation, and installing air cleaning devices. Often a resident can take the appropriate action to improve the indoor air quality by removing a source, altering an activity, unblocking an air supply vent, or opening a window to temporarily increase the ventilation; in other cases, however, only the building owner or manager is in a position to remedy the problem. You can encourage building management to follow guidance in the EPA's [Environmental Protection Agency] "IAQ Building Education and Assessment Model" (I-BEAM), found at www.epa.gov/iaq/largebldgs/i-beam/index.html. I-BEAM updates and expands EPA's existing Building Air Quality guidance and is designed to be comprehensive state-of-the-art guidance for managing IAQ [indoor air quality] in commercial buildings. This guidance was designed to be used by building professionals and others interested in indoor air quality in commercial buildings. I-BEAM contains text, animation/visual, and interactive/calculation components that can be used to perform a number of diverse tasks. You can also encourage building management to follow guidance in EPA and NIOSH's [National Institute for Occupational Safety and Health] "Building Air Quality: A Guide for Building Owners and Facility Managers." (The BAQ is available at www.epa.gov/iaq/largebldgs/baqtoc.html as PDF files that can be downloaded and viewed individually or as a single file with all of the PDF files).

Improving the Air Quality in Your Home

Indoor Air and Your Health

Health effects from indoor air pollutants may be experienced soon after exposure or, possibly, years later.

Immediate effects may show up after a single exposure or repeated exposures. These include irritation of the eyes, nose, and throat; headaches; dizziness; and fatigue. Such immediate effects are usually short-term and treatable. Sometimes the treatment is simply eliminating the person's exposure to the source of the pollution, if it can be identified. Symptoms of some diseases, including asthma, hypersensitivity pneumonitis, and humidifier fever, may also show up soon after exposure to some indoor air pollutants.

The likelihood of immediate reactions to indoor air pollutants depends on several factors. Age and preexisting medical conditions are two important influences. In other cases, whether a person reacts to a pollutant depends on individual sensitivity, which varies tremendously from person to person. Some people can become sensitized to biological pollutants after repeated exposures, and it appears that some people can become sensitized to chemical pollutants as well.

Certain immediate effects are similar to those from colds or other viral diseases, so it is often difficult to determine if the symptoms are a result of exposure to indoor air pollution. For this reason, it is important to pay attention to the time and place the symptoms occur. If the symptoms fade or go away when a person is away from the home and return when the person returns, an effort should be made to identify indoor air sources that may be possible causes. Some effects may be made worse by an inadequate supply of outdoor air or from the heating, cooling, or humidity conditions prevalent in the home.

Other health effects may show up either years after exposure has occurred or only after long or repeated periods of exposure. These effects, which include some respiratory diseases, heart disease, and cancer, can be severely debilitating or fatal. It is prudent to try to improve the indoor air quality in your home even if symptoms are not noticeable.

While pollutants commonly found in indoor air are responsible for many harmful effects, there is considerable uncertainty about what concentrations or periods of exposure are necessary to produce specific health problems. People also react very differently to exposure to indoor air pollutants. Further research is needed to better understand which health effects occur after exposure to the average pollutant concentrations found in homes and which occur from the higher concentrations that occur for short periods of time.

Identifying Air Quality Problems

Some health effects can be useful indicators of an indoor air quality problem, especially if they appear after a person moves to a new residence, remodels or refurnishes a home, or treats a home with pesticides. If you think that you have symptoms that may be related to your home environment, discuss them with your doctor or your local health department to see if they could be caused by indoor air pollution. You may also want to consult a board-certified allergist or an occupational medicine specialist for answers to your questions.

Another way to judge whether your home has or could develop indoor air problems is to identify potential sources of indoor air pollution. Although the presence of such sources does not necessarily mean that you have an indoor air quality problem, being aware of the type and number of potential sources is an important step toward assessing the air quality in your home.

A third way to decide whether your home may have poor indoor air quality is to look at your lifestyle and activities. Human activities can be significant sources of indoor air pollution. Finally, look for signs of problems with the ventilation in your home. Signs that can indicate your home may not have enough ventilation include moisture condensation on windows or walls, smelly or stuffy air, dirty central heating and air cooling equipment, and areas where books, shoes, or other items become moldy (see www.epa.gov/mold). To detect odors in your home, step outside for a few minutes, and then upon reentering your home, note whether odors are noticeable.

Measuring Pollutant Levels

The federal government recommends that you measure the level of radon in your home. Without measurements there is no way to tell whether radon is present because it is a colorless, odorless, radioactive gas. Inexpensive devices are available for measuring radon. EPA provides guidance as to risks associated with different levels of exposure and when the public should consider corrective action. There are specific mitigation techniques that have proven effective in reducing levels of radon in the home.

For pollutants other than radon, measurements are most appropriate when there are either health symptoms or signs of poor ventilation and specific sources or pollutants have been identified as possible causes of indoor air quality problems. Testing for many pollutants can be expensive. Before monitoring your home for pollutants besides radon, consult your state or local health department or professionals who have experience in solving indoor air quality problems in nonindustrial buildings.

Weatherizing Your Home

The federal government recommends that homes be weatherized in order to reduce the amount of energy needed for heating and cooling. While weatherization is underway, however, steps should also be taken to minimize pollution from sources inside the home. In addition, residents should be alert to the emergence of signs of inadequate ventilation, such as stuffy air, moisture condensation on cold surfaces, or mold and mildew growth. Additional weatherization measures should not be undertaken until these problems have been corrected.

Weatherization generally does not cause indoor air problems by adding new pollutants to the air. (There are a few exceptions, such as caulking, that can sometimes emit pollutants.) However, measures such as installing storm windows, weather stripping, caulking, and blown-in wall insulation can reduce the amount of outdoor air infiltrating into a home. Consequently, after weatherization, concentrations of indoor air pollutants from sources inside the home can increase.

Three Basic Strategies

Source Control: Usually the most effective way to improve indoor air quality is to eliminate individual sources of pollution or to reduce their emissions. Some sources, like those that contain asbestos, can be sealed or enclosed; others, like gas stoves, can be adjusted to decrease the amount of emissions. In many cases, source control is also a more cost-efficient approach to protecting indoor air quality than increasing ventilation because increasing ventilation can increase energy costs.

Ventilation Improvements: Another approach to lowering the concentrations of indoor air pollutants in your home is to increase the amount of outdoor air coming indoors. Most home heating and cooling systems, including forced air heating systems, do not mechanically bring fresh air into the house. Opening windows and doors, operating window or attic fans, when the weather permits, or running a window air conditioner with the vent control open increases the outdoor ventilation rate. Local bathroom or kitchen fans that exhaust outdoors remove contaminants directly from the room where the fan is located and also increase the outdoor air ventilation rate.

It is particularly important to take as many of these steps as possible while you are involved in short-term activities that can generate high levels of pollutants—for example, painting, paint stripping, heating with kerosene heaters, cooking, or engaging in maintenance and hobby activities such as welding, soldering, or sanding. You might also choose to do some of these activities outdoors, if you can and if weather permits.

Advanced designs of new homes are starting to feature mechanical systems that bring outdoor air into the home. Some of these designs include energy-efficient heat recovery ventilators (also known as air-to-air heat exchangers).

For more information about air-to-air heat exchangers, contact the U.S. Department of Energy's Energy Efficiency and Renewable Energy's Office (EERE) at www.eere.energy.gov/. You may contact the EERE Information Center with questions on EERE's products, services, and 11 technology programs by calling 877-EERE-INF (877-337-3463).

Air Cleaners: There are many types and sizes of air cleaners on the market, ranging from relatively inexpensive tabletop models to sophisticated and expensive whole-house systems. Some air cleaners are highly effective at particle removal, while others, including most tabletop models, are much less so. Air cleaners are generally not designed to remove gaseous pollutants.

The effectiveness of an air cleaner depends on how well it collects pollutants from indoor air (expressed as a percentage efficiency rate) and how much air it draws through the cleaning or filtering element (expressed in cubic feet per minute). A very efficient collector with a low air-circulation rate will not be effective, nor will a cleaner with a high air-circulation rate but a less efficient collector. The long-term performance of any air cleaner depends on maintaining it according to the manufacturer's directions.

Another important factor in determining the effectiveness of an air cleaner is the strength of the pollutant source. Tabletop air cleaners, in particular, may not remove satisfactory amounts of pollutants from strong nearby sources. People with a sensitivity to particular sources may find that air cleaners are helpful only in conjunction with concerted efforts to remove the source.

Over the past few years, there has been some publicity suggesting that houseplants have been shown to reduce levels of some chemicals in laboratory experiments. There is currently no evidence, however, that a reasonable number of houseplants remove significant quantities of pollutants in homes and offices. Indoor houseplants should not be overwatered because overly damp soil may promote the growth of microorganisms that can affect allergic individuals.

At present, EPA does not recommend using air cleaners to reduce levels of radon and its decay products. The effectiveness of these devices is uncertain because they only partially remove the radon decay products and do not diminish the amount of radon entering the home. EPA plans to do additional research on whether air cleaners are, or could become, a reliable means of reducing the health risk from radon. EPA's booklet, "Residential Air-Cleaning Devices" (www.epa.gov/iaq/pubs/residair.html), provides further information on air-cleaning devices to reduce indoor air pollutants.

"Ozone Generators That Are Sold as Air Cleaners" (www.epa.gov/iaq/pubs/ozonegen.html) was prepared by EPA to provide accurate information regarding the use of ozone-generating devices in indoor occupied spaces. This information is based on the most credible scientific evidence currently available.

"Should You Have The Air Ducts in Your Home Cleaned?" (www.epa.gov/iaq/pubs/airduct.html) was prepared by EPA to assist consumers in answering this often confusing question. The document explains what air duct cleaning is, provides guidance to help consumers decide whether to have the service performed in their home, and provides helpful information for choosing a duct cleaner, determining if duct cleaning was done properly, and how to prevent contamination of air ducts.

Chapter 24

Harmful Agents in Indoor Air

Chapter Contents

Section 24.1

Biological Contaminants

This section excerpted from "The Inside Story: A Guide to Indoor Air Quality," Consumer Product Safety Commission (www.cpsc.gov), April 2009.

Biological contaminants include bacteria, molds, mildew, viruses, animal dander and cat saliva, house dust mites, cockroaches, and pollen. There are many sources of these pollutants. Pollens originate from plants; viruses are transmitted by people and animals; bacteria are carried by people, animals, and soil and plant debris; and household pets are sources of saliva and animal dander. The protein in urine from rats and mice is a potent allergen. When it dries, it can become airborne. Contaminated central air handling systems can become breeding grounds for mold, mildew, and other sources of biological contaminants and can then distribute these contaminants through the home.

By controlling the relative humidity level in a home, the growth of some sources of biologicals can be minimized. A relative humidity of 30–50% is generally recommended for homes. Standing water, water-damaged materials, or wet surfaces also serve as a breeding ground for molds, mildews, bacteria, and insects. House dust mites, the source of one of the most powerful biological allergens, grow in damp, warm environments.

Health Effects from Biological Contaminants

Some biological contaminants trigger allergic reactions, including hypersensitivity pneumonitis, allergic rhinitis, and some types of asthma. Infectious illnesses, such as influenza, measles, and chicken pox, are transmitted through the air. Molds and mildews release disease-causing toxins. Symptoms of health problems caused by biological pollutants include sneezing, watery eyes, coughing, shortness of breath, dizziness, lethargy, fever, and digestive problems.

Allergic reactions occur only after repeated exposure to a specific biological allergen. However, that reaction may occur immediately upon re-exposure or after multiple exposures over time. As a result, people who have noticed only mild allergic reactions, or no reactions at all, may suddenly find themselves very sensitive to particular allergens.

Some diseases, like humidifier fever, are associated with exposure to toxins from microorganisms that can grow in large building ventilation systems. However, these diseases can also be traced to microorganisms that grow in home heating and cooling systems and humidifiers. Children, elderly people, and people with breathing problems, allergies, and lung diseases are particularly susceptible to disease-causing biological agents in the indoor air.

Reducing Exposure to Biological Contaminants

Install and use exhaust fans that are vented to the outdoors in kitchens and bathrooms and vent clothes dryers outdoors. These actions can eliminate much of the moisture that builds up from everyday activities. There are exhaust fans on the market that produce little noise, an important consideration for some people. Another benefit to using kitchen and bathroom exhaust fans is that they can reduce levels of organic pollutants that vaporize from hot water used in showers and dishwashers.

Ventilate the attic and crawl spaces to prevent moisture buildup. Keeping humidity levels in these areas below 50% can prevent water condensation on building materials.

If using cool mist or ultrasonic humidifiers, clean appliances according to manufacturer's instructions and refill with fresh water daily. Because these humidifiers can become breeding grounds for biological contaminants, they have the potential for causing diseases such as hypersensitivity pneumonitis and humidifier fever. Evaporation trays in air conditioners, dehumidifiers, and refrigerators should also be cleaned frequently.

Thoroughly clean and dry water-damaged carpets and building materials (within 24 hours if possible) or consider removal and replacement. Water-damaged carpets and building materials can harbor mold and bacteria. It is very difficult to completely rid such materials of biological contaminants.

Keep the house clean. House dust mites, pollens, animal dander, and other allergy-causing agents can be reduced, although not eliminated, through regular cleaning. People who are allergic to these pollutants should use allergen-proof mattress encasements, wash bedding in hot (130° F) water, and avoid room furnishings that accumulate dust, especially if they cannot be washed in hot water. Allergic individuals should also leave the house while it is being vacuumed because vacuuming can actually increase airborne levels of mite allergens and other biological contaminants. Using central vacuum systems that are vented to the outdoors or vacuums with high efficiency filters may also be of help.

Take steps to minimize biological pollutants in basements. Clean and disinfect the basement floor drain regularly. Do not finish a basement below ground level unless all water leaks are patched and outdoor ventilation and adequate heat to prevent condensation are provided. Operate a dehumidifier in the basement if needed to keep relative humidity levels between 30–50%.

Section 24.2

Carbon Monoxide

"An Introduction to Indoor Air Quality: Carbon Monoxide (CO)," Environmental Protection Agency (www.epa.gov), January 28, 2009.

Carbon monoxide is an odorless, colorless, and toxic gas. Because it is impossible to see, taste, or smell the toxic fumes, CO can kill you before you are aware it is in your home. At lower levels of exposure, CO causes mild effects that are often mistaken for the flu. These symptoms include headaches, dizziness, disorientation, nausea, and fatigue. The effects of CO exposure can vary greatly from person to person depending on age, overall health, and the concentration and length of exposure.

Sources of Carbon Monoxide

Sources of carbon monoxide are the following: unvented kerosene and gas space heaters; leaking chimneys and furnaces; backdrafting from furnaces, gas water heaters, wood stoves, and fireplaces; gas stoves; generators and other gasoline-powered equipment; automobile exhaust from attached garages; and tobacco smoke. Incomplete oxidation during combustion in gas ranges and unvented gas or kerosene heaters may cause high concentrations of CO in indoor air. Worn or poorly adjusted and maintained combustion devices (e.g., boilers, furnaces) can be significant sources, or if the flue is improperly sized, blocked, disconnected, or is leaking. Auto, truck, or bus exhaust from attached garages, nearby roads, or parking areas can also be a source.

Health Effects Associated with Carbon Monoxide

At low concentrations, CO causes fatigue in healthy people and chest pain in people with heart disease. At higher concentrations, it causes impaired vision and coordination, headaches, dizziness, confusion, and nausea. CO can cause flu-like symptoms that clear up after leaving home. Acute effects are due to the formation of carboxyhemoglobin in the blood, which inhibits oxygen intake. At moderate concentrations, angina, impaired vision, and reduced brain function may result. At higher concentrations, CO exposure can be fatal.

Levels in Homes

Average levels in homes without gas stoves vary from 0.5 to 5 parts per million (ppm). Levels near properly adjusted gas stoves are often 5 to 15 ppm and those near poorly adjusted stoves may be 30 ppm or higher.

Steps to Reduce Exposure to Carbon Monoxide

It is most important to be sure combustion equipment is maintained and properly adjusted. Vehicular use should be carefully managed adjacent to buildings and in vocational programs. Additional ventilation can be used as a temporary measure when high levels of CO are expected for short periods of time.

- Keep gas appliances properly adjusted.
- Consider purchasing a vented space heater when replacing an unvented one.
- Use proper fuel in kerosene space heaters.
- Install and use an exhaust fan vented to outdoors over gas stoves.
- Open flues when fireplaces are in use.
- Choose properly sized wood stoves that are certified to meet Environmental Protection Agency (EPA) emission standards. Make certain that doors on all wood stoves fit tightly.
- Have a trained professional inspect, clean, and tune-up central heating system (furnaces, flues, and chimneys) annually. Repair any leaks promptly.
- Do not idle the car inside garage.

Measurement Methods

Some relatively high-cost infrared radiation adsorption and electrochemical instruments do exist. Moderately priced real-time measuring devices are also available. A passive monitor is currently under development.

Standards or Guidelines

No standards for CO have been agreed upon for indoor air. The U.S. National Ambient Air Quality Standards for outdoor air are 9 ppm (40,000 micrograms per meter cubed) for eight hours, and 35 ppm for one hour.

Section 24.3

Combustion Pollutants

This section excerpted from "The Inside Story: A Guide to Indoor Air Quality," Consumer Product Safety Commission (www.cpsc.gov), April 2009.

In addition to environmental tobacco smoke, other sources of combustion products are unvented kerosene and gas space heaters, woodstoves, fireplaces, and gas stoves. The major pollutants released are carbon monoxide, nitrogen dioxide, and particles. Unvented kerosene heaters may also generate acid aerosols.

Combustion gases and particles also come from chimneys and flues that are improperly installed or maintained and cracked furnace heat exchangers. Pollutants from fireplaces and woodstoves with no dedicated outdoor air supply can be "back-drafted" from the chimney into the living space, particularly in weatherized homes.

Health Effects of Combustion Products

Carbon monoxide (CO) is a colorless, odorless gas that interferes with the delivery of oxygen throughout the body. At high concentrations it can cause unconsciousness and death. Lower concentrations can cause a range of symptoms from headaches, dizziness, weakness, nausea, confusion, and disorientation, to fatigue in healthy people and episodes of increased chest pain in people with chronic heart disease. The symptoms of carbon monoxide poisoning are sometimes confused with the flu or food poisoning. Fetuses, infants, elderly people, and people with anemia or with a history of heart or respiratory disease can be especially sensitive to carbon monoxide exposures.

Nitrogen dioxide (NO_2) is a reddish-brown, irritating odor gas that irritates the mucous membranes in the eye, nose, and throat and causes shortness of breath after exposure to high concentrations. There is evidence that high concentrations or continued exposure to low levels of nitrogen dioxide increases the risk of respiratory infection; there is also evidence from animal studies that repeated exposures to elevated nitrogen dioxide levels may lead, or contribute, to the development of lung disease such as emphysema. People at particular risk from exposure to nitrogen dioxide include children and individuals with asthma and other respiratory diseases.

Particles, released when fuels are incompletely burned, can lodge in the lungs and irritate or damage lung tissue. A number of pollutants, including radon and benzo(a)pyrene, both of which can cause cancer, attach to small particles that are inhaled and then carried deep into the lung.

Reducing Exposure to Combustion Products in Homes

Take special precautions when operating fuel-burning unvented space heaters. Consider potential effects of indoor air pollution if you use an unvented kerosene or gas space heater. Follow the manufacturer's directions, especially instructions on the proper fuel and keeping the heater properly adjusted. A persistent yellow-tipped flame is generally an indicator of maladjustment and increased pollutant emissions. While a space heater is in use, open a door from the room where the heater is located to the rest of the house and open a window slightly.

Install and use exhaust fans over gas cooking stoves and ranges and keep the burners properly adjusted. Using a stove hood with a fan vented to the outdoors greatly reduces exposure to pollutants during cooking. Improper adjustment, often indicated by a persistent yellow-tipped flame, causes increased pollutant emissions. Ask your gas company to adjust the burner so that the flame tip is blue. If you purchase a new gas stove or range, consider buying one with pilotless ignition because it does not have a pilot light that burns continuously. Never use a gas stove to heat your home. Always make certain the flue in your gas fireplace is open when the fireplace is in use.

Keep woodstove emissions to a minimum. Choose properly sized new stoves that are certified as meeting EPA emission standards. Make certain that doors in old woodstoves are tight fitting.

Use aged or cured (dried) wood only and follow the manufacturer's directions for starting, stoking, and putting out the fire in woodstoves. Chemicals are used to pressure-treat wood; such wood should never be burned indoors. (Because some old gaskets in woodstove doors contain asbestos, when replacing gaskets refer to the instructions in the booklet "Asbestos in Your Home," at www.epa.gov/asbestos/pubs/ashome.html, to avoid creating an asbestos problem. New gaskets are made of fiberglass.)

Have central air handling systems, including furnaces, flues, and chimneys, inspected annually and promptly repair cracks or damaged parts. Blocked, leaking, or damaged chimneys or flues release harmful combustion gases and particles and even fatal concentrations of carbon monoxide. Strictly follow all service and maintenance procedures recommended by the manufacturer, including those that tell you how frequently to change the filter. If manufacturer's instructions are not readily available, change filters once every month or two during periods of use. Proper maintenance is important even for new furnaces because they can also corrode and leak combustion gases, including carbon monoxide.

Read the booklet "What You Should Know about Combustion Appliances and Indoor Air Pollution" (www.epa.gov/iaq/pubs/combust.html) to learn more about combustion pollutants.

Section 24.4

Flame Retardants (Polybrominated Diphenyl Ethers, or PBDEs)

This section begins with three questions and answers excerpted from "Polybrominated diphenylethers (PBDEs)," Environmental Protection Agency (www.epa.gov), December 23, 2008; it continues with excerpts from "ToxFAQs™ for Polybrominated Diphenyl Ethers (PBDEs)," Centers for Disease Control and Prevention (www.cdc.gov), 2004.

What are PBDEs?

Polybrominated diphenyl ethers (PBDEs) are flame-retardant chemicals that are added to plastics and foam products to make them difficult to burn. There are different kinds of PBDEs; some have only a few bromine atoms attached, while some have as many as 10 bromine attached to the central molecule.

PBDEs exist as mixtures of similar chemicals called congeners. Because they are mixed into plastics and foams rather than bound to them, PBDEs can leave the products that contain them and enter the environment.

What are PBDEs used for?

These chemicals are major components of commercial formulations often used as flame retardants in furniture foam (pentaBDE), plastics for TV cabinets, consumer electronics, wire insulation, back coatings for draperies and upholstery (decaBDE), and plastics for personal computers and small appliances (octaBDE). The benefit of these chemicals is their ability to slow ignition and rate of fire growth, and as a result increase available escape time in the event of a fire.

What are concerns associated with PBDEs?

Although use of flame retardants saves lives and property, there have been unintended consequences. There is growing evidence that PBDEs persist in the environment and accumulate in living organisms, as well as toxicological testing that indicates these chemicals may cause liver toxicity, thyroid toxicity, and neurodevelopmental toxicity. Environmental monitoring programs in Europe, Asia, North America, and the Arctic have found traces of several PBDEs in human breast milk, fish, aquatic birds, and elsewhere in the environment. Particular congeners, tetra- to hexabrominated diphenyl ethers, are the forms most frequently detected in wildlife and humans. The mechanisms or pathways through which PBDEs get into the environment and humans are not known yet, but could include releases from manufacturing or processing of the chemicals into products like plastics or textiles, aging and wear of the end consumer products, and direct exposure during use (e.g., from furniture).

What happens to PBDEs when they enter the environment?

- PBDEs enter air, water, and soil during their manufacture and use in consumer products.
- In air, PBDEs can be present as particles, but eventually settle to soil or water.
- Sunlight can degrade some PBDEs.
- PBDEs do not dissolve easily in water, but stick to particles and settle to the bottom of rivers or lakes.
- Some PBDEs can accumulate in fish but usually at low concentrations.

How might I be exposed to PBDEs?

- The concentrations of PBDEs in human blood, breast milk, and body fat indicate that most people are exposed to low levels of PBDEs.
- You may be exposed to PBDEs from eating foods or breathing air contaminated with PBDEs.
- Workers involved in the manufacture of PBDEs or products that contain PBDEs may be exposed to higher levels than usual.
- Occupational exposure can also occur in people who work in enclosed spaces where PBDE-containing products are repaired or recycled.

How can PBDEs affect my health?

There is no definite information on health effects of PBDEs in people. Rats and mice that ate food with moderate amounts of PBDEs for a few days had effects on the thyroid gland. Those that ate smaller amounts for weeks or months had effects on the thyroid and the liver. Large differences in effects are seen between highly brominated and less brominated PBDEs in animal studies.

Preliminary evidence suggests that high concentrations of PBDEs may cause neurobehavioral alterations and affect the immune system in animals.

How likely are PBDEs to cause cancer?

We do not know whether PBDEs can cause cancer in humans. Rats and mice that ate food with decabromodiphenyl ether (one type of PBDE) throughout their lives developed liver tumors. Based on this evidence, the EPA has classified decabromodiphenyl ether as a possible human carcinogen. PBDEs with fewer bromine atoms than decabromodiphenyl ether are listed by the EPA as not classifiable as to human carcinogenicity due to the lack of human and animal cancer studies.

How can PBDEs affect children?

Children are exposed to PBDEs in generally the same way as adults, mainly by eating contaminated food. Because PBDEs dissolve readily in fat, they can accumulate in breast milk and may be transferred to babies and young children.

Exposure to PBDEs in the womb and through nursing has caused thyroid effects and neurobehavioral alterations in newborn animals, but not birth defects. It is not known if PBDEs can cause birth defect in children.

How can families reduce the risk of exposure to PBDEs?

- Children living near hazardous waste sites should be discouraged from playing in the dirt near these sites. Children should also be discouraged from eating dirt and should wash their hands frequently.
- People who are exposed to PBDEs at work should shower and change clothes before going home each day. Work clothes should be stored and laundered separately from the rest of your family's clothes.

Is there a medical test to show whether I've been exposed to PBDEs?

There are tests that can detect PBDEs in blood, body fat, and breast milk. These tests can tell whether you have been exposed to high levels of the chemicals, but cannot tell the exact amount or type of PBDE you were exposed to, or whether harmful effects will occur. Blood tests are the easiest and safest for detecting recent exposures to large amounts of PBDEs. These tests are not routinely available at the doctor's office, but samples can be sent to laboratories that have the appropriate equipment.

Has the federal government made recommendations to protect human health?

The EPA requires that companies that transport, store, or dispose p-bromodiphenyl ether (a particular PBDE compound) follow the rules and regulations of the federal hazardous waste management program. The EPA requires that industry tell the National Response Center each time 100 pounds or more of p-bromodiphenyl ether are released to the environment.

Section 24.5

Formaldehyde

This section excerpted from "The Inside Story: A Guide to Indoor Air Quality," Consumer Product Safety Commission (www.cpsc.gov), April 2009.

Formaldehyde is an important chemical used widely by industry to manufacture building materials and numerous household products. It is also a by-product of combustion and certain other natural processes. Thus, it may be present in substantial concentrations both indoors and outdoors.

Sources of formaldehyde in the home include building materials, smoking, household products, and the use of unvented, fuel-burning appliances, like gas stoves or kerosene space heaters. Formaldehyde, by itself or in combination with other chemicals, serves a number of purposes in manufactured products. For example, it is used to add permanent-press qualities to clothing and draperies, as a component of glues and adhesives, and as a preservative in some paints and coating products.

In homes, the most significant sources of formaldehyde are likely to be pressed wood products made using adhesives that contain urea-formaldehyde (UF) resins. Pressed wood products made for indoor use include: particleboard (used as subflooring and shelving and in cabinetry and furniture); hardwood plywood paneling (used for decorative wall covering and used in cabinets and furniture); and medium density fiberboard (used for drawer fronts, cabinets, and furniture tops). Medium density fiberboard contains a higher resin-to-wood ratio than any other UF pressed wood product and is generally recognized as being the highest formaldehyde-emitting pressed wood product.

Other pressed wood products, such as softwood plywood and flake or oriented strandboard, are produced for exterior construction use and contain the dark, or red/black-colored, phenol-formaldehyde (PF) resin. Although formaldehyde is present in both types of resins, pressed woods that contain PF resin generally emit formaldehyde at considerably lower rates than those containing UF resin.

Since 1985, the Department of Housing and Urban Development (HUD) has permitted only the use of plywood and particleboard that conform to specified formaldehyde emission limits in the construction of prefabricated and mobile homes. In the past, some of these homes had elevated levels of formaldehyde because of the large amount of high-emitting pressed wood products used in their construction and because of their relatively small interior space.

The rate at which products like pressed wood or textiles release formaldehyde can change. Formaldehyde emissions will generally decrease as products age. When the products are new, high indoor temperatures or humidity can cause increased release of formaldehyde from these products.

During the 1970s, many homeowners had urea-formaldehyde foam insulation (UFFI) installed in the wall cavities of their homes as an energy conservation measure. However, many of these homes were found to have relatively high indoor concentrations of formaldehyde soon after the UFFI installation. Few homes are now being insulated with this product. Studies show that formaldehyde emissions from UFFI decline with time; therefore, homes in which UFFI was installed many years ago are unlikely to have high levels of formaldehyde now.

Health Effects of Formaldehyde

Formaldehyde, a colorless, pungent-smelling gas, can cause watery eyes, burning sensations in the eyes and throat, nausea, and difficulty in breathing in some humans exposed at elevated levels (above 0.1 parts per million). High concentrations may trigger attacks in people with asthma. There is evidence that some people can develop a sensitivity to formaldehyde. It has also been shown to cause cancer in animals and may cause cancer in humans.

Reducing Exposure to Formaldehyde in Homes

Ask about the formaldehyde content of pressed wood products, including building materials, cabinetry, and furniture, before you purchase them. If you experience adverse reactions to formaldehyde, you may want to avoid the use of pressed wood products and other formaldehyde-emitting goods. Even if you do not experience such reactions, you may wish to reduce your exposure as much as possible by purchasing exterior-grade products, which emit less formaldehyde. For further information on formaldehyde and consumer products, call the EPA Toxic Substance Control Act (TSCA) assistance line (202-554-1404).

Some studies suggest that coating pressed wood products with polyurethane may reduce formaldehyde emissions for some period of time. To be effective, any such coating must cover all surfaces and edges and remain intact. Increase the ventilation and carefully follow the manufacturer instructions while applying these coatings. (If you are sensitive to formaldehyde, check the label contents before purchasing coating products to avoid buying products that contain formaldehyde, as they will emit the chemical for a short time after application.) Maintain moderate temperature and humidity levels and provide adequate ventilation. The rate at which formaldehyde is released is accelerated by heat and may also depend somewhat on the humidity level. Therefore, the use of dehumidifiers and air conditioning to control humidity and to maintain a moderate temperature can help reduce formaldehyde emissions. (Drain and clean dehumidifier collection trays frequently so that they do not become a breeding ground for microorganisms.) Increasing the rate of ventilation in your home will also help in reducing formaldehyde levels.

Section 24.6

Household Chemicals

This section excerpted from "The Inside Story: A Guide to Indoor Air Quality," Consumer Product Safety Commission (www.cpsc.gov), April 2009.

Organic chemicals are widely used as ingredients in household products. Paints, varnishes, and wax all contain organic solvents, as do many cleaning, disinfecting, cosmetic, degreasing, and hobby products. Fuels are made up of organic chemicals. All of these products can release organic compounds while you are using them, and, to some degree, when they are stored.

EPA's Total Exposure Assessment Methodology (TEAM) studies found levels of about a dozen common organic pollutants to be two to five times higher inside homes than outside, regardless of whether the homes were located in rural or highly industrial areas. Additional TEAM studies indicate that while people are using products containing organic chemicals, they can expose themselves and others to very high pollutant levels, and elevated concentrations can persist in the air long after the activity is completed.

Health Effects of Household Chemicals

The ability of organic chemicals to cause health effects varies greatly, from those that are highly toxic, to those with no known health effect. As with other pollutants, the extent and nature of the health effect will depend on many factors including level of exposure and length of time exposed. Eye and respiratory tract irritation, headaches, dizziness, visual disorders, and memory impairment are among the immediate symptoms that some people have experienced soon after exposure to some organics. At present, not much is known about what health effects occur from the levels of organics usually found in homes. Many organic compounds are known to cause cancer in animals; some are suspected of causing, or are known to cause, cancer in humans.

Reducing Exposure to Household Chemicals

Follow label instructions carefully. Potentially hazardous products often have warnings aimed at reducing exposure of the user. For example, if a label says to use the product in a well-ventilated area, go outdoors or in areas equipped with an exhaust fan to use it. Otherwise, open up windows to provide the maximum amount of outdoor air possible.

Throw away partially full containers of old or unneeded chemicals safely. Because gases can leak even from closed containers, this single step could help lower concentrations of organic chemicals in your home. (Be sure that materials you decide to keep are stored not only in a well-ventilated area but are also safely out of reach of children.) Do not simply toss these unwanted products in the garbage can. Find out if your local government or any organization in your community sponsors special days for the collection of toxic household wastes. If such days are available, use them to dispose of the unwanted containers safely. If no such collection days are available, think about organizing one.

Buy limited quantities. If you use products only occasionally or seasonally, such as paints, paint strippers, and kerosene for space heaters or gasoline for lawn mowers, buy only as much as you will use right away.

Keep exposure to emissions from products containing methylene chloride to a minimum. Consumer products that contain methylene chloride include paint strippers, adhesive removers, and aerosol spray paints. Methylene chloride is known to cause cancer in animals. Also, methylene chloride is converted to carbon monoxide in the body and can cause symptoms associated with exposure to carbon monoxide. Carefully read the labels containing health hazard information and cautions on the proper use of these products. Use products that contain methylene chloride outdoors when possible; use indoors only if the area is well ventilated.

Keep exposure to benzene to a minimum. Benzene is a known human carcinogen. The main indoor sources of this chemical are environmental tobacco smoke, stored fuels and paint supplies, and automobile emissions in attached garages. Actions that will reduce benzene exposure include eliminating smoking within the home, providing for maximum ventilation during painting, and discarding paint supplies and special fuels that will not be used immediately.

Keep exposure to perchloroethylene emissions from newly dry-cleaned materials to a minimum. Perchloroethylene is the chemical most widely used in dry cleaning. In laboratory studies, it has been shown to cause cancer in animals. Recent studies indicate that people breathe low levels of this chemical both in homes where dry-cleaned goods are stored and as they wear dry-cleaned clothing. Dry cleaners recapture the perchloroethylene during the dry-cleaning process so they can save money by reusing it, and they remove more of the chemical during the pressing and finishing processes. Some dry cleaners, however, do not remove as much perchloroethylene as possible all of the time. Taking steps to minimize your exposure to this chemical is prudent. If dry-cleaned goods have a strong chemical odor when you pick them up, do not accept them until they have been properly dried. If goods with a chemical odor are returned to you on subsequent visits, try a different dry cleaner.

Section 24.7

Pesticides

This section excerpted from "The Inside Story: A Guide to Indoor Air Quality," Consumer Product Safety Commission (www.cpsc.gov), April 2009.

According to a recent survey, 75% of U.S. households used at least one pesticide product indoors during the past year. Products used most often are insecticides and disinfectants. Another study suggests that 80% of most people's exposure to pesticides occurs indoors and that measurable levels of up to a dozen pesticides have been found in the air inside homes. The amount of pesticides found in homes appears to be greater than can be explained by recent pesticide use in those households; other possible sources include contaminated soil or dust that floats or is tracked in from outside, stored pesticide containers, and household surfaces that collect and then release the pesticides. Pesticides used in and around the home include products to control insects (insecticides), termites (termiticides), rodents (rodenticides), fungi (fungicides), and microbes (disinfectants). They are sold as sprays, liquids, sticks, powders, crystals, balls, and foggers.

In 1990, the American Association of Poison Control Centers reported that some 79,000 children were involved in common household pesticide poisonings or exposures. In households with children under five years old, almost one-half stored at least one pesticide product within reach of children.

EPA registers pesticides for use and requires manufacturers to put information on the label about when and how to use the pesticide. It is important to remember that the "-cide" in pesticides means "to kill." These products can be dangerous if not used properly.

In addition to the active ingredient, pesticides are also made up of ingredients that are used to carry the active agent. These carrier agents are called "inerts" in pesticides because they are not toxic to the targeted pest; nevertheless, some inerts are capable of causing health problems.

Health Effects from Pesticides

Both the active and inert ingredients in pesticides can be organic compounds; therefore, both could add to the levels of airborne organics inside homes. Both types of ingredients can cause the effects discussed in this chapter under "Household Chemicals," however, as with other household products, there is insufficient understanding at present about what pesticide concentrations are necessary to produce these effects.

Exposure to high levels of cyclodiene pesticides, commonly associated with misapplication, has produced various symptoms, including headaches, dizziness, muscle twitching, weakness, tingling sensations, and nausea. In addition, EPA is concerned that cyclodienes might cause long-term damage to the liver and the central nervous system, as well as an increased risk of cancer.

There is no further sale or commercial use permitted for the following cyclodiene or related pesticides: chlordane, aldrin, dieldrin, and heptachlor. The only exception is the use of heptachlor by utility companies to control fire ants in underground cable boxes.

Reducing Exposure to Pesticides in Homes

Read the label and follow the directions. It is illegal to use any pesticide in any manner inconsistent with the directions on its label. Unless you have had special training and are certified, never use a pesticide that is restricted to use by state-certified pest control operators. Such pesticides are simply too dangerous for application by a noncertified person. Use only the pesticides approved for use by the general public and then only in recommended amounts; increasing the amount does not offer more protection against pests and can be harmful to you and your plants and pets.

Ventilate the area well after pesticide use. Mix or dilute pesticides outdoors or in a well-ventilated area and only in the amounts that will be immediately needed. If possible, take plants and pets outside when applying pesticides to them.

Use nonchemical methods of pest control when possible. Since pesticides can be found far from the site of their original application, it is prudent to reduce the use of chemical pesticides outdoors as well as indoors. Depending on the site and pest to be controlled, one or more of the following steps can be effective: use of biological pesticides, such as *Bacillus thuringiensis*, for the control of gypsy moths;

selection of disease-resistant plants; and frequent washing of indoor plants and pets. Termite damage can be reduced or prevented by making certain that wooden building materials do not come into direct contact with the soil and by storing firewood away from the home. By appropriately fertilizing, watering, and aerating lawns, the need for chemical pesticide treatments of lawns can be dramatically reduced.

If you decide to use a pest control company, choose one carefully. Ask for an inspection of your home and get a written control program for evaluation before you sign a contract. The control program should list specific names of pests to be controlled and chemicals to be used; it should also reflect any of your safety concerns. Insist on a proven record of competence and customer satisfaction.

Dispose of unwanted pesticides safely. If you have unused or partially used pesticide containers you want to get rid of, dispose of them according to the directions on the label or on special household hazardous waste collection days. If there are no such collection days in your community, work with others to organize them.

Keep exposure to moth repellents to a minimum. One pesticide often found in the home is paradichlorobenzene, a commonly used active ingredient in moth repellents. This chemical is known to cause cancer in animals, but substantial scientific uncertainty exists over the effects, if any, of long-term human exposure to paradichlorobenzene. EPA requires that products containing paradichlorobenzene bear warnings such as "avoid breathing vapors" to warn users of potential short-term toxic effects. Where possible, paradichlorobenzene, and items to be protected against moths, should be placed in trunks or other containers that can be stored in areas that are separately ventilated from the home, such as attics and detached garages. Paradichlorobenzene is also the key active ingredient in many air fresheners (in fact, some labels for moth repellents recommend that these same products be used as air fresheners or deodorants). Proper ventilation and basic household cleanliness will go a long way toward preventing unpleasant odors.

National Pesticide Information Center (NPIC)

EPA sponsors the NPIC (800-858-PEST/800-858-7378, npic.orst.edu/) to answer your questions about pesticides and to provide selected EPA publications on pesticides.

Section 24.8

Radon

This section excerpted from "The Inside Story: A Guide to Indoor Air Quality," Consumer Product Safety Commission (www.cpsc.gov), April 2009.

The most common source of indoor radon is uranium in the soil or rock on which homes are built. As uranium naturally breaks down, it releases radon gas which is a colorless, odorless, radioactive gas. Radon gas enters homes through dirt floors, cracks in concrete walls and floors, floor drains, and sumps. When radon becomes trapped in buildings and concentrations build up indoors, exposure to radon becomes a concern.

Any home may have a radon problem. This means new and old homes, well-sealed and drafty homes, and homes with or without basements.

Sometimes radon enters the home through well water. In a small number of homes, the building materials can give off radon, too. However, building materials rarely cause radon problems by themselves.

Health Effects of Radon

The predominant health effect associated with exposure to elevated levels of radon is lung cancer. Research suggests that swallowing water with high radon levels may pose risks, too, although these are believed to be much lower than those from breathing air containing radon. Major health organizations (like the Centers for Disease Control and Prevention, the American Lung Association, and the American Medical Association) agree with estimates that radon causes thousands of preventable lung cancer deaths each year. EPA estimates that radon causes about 14,000 deaths per year in the United States—however, this number could range from 7,000 to 30,000 deaths per year. If you smoke and your home has high radon levels, your risk of lung cancer is especially high.

Reducing Exposure to Radon in Homes

Measure levels of radon in your home. You can't see radon, but it's not hard to find out if you have a radon problem in your home.

Testing is easy and should only take a little of your time. There are many kinds of inexpensive, do-it-yourself radon test kits you can get through the mail and in hardware stores and other retail outlets. EPA recommends that consumers use test kits that are state-certified or have met the requirements of some national radon proficiency program. If you prefer, or if you are buying or selling a home, you can hire a trained contractor to do the testing for you (see www.epa.gov/radon/radontest.html). You should call your state radon office to obtain a list of qualified contractors in your area. You can also contact either the National Environmental Health Association's (NEHA) National Radon Proficiency Program (NRPP) at www.neha-nrpp.org or the National Radon Safety Board (NRSB) at www.nrsb.org for a list of proficient radon measurement and/or mitigation contractors.

Refer to the EPA guidelines on how to test and interpret your test results. You can learn more about radon through EPA's publications, including "A Citizen's Guide to Radon: The Guide to Protecting Yourself and Your Family from Radon" (www.epa.gov/radon/pubs/citguide.html) and "Home Buyer's and Seller's Guide to Radon" (www.epa.gov/radon/pubs/hmbyguid.html).

Learn about radon reduction methods. Ways to reduce radon in your home are discussed in EPA's "Consumer's Guide to Radon Reduction." There are simple solutions to radon problems in homes. Thousands of homeowners have already fixed radon problems. Lowering high radon levels requires technical knowledge and special skills. You should use a contractor who is trained to fix radon problems.

A trained radon-reduction contractor can study the problem in your home and help you pick the correct treatment method. Check with your state radon office for names of qualified or state-certified radon-reduction contractors in your area.

Stop smoking and discourage smoking in your home. Scientific evidence indicates that smoking combined with radon is an especially serious health risk. Stop smoking and lower your radon level to reduce lung cancer risk.

Treat radon-contaminated well water. While radon in water is not a problem in homes served by most public water supplies, it has been found in well water. If you've tested the air in your home and found a radon problem, and you have a well, contact a lab certified to measure radiation in water to have your water tested. Radon problems in water can be readily fixed. Call your state radon office or the EPA Drinking Water Hotline (800-426-4791) for more information.

Section 24.9

Secondhand Smoke

This section excerpted from "The Inside Story: A Guide to Indoor Air Quality," Consumer Product Safety Commission (www.cpsc.gov), April 2009.

Environmental tobacco smoke (ETS) is the mixture of smoke that comes from the burning end of a cigarette, pipe, or cigar, and smoke exhaled by the smoker. It is a complex mixture of over 4,000 compounds, more than 40 of which are known to cause cancer in humans or animals and many of which are strong irritants. ETS is often referred to as "secondhand smoke" and exposure to ETS is often called "passive smoking."

Health Effects of Environmental Tobacco Smoke

In 1992, EPA completed a major assessment of the respiratory health risks of ETS ("Respiratory Health Effects of Passive Smoking: Lung Cancer and Other Disorders" EPA/600/6-90/006F). The report concludes that exposure to ETS is responsible for approximately 3,000 lung cancer deaths each year in nonsmoking adults and impairs the respiratory health of hundreds of thousands of children.

Infants and young children whose parents smoke in their presence are at increased risk of lower respiratory tract infections (pneumonia and bronchitis) and are more likely to have symptoms of respiratory irritation like cough, excess phlegm, and wheeze. EPA estimates that passive smoking annually causes between 150,000 and 300,000 lower respiratory tract infections in infants and children under 18 months of age, resulting in between 7,500 and 15,000 hospitalizations each year. These children may also have a buildup of fluid in the middle ear, which can lead to ear infections. Older children who have been exposed to secondhand smoke may have slightly reduced lung function.

Asthmatic children are especially at risk. EPA estimates that exposure to secondhand smoke increases the number of episodes and severity of symptoms in hundreds of thousands of asthmatic children, and may cause thousands of non-asthmatic children to develop the disease each year. EPA estimates that between 200,000 and 1,000,000 asthmatic children have their condition made worse by exposure to secondhand smoke each year. Exposure to secondhand smoke causes eye, nose, and throat irritation. It may affect the cardiovascular system and some studies have linked exposure to secondhand smoke with the onset of chest pain.

Reducing Exposure to Environmental Tobacco Smoke

Don't smoke at home or permit others to do so. Ask smokers to smoke outdoors. The 1986 Surgeon General's report concluded that physical separation of smokers and nonsmokers in a common air space, such as different rooms within the same house, may reduce—but will not eliminate—nonsmokers' exposure to environmental tobacco smoke.

If smoking indoors cannot be avoided, increase ventilation in the area where smoking takes place. Open windows or use exhaust fans. Ventilation, a common method of reducing exposure to indoor air pollutants, also will reduce but not eliminate exposure to environmental tobacco smoke. Because smoking produces such large amounts of pollutants, natural or mechanical ventilation techniques do not remove them from the air in your home as quickly as they build up. In addition, the large increases in ventilation it takes to significantly reduce exposure to environmental tobacco smoke can also increase energy costs substantially. Consequently, the most effective way to reduce exposure to environmental tobacco smoke in the home is to eliminate smoking there.

Do not smoke if children are present, particularly infants and toddlers. Children are particularly susceptible to the effects of passive smoking. Do not allow babysitters or others who work in your home to smoke indoors. Discourage others from smoking around children. Find out about the smoking policies of the day care center providers, schools, and other care givers for your children. The policy should protect children from exposure to ETS.

Chapter 25

Mold

About Mold and Moisture

Molds are living organisms that grow in damp places in your home. They stain or discolor surfaces and smell musty. There are hundreds of thousands of different types of mold.

Mold can grow almost anywhere: on walls, ceilings, carpets, or furniture. Humidity or wetness, caused by water leaks; spills from bathtubs or showers; or condensation can cause mold to grow in your home.

Mold spores are tiny particles that float through the air. These can sometimes cause health problems. Mold does not affect everyone, and different people are affected differently when mold is breathed or inhaled.

People with allergies to mold may have the following symptoms:

- Watery eyes
- Runny or stuffed noses
- Itching
- Headaches
- Difficulty breathing

Mold can also trigger asthma attacks. Some molds produce toxins (poisons) that may be hazardous if people are exposed to large amounts of these molds. Mold spores and related mycotoxins can also pose a serious health threat to individuals who have compromised immune systems.

This section includes "About Mold and Moisture," U.S. Department of Housing and Urban Development (www.hud.gov), October 20, 2007, and excerpts from "Facts about *Stachybotrys Chartarum* and Other Molds," Centers for Disease Control and Prevention (www.cdc.gov), November 2004.

What can you do?

Take the following steps to prevent and get rid of mold:

- Keep your house clean and dry.
- Fix water problems such as roof leaks, wet basements, and leaking pipes or faucets.
- Make sure your home is well ventilated and always use ventilation fans in bathrooms and kitchens.
- If possible, keep humidity in your house below 50% by using an air conditioner or dehumidifier.
- Avoid using carpeting in areas of the home that may become wet, such as kitchens, bathrooms, and basements.
- Dry floor mats regularly.

To find mold that might be growing in your home, do the following:

- Search for moisture in areas that have a damp or moldy smell, especially in basements, kitchens, and bathrooms.
- Look for water stains or colored, fuzzy growth on and around ceilings, walls, floors, windowsills, and pipes.
- If you smell a musty odor, search behind and underneath materials such as carpeting, furniture, or stored items.
- Inspect kitchens, bathrooms, and basements for standing water, water stains, and patches of out-of-place color.

To control moisture problems and mold take the following steps:

- Fix any water problems immediately and clean or remove wet materials, furnishings, or mold.
- Clean up spills or floods within one day. If practical, take furniture that has been wet outside to dry and clean. Direct sunlight prevents mold growth.
- Dry all surfaces and fix the problem or leak to prevent further damage.
- Install a dehumidifier when a moisture problem is evident or when the humidity is high.

Facts about Stachybotrys Chartarum *and Other Molds*

I heard about "toxic molds" that grow in homes and other buildings. Should I be concerned about a serious health risk to me and my family?

The term "toxic mold" is not accurate. While certain molds are toxigenic, meaning they can produce toxins (specifically mycotoxins), the molds themselves are not toxic, or poisonous. Hazards presented by molds that may produce mycotoxins should be considered the same as other common molds which can grow in your house. There is always a little mold everywhere—in the air and on many surfaces. There are very few reports that toxigenic molds found inside homes can cause unique or rare health conditions such as pulmonary hemorrhage or memory loss. These case reports are rare, and a causal link between the presence of the toxigenic mold and these conditions has not been proven. A commonsense approach should be used for any mold contamination existing inside buildings and homes. The common health concerns from molds include hay fever–like allergic symptoms. Certain individuals with chronic respiratory disease (chronic obstructive pulmonary disorder [COPD] or asthma) may experience difficulty breathing. Individuals with immune suppression may be at increased risk for infection from molds. If you or your family members have these conditions, a qualified medical clinician should be consulted for diagnosis and treatment. For the most part, one should take routine measures to prevent mold growth in the home.

How common is mold, including Stachybotrys chartarum *(also known by its synonym* Stachybotrys atra*) in buildings?*

Molds are very common in buildings and homes and will grow anywhere indoors where there is moisture. The most common indoor molds are *Cladosporium, Penicillium, Aspergillus,* and *Alternaria*. We do not have precise information about how often *Stachybotrys chartarum* is found in buildings and homes. While it is less common than other mold species, it is not rare.

How do molds get in the indoor environment and how do they grow?

Mold spores occur in the indoor and outdoor environments. Mold spores may enter your house from the outside through open doorways;

windows; and heating, ventilation, and air conditioning systems with outdoor air intakes. Spores in the air outside also attach themselves to people and animals, making clothing, shoes, bags, and pets convenient vehicles for carrying mold indoors.

When mold spores drop on places where there is excessive moisture, such as where leakage may have occurred in roofs, pipes, walls, plant pots, or where there has been flooding, they will grow. Many building materials provide suitable nutrients that encourage mold to grow. Wet cellulose materials, including paper and paper products, cardboard, ceiling tiles, wood, and wood products, are particularly conducive for the growth of some molds. Other materials such as dust, paints, wallpaper, insulation materials, drywall, carpet, fabric, and upholstery commonly support mold growth.

What is Stachybotrys chartarum (Stachybotrys atra)*?*

Stachybotrys chartarum is a greenish-black mold. It can grow on material with a high cellulose and low nitrogen content, such as fiberboard, gypsum board, paper, dust, and lint. Growth occurs when there is moisture from water damage, excessive humidity, water leaks, condensation, water infiltration, or flooding. Constant moisture is required for its growth. It is not necessary, however, to determine what type of mold you may have. All molds should be treated the same with respect to potential health risks and removal.

Who are the people who are most at risk for health problems associated with exposure to mold?

People with allergies may be more sensitive to molds. People with immune suppression or underlying lung disease are more susceptible to fungal infections.

How do you know if you have a mold problem?

Large mold infestations can usually be seen or smelled.

Does Stachybotrys chartarum (Stachybotrys atra) *cause acute idiopathic pulmonary hemorrhage among infants?*

To date, a possible association between acute idiopathic pulmonary hemorrhage among infants and *Stachybotrys chartarum* has not been proved. Further studies are needed to determine what causes acute idiopathic hemorrhage.

What are the potential health effects of mold in buildings and homes?

Mold exposure does not always present a health problem indoors. However some people are sensitive to molds. These people may experience symptoms such as nasal stuffiness, eye irritation, wheezing, or skin irritation when exposed to molds. Some people may have more severe reactions to molds. Severe reactions may occur among workers exposed to large amounts of molds in occupational settings, such as farmers working around moldy hay. Severe reactions may include fever and shortness of breath. Immunocompromised persons and persons with chronic lung diseases like COPD are at increased risk for opportunistic infections and may develop fungal infections in their lungs.

How do you get the molds out of buildings, including homes, schools, and places of employment?

In most cases mold can be removed from hard surfaces by a thorough cleaning with commercial products, soap and water, or a bleach solution of no more than one cup of bleach in one gallon of water. Absorbent or porous materials like ceiling tiles, drywall, and carpet may have to be thrown away if they become moldy. If you have an extensive amount of mold and you do not think you can manage the cleanup on your own, you may want to contact a professional who has experience in cleaning mold in buildings and homes. It is important to properly clean and dry the area as you can still have an allergic reaction to parts of the dead mold and mold contamination may recur if there is still a source of moisture.

Take the following precautions if you choose to use bleach to clean up mold:

- Never mix bleach with ammonia or other household cleaners. Mixing bleach with ammonia or other cleaning products will produce dangerous, toxic fumes.
- Open windows and doors to provide fresh air.
- Wear nonporous gloves and protective eye wear.
- If the area to be cleaned is more than 10 square feet, consult the U.S. Environmental Protection Agency (EPA) guide titled "Mold Remediation in Schools and Commercial Buildings." Although focused on schools and commercial buildings, this document also applies to other building types. You can get it free by calling the

EPA Indoor Air Quality Information Clearinghouse at 800-438-4318 or by going to the EPA website at www.epa.gov/mold/mold_remediation.html.

- Always follow the manufacturer's instructions when using bleach or any other cleaning product.

What should people to do if they determine they have **Stachybotrys chartarum (Stachybotrys atra)** *in their buildings or homes?*

Mold growing in homes and buildings, whether it is *Stachybotrys chartarum* or other molds, indicates that there is a problem with water or moisture. This is the first problem that needs to be addressed. Mold growth can be removed from hard surfaces with commercial products, soap and water, or a bleach solution of no more than one cup of bleach in one gallon of water. Mold in or under carpets typically requires that the carpets be removed. Once mold starts to grow in insulation or wallboard, the only way to deal with the problem is by removal and replacement. We do not believe that one needs to take any different precautions with *Stachybotrys chartarum* than with other molds. In areas where flooding has occurred, prompt drying out of materials and cleaning of walls and other flood-damaged items with commercial products, soap and water, or a bleach solution of no more than one cup of bleach in one gallon of water is necessary to prevent mold growth. Never mix bleach with ammonia or other household cleaners. If a home has been flooded, it also may be contaminated with sewage. Moldy items should be removed from living areas.

How do you keep mold out of buildings and homes?

As part of routine building maintenance, buildings should be inspected for evidence of water damage and visible mold. The conditions causing mold (such as water leaks, condensation, infiltration, or flooding) should be corrected to prevent mold from growing.

- Keep humidity level in house between 40% and 60%.
- Use an air conditioner or a dehumidifier during humid months.
- Be sure the home has adequate ventilation, including exhaust fans in kitchen and bathrooms.
- Use mold inhibitors, which can be added to paints.

- Clean bathroom with mold-killing products.
- Do not carpet bathrooms.
- Remove and replace flooded carpets.

I found mold growing in my home; how do I test the mold?

Generally, it is not necessary to identify the species of mold growing in a residence, and CDC does not recommend routine sampling for molds. Current evidence indicates that allergies are the type of diseases most often associated with molds. Since the reaction of individuals can vary greatly either because of the person's susceptibility or type and amount of mold present, sampling and culturing are not reliable in determining your health risk. If you are susceptible to mold and mold is seen or smelled, there is a potential health risk; therefore, no matter what type of mold is present, you should arrange for its removal. Furthermore, reliable sampling for mold can be expensive, and standards for judging what is and what is not an acceptable or tolerable quantity of mold have not been established.

Chapter 26

Asbestos

What Is Asbestos?

Asbestos is a mineral fiber. It can be positively identified only with a special type of microscope. There are several types of asbestos fibers. In the past, asbestos was added to a variety of products to strengthen them and to provide heat insulation and fire resistance.

How Can Asbestos Affect My Health?

From studies of people who were exposed to asbestos in factories and shipyards, we know that breathing high levels of asbestos fibers can lead to an increased risk of the following:

- Lung cancer
- Mesothelioma, a cancer of the lining of the chest and the abdominal cavity
- Asbestosis, in which the lungs become scarred with fibrous tissue

The risk of lung cancer and mesothelioma increases with the number of fibers inhaled. The risk of lung cancer from inhaling asbestos fibers is also greater if you smoke. People who get asbestosis have usually been exposed to high levels of asbestos for a long time. The

---

This section excerpted from "Asbestos in Your Home," Environmental Protection Agency (www.epa.gov), 2008.

symptoms of these diseases do not usually appear until about 20 to 30 years after the first exposure to asbestos.

Most people exposed to small amounts of asbestos, as we all are in our daily lives, do not develop these health problems. However, if disturbed, asbestos material may release asbestos fibers, which can be inhaled into the lungs. The fibers can remain there for a long time, increasing the risk of disease. Asbestos material that would crumble easily if handled, or that has been sawed, scraped, or sanded into a powder, is more likely to create a health hazard.

Where Can I Find Asbestos and When Can It Be a Problem?

Most products made today do not contain asbestos. Those few products made which still contain asbestos that could be inhaled are required to be labeled as such. However, until the 1970s, many types of building products and insulation materials used in homes contained asbestos. Common products that might have contained asbestos in the past, and conditions which may release fibers, include the following:

- Steam pipes, boilers, and furnace ducts insulated with an asbestos blanket or asbestos paper tape. These materials may release asbestos fibers if damaged, repaired, or removed improperly.
- Resilient floor tiles (vinyl asbestos, asphalt, and rubber), the backing on vinyl sheet flooring, and adhesives used for installing floor tile. Sanding tiles can release fibers. So may scraping or sanding the backing of sheet flooring during removal.
- Cement sheet, millboard, and paper used as insulation around furnaces and wood-burning stoves. Repairing or removing appliances may release asbestos fibers. So may cutting, tearing, sanding, drilling, or sawing insulation.
- Door gaskets in furnaces, wood stoves, and coal stoves. Worn seals can release asbestos fibers during use.
- Soundproofing or decorative material sprayed on walls and ceilings. Loose, crumbly, or water-damaged material may release fibers. So will sanding, drilling, or scraping the material.
- Patching and joint compounds for walls and ceilings, and textured paints. Sanding, scraping, or drilling these surfaces may release asbestos.

- Asbestos cement roofing, shingles, and siding. These products are not likely to release asbestos fibers unless sawed, drilled, or cut.
- Artificial ashes and embers sold for use in gas-fired fireplaces. Also, other older household products such as fireproof gloves, stove-top pads, ironing board covers, and certain hairdryers.
- Automobile brake pads and linings, clutch facings, and gaskets.

What Should Be Done about Asbestos in the Home?

If you think asbestos may be in your home, don't panic. Usually the best thing is to leave asbestos material that is in good condition alone.

Generally, material in good condition will not release asbestos fibers. There is no danger unless fibers are released and inhaled into the lungs.

Check material regularly if you suspect it may contain asbestos. Don't touch it, but look for signs of wear or damage such as tears, abrasions, or water damage. Damaged material may release asbestos fibers. This is particularly true if you often disturb it by hitting, rubbing, or handling it, or if it is exposed to extreme vibration or air flow.

Sometimes, the best way to deal with slightly damaged material is to limit access to the area and not touch or disturb it. Discard damaged or worn asbestos gloves, stove-top pads, or ironing board covers. Check with local health, environmental, or other appropriate officials to find out proper handling and disposal procedures.

If asbestos material is more than slightly damaged, or if you are going to make changes in your home that might disturb it, repair or removal by a professional is needed. Before you have your house remodeled, find out whether asbestos materials are present.

How to Identify Materials That Contain Asbestos

You can't tell whether a material contains asbestos simply by looking at it, unless it is labeled. If in doubt, treat the material as if it contains asbestos or have it sampled and analyzed by a qualified professional. A professional should take samples for analysis, since a professional knows what to look for, and because there may be an increased health risk if fibers are released. In fact, if done incorrectly, sampling can be more hazardous than leaving the material alone. Taking samples yourself is not recommended. Material that is in good condition and will not be disturbed (by remodeling, for example) should be left alone. Only material that is damaged or will be disturbed should be sampled.

How to Manage an Asbestos Problem

If the asbestos material is in good shape and will not be disturbed, do nothing. If it is a problem, there are two types of corrections: repair and removal.

Repair usually involves either sealing or covering asbestos material.

- Sealing (encapsulation) involves treating the material with a sealant that either binds the asbestos fibers together or coats the material so fibers are not released. Pipe, furnace, and boiler insulation can sometimes be repaired this way. This should be done only by a professional trained to handle asbestos safely.

- Covering (enclosure) involves placing something over or around the material that contains asbestos to prevent release of fibers. Exposed insulated piping may be covered with a protective wrap or jacket.

With any type of repair, the asbestos remains in place. Repair is usually cheaper than removal, but it may make later removal of asbestos, if necessary, more difficult and costly. Repairs can either be major or minor.

Asbestos Dos and Don'ts for the Homeowner

- Do keep activities to a minimum in any areas having damaged material that may contain asbestos.

- Do take every precaution to avoid damaging asbestos material.

- Do have removal and major repair done by people trained and qualified in handling asbestos. It is highly recommended that sampling and minor repair also be done by asbestos professionals.

- Don't dust, sweep, or vacuum debris that may contain asbestos.

- Don't saw, sand, scrape, or drill holes in asbestos materials.

- Don't use abrasive pads or brushes on power strippers to strip wax from asbestos flooring. Never use a power stripper on a dry floor.

- Don't sand or try to level asbestos flooring or its backing. When asbestos flooring needs replacing, install new floor covering over it, if possible.

- Don't track material that could contain asbestos through the house. If you cannot avoid walking through the area, have it cleaned with a wet mop. If the material is from a damaged area, or if a large area must be cleaned, call an asbestos professional.

Major repairs must be done only by a professional trained in methods for safely handling asbestos.

Minor repairs should also be done by professionals since there is always a risk of exposure to fibers when asbestos is disturbed.

Doing minor repairs yourself is not recommended since improper handling of asbestos materials can create a hazard where none existed.

Removal is usually the most expensive method and, unless required by state or local regulations, should be the last option considered in most situations. This is because removal poses the greatest risk of fiber release. However, removal may be required when remodeling or making major changes to your home that will disturb asbestos material. Also, removal may be called for if asbestos material is damaged extensively and cannot be otherwise repaired. Removal is complex and must be done only by a contractor with special training. Improper removal may actually increase the health risks to you and your family.

Asbestos Professionals: Who Are They and What Can They Do?

Asbestos professionals are trained in handling asbestos material. The type of professional will depend on the type of product and what needs to be done to correct the problem. You may hire a general asbestos contractor or, in some cases, a professional trained to handle specific products containing asbestos.

Asbestos professionals can conduct home inspections, take samples of suspected material, assess its condition, and advise about what corrections are needed and who is qualified to make these corrections. Once again, material in good condition need not be sampled unless it is likely to be disturbed. Professional correction or abatement contractors repair or remove asbestos materials.

Some firms offer combinations of testing, assessment, and correction. A professional hired to assess the need for corrective action should not be connected with an asbestos-correction firm. It is better to use two different firms so there is no conflict of interest. Services vary from one area to another around the country.

The federal government has training courses for asbestos professionals around the country. Some state and local governments also have or require training or certification courses. Ask asbestos professionals to document their completion of federal- or state-approved training. Each person performing work in your home should provide proof of training and licensing in asbestos work, such as completion of EPA-approved training. State and local health departments or EPA regional offices may have listings of licensed professionals in your area.

If you have a problem that requires the services of asbestos professionals, check their credentials carefully. Hire professionals who are trained, experienced, reputable, and accredited—especially if accreditation is required by state or local laws. Before hiring a professional, ask for references from previous clients. Find out if they were satisfied. Ask whether the professional has handled similar situations. Get cost estimates from several professionals, as the charges for these services can vary.

Though private homes are usually not covered by the asbestos regulations that apply to schools and public buildings, professionals should still use procedures described during federal- or state-approved training. Homeowners should be alert to the chance of misleading claims by asbestos consultants and contractors. There have been reports of firms incorrectly claiming that asbestos materials in homes must be replaced. In other cases, firms have encouraged unnecessary removals or performed them improperly. Unnecessary removals are a waste of money. Improper removals may actually increase the health risks to you and your family. To guard against this, know what services are available and what procedures and precautions are needed to do the job properly.

In addition to general asbestos contractors, you may select a roofing, flooring, or plumbing contractor trained to handle asbestos when it is necessary to remove and replace roofing, flooring, siding, or asbestos-cement pipe that is part of a water system. Normally, roofing and flooring contractors are exempt from state and local licensing requirements because they do not perform any other asbestos-correction work. Call 800-USA-ROOF for names of qualified roofing contractors in your area.

Asbestos-containing automobile brake pads and linings, clutch facings, and gaskets should be repaired and replaced only by a professional using special protective equipment. Many of these products are now available without asbestos.

If You Hire a Professional Asbestos Inspector

- Make sure that the inspection will include a complete visual examination and the careful collection and lab analysis of samples. If asbestos is present, the inspector should provide a written evaluation describing its location and extent of damage, and give recommendations for correction or prevention.

- Make sure an inspecting firm makes frequent site visits if it is hired to assure that a contractor follows proper procedures and requirements. The inspector may recommend and perform checks after the correction to assure the area has been properly cleaned.

If You Hire a Corrective-Action Contractor

- Check with your local air pollution control board, the local agency responsible for worker safety, and the Better Business Bureau. Ask if the firm has had any safety violations. Find out if there are legal actions filed against it.

- Insist that the contractor use the proper equipment to do the job. The workers must wear approved respirators, gloves, and other protective clothing.

- Before work begins, get a written contract specifying the work plan, cleanup, and the applicable federal, state, and local regulations which the contractor must follow (such as notification requirements and asbestos disposal procedures). Contact your state and local health departments, EPA's regional office, and the Occupational Safety and Health Administration's regional office to find out what the regulations are. Be sure the contractor follows local asbestos removal and disposal laws. At the end of the job, get written assurance from the contractor that all procedures have been followed.

- Assure that the contractor avoids spreading or tracking asbestos dust into other areas of your home. They should seal the work area from the rest of the house using plastic sheeting and duct tape, and also turn off the heating and air conditioning system. For some repairs, such as pipe insulation removal, plastic glove bags may be adequate. They must be sealed with tape and properly disposed of when the job is complete.

- Make sure the work site is clearly marked as a hazard area. Do not allow household members and pets into the area until work is completed.

- Insist that the contractor apply a wetting agent to the asbestos material with a hand sprayer that creates a fine mist before removal. Wet fibers do not float in the air as easily as dry fibers and will be easier to clean up.

- Make sure the contractor does not break removed material into small pieces. This could release asbestos fibers into the air. Pipe insulation was usually installed in preformed blocks and should be removed in complete pieces.

- Upon completion, assure that the contractor cleans the area well with wet mops, wet rags, sponges, or HEPA (high efficiency particulate air) vacuum cleaners. A regular vacuum cleaner must never be used. Wetting helps reduce the chance of spreading asbestos fibers in the air. All asbestos materials and disposable equipment and clothing used in the job must be placed in sealed, leakproof, and labeled plastic bags. The work site should be visually free of dust and debris. Air monitoring (to make sure there is no increase of asbestos fibers in the air) may be necessary to assure that the contractor's job is done properly. This should be done by someone not connected with the contractor.

Caution! Do not dust, sweep, or vacuum debris that may contain asbestos. These steps will disturb tiny asbestos fibers and may release them into the air. Remove dust by wet mopping or with a special HEPA vacuum cleaner used by trained asbestos contractors.

Chapter 27

Lead Paint

What is lead poisoning and who is affected?

Lead is a highly toxic substance, exposure to which can produce a wide range of adverse health effects. Both adults and children can suffer from the effects of lead poisoning, but childhood lead poisoning is much more frequent. Over the many years since we have known about the hazards of lead, tens of millions of children have suffered its health effects. Even today, in 2008, there are still an estimated 310,000 children under the age of six who have too much lead in their blood.

Where is it found?

There are many ways in which humans are exposed to lead: through deteriorating paint, household dust, bare soil, air, drinking water, food, ceramics, home remedies, hair dyes, and other cosmetics. Much of this lead is of microscopic size, invisible to the naked eye. More often than not, children with elevated blood lead levels are exposed to lead in their own home.

By far the biggest source of concern is the lead paint that is found in much of our nation's older housing. Until 1978, lead paint was commonly used on the interiors and exteriors of our homes. Today, the U.S. Department of Housing and Urban Development (HUD) estimates

---

"Lead Poisoning," © 2008. Permission to reprint granted by the National Safety Council, a membership organization dedicated to protecting life and promoting health.

that about 38 million homes in the U.S. still contain some lead paint. While lead paint that is in intact condition does not pose an immediate concern, lead paint that is allowed to deteriorate creates a lead-based paint hazard. It can contaminate household dust as well as bare soil around the house, where children may play. In either situation, a child who comes into contact with lead-contaminated dust or soil is easily poisoned. All it takes is hand-to-mouth activity, which is perfectly normal for young children to engage in. All it takes is the lead dust equivalent of a single grain of salt for a child to register an elevated blood lead level.

According to HUD, about 25% of the nation's housing stock—some 24 million homes—contains significant lead-based paint hazards, i.e. deteriorating lead paint or lead-contaminated dust. These are the homes producing the vast majority of the childhood lead poisoning cases we see today.

Children and adults too can get seriously lead poisoned when renovation and remodeling activities take place in a home that contains lead paint. Anytime a surface containing lead paint is worked on, the debris and the dust created by the work must be contained and thoroughly cleaned up, and those doing the work must have adequate personal protection to prevent them from breathing in any lead dust generated by the work. It is therefore of critical importance that lead-painted surfaces be identified prior to the commencement of any renovation or remodeling work, and that lead-safe work practices are used during such activities. Of course, steps must also be taken to ensure that children, pets, and personal belongings including furniture are protected from exposure to lead while work is ongoing, as well.

The past use of leaded gasoline, only recently banned in this country, contributed greatly to the number of cases of childhood lead poisoning in the U.S. during the last 60 years or so. The lead produced by vehicle emissions continues even today to present a hazard, as much of that lead now remains in soil where it was deposited over the years, especially near well-traveled roads and highways. Children who play in dirt contaminated by lead (whether that lead is from gasoline emissions or from deteriorated house paint) can end up with lead-contaminated soil under their fingernails or on their toys, or they can track it into their homes. Even pets can come into contact with lead-contaminated soil and cause human exposure to lead. In each such case, an elevated blood lead level can easily result.

Drinking water can also sometimes contribute to elevated blood lead levels. Lead can leach into drinking water from certain types of plumbing materials (lead pipes, copper pipes with lead solder, and brass faucets). While water is usually not the primary source of exposure to lead for children with elevated blood lead levels, it is nevertheless important to note that formula-fed infants are at special risk of lead poisoning, if their formula is made with lead-contaminated water.

What are the health effects?

There are many different health effects associated with elevated blood lead levels. Young children under the age of six are especially vulnerable to lead's harmful health effects, because their brains and central nervous system are still being formed. For them, even very low levels of exposure can result in reduced IQ, learning disabilities, attention deficit disorders, behavioral problems, stunted growth, impaired hearing, and kidney damage. At high levels of exposure, a child may become mentally retarded, fall into a coma, and even die from lead poisoning. Within the last 10 years, children have died from lead poisoning in New Hampshire and in Alabama. Lead poisoning has also been associated with juvenile delinquency and criminal behavior.

In adults, lead can increase blood pressure and cause fertility problems, nerve disorders, muscle and joint pain, irritability, and memory or concentration problems. It takes a significantly greater level of exposure to lead for adults than it does for kids to sustain adverse health effects. Most adults who are lead poisoned get exposed to lead at work. Occupations related to house painting, welding, renovation and remodeling activities, smelters, firing ranges, the manufacture and disposal of car batteries, and the maintenance and repair of bridges and water towers are particularly at risk for lead exposure. Workers in these occupations must also take care not to leave their work site with potentially contaminated clothing, tools, and facial hair, or with unwashed hands. Otherwise, they can spread the lead to their family vehicles and ultimately to other family members.

When a pregnant woman has an elevated blood lead level, that lead can easily be transferred to the fetus, as lead crosses the placenta. In fact, pregnancy itself can cause lead to be released from the bone, where lead is stored—often for decades—after it first enters the blood stream. (The same process can occur with the onset of menopause.) Once the lead is released from the mother's bones, it re-enters the blood stream and can end up in the fetus. In other words, if a woman had been exposed to enough lead as a child for some of the lead to have been stored in her bones, the mere fact of pregnancy can trigger the release of that lead and can cause the fetus to be exposed. In such cases, the baby is born with an elevated blood lead level.

Exposure to lead is estimated by measuring levels of lead in the blood (in micrograms of lead per deciliter of blood). The U.S. Centers for Disease Control and Prevention (CDC) has set a "level of concern" for children at 10 micrograms per deciliter. At this level, it is generally accepted that adverse health effects can begin to set in. However, recent research published in the *New England Journal of Medicine* provides new evidence that there could well be very harmful effects occurring at even lower levels of exposure, even as low as five micrograms of lead per deciliter of blood. In other words, science is now telling us that there is in fact no level of lead exposure that can be considered safe.

How can I check my home to see if it contains lead-based paint hazards?

If you live in a home built before 1960, it is very likely that it contains some lead paint. Homes built between 1960 and 1978 may also contain lead paint, but they are less and less likely to the closer you get to 1978, when the Consumer Product Safety Commission finally issued its ban against lead-based paint. If you live in a home built before 1978 that also has been allowed to deteriorate for a few years, you may have a lead-contaminated dust problem. To find out if your home contains lead paint or a lead-based paint hazard, you should hire a professional.

If all you want to do is find out if there is lead paint in your home, you should hire a lead inspector to test all the paint. Depending on the size of your home, this normally takes between one and four hours. You will know the results of the inspection on the spot. The inspector will be able to tell you whether or not there is lead paint in the home, where it is, and the concentration of lead in the paint. (Older homes contain higher concentrations of lead in paint than homes built after the early 1950s. The higher the concentration, the greater the hazard once the paint deteriorates.)

If you also want to find out if your home contains any lead-contaminated dust, which is the most dangerous of all lead-based paint hazards, you should hire either a risk assessor or a sampling technician. They will take samples of dust throughout your home and then send them to a laboratory for analysis. You should be able to learn the results within three to seven days. You will learn whether there is any lead-contaminated dust in your home and where it was found. A risk assessor can also tell you what you should do next to take care of the problem. Alternatively, you can buy a dust sampling kit and carefully do the sampling yourself, send the samples to an appropriate laboratory for analysis, and get the results directly from the lab. This is a less expensive way to find out about lead-contaminated dust in your home. The National Safety Council offers a lead dust test kit that includes everything a consumer needs to determine the presence of lead dust in their home, including detailed instructions and a prestamped, preaddressed envelope to the lab for sample analysis. Download an order form at downloads.nsc.org/pdf/OrderFormLeadKits.pdf.

Various manufacturers also offer what is called a "spot test kit," basically a sampling tool that uses a chemical process to help consumers figure out if there is lead present in household paint, or even on ceramic ware or on toys. However, spot test kits are not considered completely reliable tools in terms of their accuracy, and they should not be relied upon for definitive answers regarding the presence of lead paint.

To locate a lead inspector, a risk assessor, or another certified professional in lead hazard evaluation and control activities, go to the Lead Listing at www.leadlisting.org.

What are some simple steps to take to prevent or reduce lead exposure?

Maintain the paint in your home and clean up any lead dust. If you live in a home built before 1978, the most important step to take to reduce the risk of exposure to lead is to make sure that the paint is well maintained. Whenever repainting, renovation, or other work is undertaken that may end up disturbing a painted surface, it is critical to moisten the surface first, in order to prevent the work from generating dust. Similarly, all painted debris from the work should be contained, in other words prevented from spreading beyond the area where the debris can be carefully gathered and then safely disposed of.

If you think you may have a lead dust problem, you can clean up lead-contaminated dust yourself by carefully and thoroughly washing the area, using soapy water and a mop. A three-bucket system is ideal, with one bucket holding the soapy water (a general all-purpose cleaner is adequate, but dishwasher soap containing phosphates or a lead-specific detergent may be more effective), a second bucket serving as the rinse bucket, and the third containing only clean water. After you wash a section of floor with the soapy water, rinse the mop in the rinse bucket, then dunk it in the clean water bucket, and finally dip it back in the soapy water bucket before cleaning the next area. For smaller areas such as window sills, a rag should be used instead of a mop. Once done, throw the mop or rag away. Whenever cleaning lead-contaminated dust, vigorous wiping is most effective in removing the lead. However, wiping should never be done in a back-and-forth manner, but rather from left to right (or vice versa), or from the top of a wall downwards.

Once cleaning has been completed for a given room, it is time to rinse, using only clean water and preferably a new mop head.

Remember that if you do have a lead dust problem, you will also need to address the source of the lead dust. In many instances, lead dust particles are generated by friction caused by the opening and shutting of old windows. With old, deteriorating windows, outright window replacement may be the best option. In addition to solving your lead dust problem, this also typically results in significantly increased energy efficiency, higher property values, and lower heating and cooling bills.

If you have a young child in your home and you suspect there may be a lead problem, take the recommended steps to eliminate any lead-contaminated dust, and make sure the child washes his/her hands frequently. Also make sure to clean any toys that have been lying about in areas that you suspect may contain lead-contaminated dust.

Check the water. To ensure your drinking water does not contain a hazardous level of lead, test the water at your faucets. Call the EPA [Environmental Protection Agency] Safe Drinking Water Hotline at 800-426-4791 for more information. Kits for testing water, along with the instructions for doing so, are available from a number of providers.

Eat right. The amount of lead the human body retains can be reduced if you make sure your child's diet includes plenty of foods that contain iron, calcium, and zinc. Foods rich in iron include eggs, raisins, greens, beans, peas, and other legumes. Dairy products such as milk, cheese, and yogurt are recommended for their high calcium content. Lean red meat and oysters are examples of foods that contain zinc. Avoid giving children fried or fatty foods—although remember that a certain amount of dietary fat is vital for children under two years of age. And make sure your children always wash their hands before eating.

Check your ceramic ware. Some pottery may contain lead that can leach into food and drinks. Avoid eating off any colorfully painted ceramic plates, and avoid drinking from any ceramic mugs unless you know they do not leach lead. This is particularly important if the pottery was made in Mexico or another Latin America country, or in Asia. Generally, pottery made in the U.S., in Canada, or in Western Europe tends to be safe.

Do not store alcohol in crystal containers. Crystal decanters and glasses are often made with lead. When an acidic substance or alcohol is left in these containers for longer than just a few hours, there is a risk that the lead could leach into the liquid.

Cover bare soil play areas. You should ensure your child avoids playing in bare soil areas unless you know they are lead free. Often, bare soil will contain some lead, either deposited there by vehicle emissions from leaded gasoline days, or from deteriorated exterior paint. This is frequently the case in vacant lots, where old buildings once stood, or in a neighborhood where extensive renovation work may have occurred. If you have a bare soil problem, the easiest way to reduce the risk is to cover the soil with mulch (for instance, pebbles, shrubbery, or grass). A child who plays in lead-contaminated bare soil is likely to get some under his/her fingernails, which will eventually find their way into his/her mouth, or on toys, or on their shoes, which could track the lead into the home. Similarly, a dog that rolls around in lead-contaminated bare soil may end up transporting some of that lead into the home.

What laws help prevent lead poisoning?

At the Federal level, the Lead-Based Paint Hazard Reduction Act of 1992, known as Title X (Title 10), is the source of much of the law of the land on lead paint. One of its most important requirements is the disclosure of known lead hazards at the time of the sale or lease of a home built before 1978. Sellers and landlords must also provide a pamphlet on lead poisoning to the buyer or renter before the pre-1978 property is sold or rented.

The Federal lead hazard disclosure laws have been vigorously enforced by HUD, the EPA, and the U.S. Department of Justice (DOJ). For the past five years, these federal agencies have been working closely together to help ensure that property owners and real estate agents comply with the Title X disclosure requirements.

Similarly, Title X also requires renovators, remodelers, and others who conduct such activities for compensation in homes built before 1978 to provide the pamphlet entitled "Protect Your Family from Lead in Your Home" to the owners and occupants of affected housing, prior to beginning the work.

At the state or local level, your state or municipality may have enacted additional laws to protect you from lead poisoning. Check with your state and local health and housing departments for details.

Code enforcement is another important legal tool that can be used to prevent lead poisoning. Most local codes already prohibit chipping, peeling paint conditions.

Generally, under what is called "common law," tenants have a right to live in safe housing, otherwise known as the implied warranty of habitability. Premises that contain lead-based paint hazards are inherently unsafe places to live. If you can demonstrate that your rented home contains a lead-based paint hazard, you should immediately contact your landlord or property manager and notify them of the presence of a lead hazard. Do it in writing and keep a dated copy for your records. If they fail to respond in a timely and effective manner to this notification, you may have legal recourse against them. Consult an attorney for further information—and take your own precautions.

Chapter 28

Volatile Organic Compounds (VOCs)

Volatile organic compounds (VOCs) are emitted as gases from certain solids or liquids. VOCs include a variety of chemicals, some of which may have short- and long-term adverse health effects. Concentrations of many VOCs are consistently higher indoors (up to 10 times higher) than outdoors. VOCs are emitted by a wide array of products numbering in the thousands. Examples include: paints and lacquers, paint strippers, cleaning supplies, pesticides, building materials and furnishings, office equipment such as copiers and printers, correction fluids and carbonless copy paper, graphics and craft materials including glues and adhesives, permanent markers, and photographic solutions.

Organic chemicals are widely used as ingredients in household products. Paints, varnishes, and wax all contain organic solvents, as do many cleaning, disinfecting, cosmetic, degreasing, and hobby products. Fuels are made up of organic chemicals. All of these products can release organic compounds while you are using them, and, to some degree, when they are stored.

U.S. Environmental Protection Agency (EPA)'s Total Exposure Assessment Methodology (TEAM) studies found levels of about a dozen common organic pollutants to be two to five times higher inside homes than outside, regardless of whether the homes were located in rural or highly industrial areas. Additional TEAM studies indicate

---

"An Introduction to Indoor Air Quality: Organic Gases (Volatile Organic Compounds—VOCs)," Environmental Protection Agency (www.epa.gov), January 26, 2009.

that while people are using products containing organic chemicals, they can expose themselves and others to very high pollutant levels, and elevated concentrations can persist in the air long after the activity is completed.

Sources

VOCs are found in household products including the following: paints, paint strippers, and other solvents; wood preservatives; aerosol sprays; cleansers and disinfectants; moth repellents and air fresheners; stored fuels and automotive products; hobby supplies; dry-cleaned clothing.

Health Effects

Health effects of VOCs include these symptoms: eye, nose, and throat irritation; headaches, loss of coordination, nausea; damage to liver, kidney, and central nervous system. Some organics can cause cancer in animals; some are suspected or known to cause cancer in humans. Key signs or symptoms associated with exposure to VOCs include conjunctival irritation, nose and throat discomfort, headache, allergic skin reaction, dyspnea, declines in serum cholinesterase levels, nausea, emesis, epistaxis, fatigue, dizziness.

The ability of organic chemicals to cause health effects varies greatly from those that are highly toxic to those with no known health effect. As with other pollutants, the extent and nature of the health effect will depend on many factors including level of exposure and length of time exposed. Eye and respiratory tract irritation, headaches, dizziness, visual disorders, and memory impairment are among the immediate symptoms that some people have experienced soon after exposure to some organics. At present, not much is known about what health effects occur from the levels of organics usually found in homes. Many organic compounds are known to cause cancer in animals; some are suspected of causing, or are known to cause, cancer in humans.

- Search EPA's Integrated Risk Information System (IRIS, a compilation of electronic reports on specific substances found in the environment and their potential to cause human health effects) at cfpub.epa.gov/ncea/iris/index.cfm.
- See Drinking Water regulations—Contaminant Specific Fact Sheets on VOCs at www.epa.gov/OGWDW/dwh/t-voc.html.

- Review information on VOCs in water sources developed by the U.S. Geology Survey's National Water-Quality Assessment (NAWQA) Program (water.usgs.gov/nawqa/vocs/) and their Toxic Substances Hydrology Program: Toxic Program Research on VOCs (toxics.usgs.gov/definitions/vocs.html).

Levels in Homes

Studies have found that levels of several organics average two to five times higher indoors than outdoors. During and for several hours immediately after certain activities, such as paint stripping, levels may be 1,000 times background outdoor levels.

Steps to Reduce Exposure

Increase ventilation when using products that emit VOCs. Meet or exceed any label precautions. Do not store opened containers of unused paints and similar materials within the school [or home]. Formaldehyde, one of the best-known VOCs, is one of the few indoor air pollutants that can be readily measured. Identify and, if possible, remove the source. If not possible to remove, reduce exposure by using a sealant on all exposed surfaces of paneling and other furnishings. Use integrated pest management techniques to reduce the need for pesticides.

- Use household products according to manufacturer's directions.
- Make sure you provide plenty of fresh air when using these products.
- Throw away unused or little-used containers safely; buy in quantities that you will use soon.
- Keep out of reach of children and pets.
- Never mix household care products unless directed on the label.

Follow label instructions carefully. Potentially hazardous products often have warnings aimed at reducing exposure of the user. For example, if a label says to use the product in a well-ventilated area, go outdoors or in areas equipped with an exhaust fan to use it. Otherwise, open up windows to provide the maximum amount of outdoor air possible.

Throw away partially full containers of old or unneeded chemicals safely. Because gases can leak even from closed containers, this single step could help lower concentrations of organic chemicals in your home. (Be sure that materials you decide to keep are stored not only in a well-ventilated area but are also safely out of reach of children.) Do not simply toss these unwanted products in the garbage can. Find out if your local government or any organization in your community sponsors special days for the collection of toxic household wastes. If such days are available, use them to dispose of the unwanted containers safely. If no such collection days are available, think about organizing one.

Buy limited quantities. If you use products only occasionally or seasonally, such as paints, paint strippers, and kerosene for space heaters or gasoline for lawn mowers, buy only as much as you will use right away.

Keep exposure to emissions from products containing methylene chloride to a minimum. Consumer products that contain methylene chloride include paint strippers, adhesive removers, and aerosol spray paints. Methylene chloride is known to cause cancer in animals. Also, methylene chloride is converted to carbon monoxide in the body and can cause symptoms associated with exposure to carbon monoxide. Carefully read the labels containing health hazard information and cautions on the proper use of these products. Use products that contain methylene chloride outdoors when possible; use indoors only if the area is well ventilated.

Keep exposure to benzene to a minimum. Benzene is a known human carcinogen. The main indoor sources of this chemical are environmental tobacco smoke, stored fuels and paint supplies, and automobile emissions in attached garages. Actions that will reduce benzene exposure include eliminating smoking within the home, providing for maximum ventilation during painting, and discarding paint supplies and special fuels that will not be used immediately.

Keep exposure to perchloroethylene emissions from newly dry-cleaned materials to a minimum. Perchloroethylene is the chemical most widely used in dry cleaning. In laboratory studies, it has been shown to cause cancer in animals. Recent studies indicate that people breathe low levels of this chemical both in homes where dry-cleaned goods are stored and as they wear dry-cleaned clothing. Dry cleaners recapture the perchloroethylene during the dry-cleaning process so they can save money by reusing it, and they remove more of the chemical during the pressing and finishing processes. Some dry cleaners, however, do not remove as much perchloroethylene as possible all of the time. Taking steps to minimize your exposure to this chemical is prudent. If dry-cleaned goods have a strong chemical odor when you pick them up, do not accept them until they have been properly dried. If goods with a chemical odor are returned to you on subsequent visits, try a different dry cleaner.

Chapter 29

Radiation Exposure from Microwaves and Cell Phones

Microwave Oven Radiation

Microwaves are used to detect speeding cars, to send telephone and television communications, and to treat muscle soreness. Industry uses microwaves to dry and cure plywood, to cure rubber and resins, to raise bread and doughnuts, and to cook potato chips. But the most common consumer use of microwave energy is in microwave ovens.

The Food and Drug Administration (FDA) has regulated the manufacture of microwave ovens since 1971. On the basis of current knowledge about microwave radiation, the agency believes that ovens that meet the FDA standard and are used according to the manufacturer's instructions are safe for use.

What Is Microwave Radiation?

Microwaves are a form of "electromagnetic" radiation; that is, they are waves of electrical and magnetic energy moving together through space. Electromagnetic radiation ranges from the energetic x-rays to the less energetic radio frequency waves used in broadcasting. Microwaves fall into the radio frequency band of electromagnetic radiation. Microwaves should not be confused with x-rays, which are more powerful.

This section includes "Microwave Oven Radiation," February 29, 2008, and "Health Issues: Do Cell Phones Pose a Health Hazard?" October 14, 2008, Food and Drug Administration (www.fda.gov).

Microwaves have three characteristics that allow them to be used in cooking: they are reflected by metal; they pass through glass, paper, plastic, and similar materials; and they are absorbed by foods.

Cooking with Microwaves

Microwaves are produced inside the oven by an electron tube called a magnetron. The microwaves are reflected within the metal interior of the oven where they are absorbed by food. Microwaves cause water molecules in food to vibrate, producing heat that cooks the food. That's why foods high in water content, like fresh vegetables, can be cooked more quickly than other foods. The microwave energy is changed to heat as it is absorbed by food, and does not make food "radioactive" or "contaminated."

Although heat is produced directly in the food, microwave ovens do not cook food from the "inside out." When thick foods are cooked, the outer layers are heated and cooked primarily by microwaves while the inside is cooked mainly by the conduction of heat from the hot outer layers.

Microwave cooking can be more energy efficient than conventional cooking because foods cook faster and the energy heats only the food, not the whole oven compartment. Microwave cooking does not reduce the nutritional value of foods any more than conventional cooking. In fact, foods cooked in a microwave oven may keep more of their vitamins and minerals, because microwave ovens can cook more quickly and without adding water.

Glass, paper, ceramic, or plastic containers are used in microwave cooking because microwaves pass through these materials. Although such containers can not be heated by microwaves, they can become hot from the heat of the food cooking inside. Some plastic containers should not be used in a microwave oven because they can be melted by the heat of the food inside. Generally, metal pans or aluminum foil should also not be used in a microwave oven, as the microwaves are reflected off these materials causing the food to cook unevenly and possibly damaging the oven. The instructions that come with each microwave oven indicate the kinds of containers to use. They also cover how to test containers to see whether or not they can be used in microwave ovens.

FDA recommends that microwave ovens not be used in home canning. It is believed that neither microwave ovens nor conventional ovens produce or maintain temperatures high enough to kill the harmful bacteria that occur in some foods while canning.

Microwave Oven Safety Standard

A Federal standard limits the amount of microwaves that can leak from an oven throughout its lifetime to five milliwatts (mW) of microwave radiation per square centimeter at approximately two inches from the oven surface. This limit is far below the level known to harm people. Microwave energy also decreases dramatically as you move away from the source of radiation. A measurement made 20 inches from an oven would be approximately one one-hundredth of value measured at two inches.

The standard also requires all ovens to have two independent interlock systems that stop the production of microwaves the moment the latch is released or the door opened. In addition, a monitoring system stops oven operation in case one or both of the interlock systems fail. The noise that many ovens continue to make after the door is open is usually the fan. The noise does not mean that microwaves are being produced. There is no residual radiation remaining after microwave production has stopped. In this regard a microwave oven is much like an electric light that stops glowing when it is turned off.

All ovens must have a label stating that they meet the safety standard. In addition, FDA requires that all ovens have a label explaining precautions for use. This requirement may be dropped if the manufacturer has proven that the oven will not exceed the allowable leakage limit even if used under the conditions cautioned against on the label.

To make sure the standard is met, FDA tests microwave ovens in its own laboratory. FDA also evaluates manufacturers' radiation testing and quality control programs at their factories.

Although FDA believes the standard assures that microwave ovens do not present any radiation hazard, the agency continues to reassess its adequacy as new information becomes available.

Microwave Ovens and Health

Much research is under way on microwaves and how they might affect the human body. It is known that microwave radiation can heat body tissue the same way it heats food. Exposure to high levels of microwaves can cause a painful burn. The lens of the eye is particularly sensitive to intense heat, and exposure to high levels of microwaves can cause cataracts. Likewise, the testes are very sensitive to changes in temperature. Accidental exposure to high levels of microwave energy can alter or kill sperm, producing temporary sterility.

But these types of injuries—burns, cataracts, temporary sterility—can only be caused by exposure to large amounts of microwave radiation, much more than the five-mW limit for microwave oven leakage.

Less is known about what happens to people exposed to low levels of microwaves. Controlled, long-term studies involving large numbers of people have not been conducted to assess the impact of low-level microwave energy on humans. Much research has been done with experimental animals, but it is difficult to translate the effects of microwaves on animals to possible effects on humans. For one thing, there are differences in the way animals and humans absorb microwaves. For another, experimental conditions can't exactly simulate the conditions under which people use microwave ovens. However, these studies do help us better understand the possible effects of radiation.

The fact that many scientific questions about exposure to low levels of microwaves are not yet answered require FDA to continue the enforcement of radiation protection requirements. Consumers should take certain common sense precautions.

Have Radiation Injuries Resulted from Microwave Ovens?

There have been allegations of radiation injury from microwave ovens, but none as a direct result of microwave exposure. The injuries known to FDA have been injuries that could have happened with any oven or cooking surface. For example, many people have been burned by the hot food, splattering grease, or steam from food cooked in a microwave oven.

Ovens and Pacemakers

At one time there was concern that leakage from microwave ovens could interfere with certain electronic cardiac pacemakers. Similar concerns were raised about pacemaker interference from electric shavers, auto ignition systems, and other electronic products. FDA does not specifically require microwave ovens to carry warnings for people with pacemakers. The problem has been largely resolved because pacemakers are now designed to be shielded against such electrical interference. However, patients with pacemakers may wish to consult their physicians if they have concerns.

Checking Ovens for Leakage

There is little cause for concern about excess microwaves leaking from ovens unless the door hinges, latch, or seals are damaged. In

FDA's experience, most ovens tested show little or no detectable microwave leakage. If there is some problem and you believe your oven might be leaking excessive microwaves, contact the oven manufacturer, a microwave oven service organization, your state health department, or the nearest FDA office.

A word of caution about the microwave testing devices being sold to consumers: FDA has tested a number of these devices and found them generally inaccurate and unreliable. If used, they should be relied on only for a very approximate reading. The sophisticated testing devices used by public health authorities to measure oven leakage are far more accurate and are periodically tested and calibrated.

Tips on Safe Microwave Oven Operation

- Follow the manufacturer's instruction manual for recommended operating procedures and safety precautions for your oven model.
- Don't operate an oven if the door does not close firmly or is bent, warped, or otherwise damaged.
- Never operate an oven if you have reason to believe it will continue to operate with the door open.
- As an added safety precaution, don't stand directly against an oven (and don't allow children to do this) for long periods of time while it is operating.
- Users should not heat water or liquids in the microwave oven for excessive amounts of time.

Do Cell Phones Pose a Health Hazard?

Many people are concerned that cell phone radiation will cause cancer or other serious health hazards. The weight of scientific evidence has not linked cell phones with any health problems.

Cell phones emit low levels of radiofrequency energy (RF). Over the past 15 years, scientists have conducted hundreds of studies looking at the biological effects of the radiofrequency energy emitted by cell phones. While some researchers have reported biological changes associated with RF energy, these studies have failed to be replicated. The majority of studies published have failed to show an association between exposure to radiofrequency from a cell phone and health problems.

The low levels of RF cell phones emit while in use are in the microwave frequency range. They also emit RF at substantially reduced time intervals when in the standby mode. Whereas high levels of RF can produce health effects (by heating tissue), exposure to low-level RF that does not produce heating effects causes no known adverse health effects.

The biological effects of radiofrequency energy should not be confused with the effects from other types of electromagnetic energy.

Very high levels of electromagnetic energy, such as is found in x-rays and gamma rays, can ionize biological tissues. Ionization is a process where electrons are stripped away from their normal locations in atoms and molecules. It can permanently damage biological tissues including DNA, the genetic material.

The energy levels associated with radiofrequency energy, including both radio waves and microwaves, are not great enough to cause the ionization of atoms and molecules. Therefore, RF energy is a type of non-ionizing radiation. Other types of non-ionizing radiation include visible light, infrared radiation (heat), and other forms of electromagnetic radiation with relatively low frequencies.

While RF energy doesn't ionize particles, large amounts can increase body temperatures and cause tissue damage. Two areas of the body, the eyes and the testes, are particularly vulnerable to RF heating because there is relatively little blood flow in them to carry away excess heat.

Chapter 30

Electric and Magnetic Field (EMF) Exposure

Key Points

- The electromagnetic spectrum encompasses both natural and human-made sources of electromagnetic fields.
- Frequency and wavelength characterize an electromagnetic field. In an electromagnetic wave, these two characteristics are directly related to each other: the higher the frequency the shorter the wavelength.
- Ionizing radiation such as X-ray and gamma-rays consists of photons which carry sufficient energy to break molecular bonds. Photons of electromagnetic waves at power and radio frequencies have much lower energy that does not have this ability.
- Electric fields exist whenever charge is present and are measured in volts per meter (V/m). Magnetic fields arise from current flow. Their flux densities are measured in microtesla (μT) or millitesla (mT).
- At radio and microwave frequencies, electric and magnetic fields are considered together as the two components of an

---

This section includes excerpts from "What are Electromagnetic Fields?" http://www.who.int/pehemf/ about/WhatisEMF/en/ and "What are Electromagnetic Fields? Summary of Health Effects," http://www.who.int/pehemf/ about/WhatisEMF/en/index 1.html.

electromagnetic wave. Power density, measured in watts per square meter (W/m^2), describes the intensity of these fields.

- Low frequency and high frequency electromagnetic waves affect the human body in different ways.
- Electrical power supplies and appliances are the most common sources of low frequency electric and magnetic fields in our living environment. Everyday sources of radiofrequency electromagnetic fields are telecommunications, broadcasting antennas, and microwave ovens.

Summary of Health Effects

What Happens When You Are Exposed to Electromagnetic Fields?

Exposure to electromagnetic fields is not a new phenomenon. However, during the 20th century, environmental exposure to man-made electromagnetic fields has been steadily increasing as growing electricity demand, ever-advancing technologies, and changes in social behavior have created more and more artificial sources. Everyone is exposed to a complex mix of weak electric and magnetic fields, both at home and at work, from the generation and transmission of electricity, domestic appliances and industrial equipment, to telecommunications and broadcasting.

Tiny electrical currents exist in the human body due to the chemical reactions that occur as part of the normal bodily functions, even in the absence of external electric fields. For example, nerves relay signals by transmitting electric impulses. Most biochemical reactions from digestion to brain activities go along with the rearrangement of charged particles. Even the heart is electrically active—an activity that your doctor can trace with the help of an electrocardiogram.

Low-frequency electric fields influence the human body just as they influence any other material made up of charged particles. When electric fields act on conductive materials, they influence the distribution of electric charges at their surface. They cause current to flow through the body to the ground.

Low-frequency magnetic fields induce circulating currents within the human body. The strength of these currents depends on the intensity of the outside magnetic field. If sufficiently large, these currents could cause stimulation of nerves and muscles or affect other biological processes.

Both electric and magnetic fields induce voltages and currents in the body but even directly beneath a high voltage transmission line, the induced currents are very small compared to thresholds for producing shock and other electrical effects.

Heating is the main biological effect of the electromagnetic fields of radiofrequency fields. In microwave ovens this fact is employed to warm up food. The levels of radiofrequency fields to which people are normally exposed are very much lower than those needed to produce significant heating. The heating effect of radio waves forms the underlying basis for current guidelines. Scientists are also investigating the possibility that effects below the threshold level for body heating occur as a result of long-term exposure. To date, no adverse health effects from low level, long-term exposure to radiofrequency or power frequency fields have been confirmed, but scientists are actively continuing to research this area.

Biological Effects or Health Effects? What Is a Health Hazard?

Biological effects are measurable responses to a stimulus or to a change in the environment. These changes are not necessarily harmful to your health. For example, listening to music, reading a book, eating an apple, or playing tennis will produce a range of biological effects. Nevertheless, none of these activities is expected to cause health effects. The body has sophisticated mechanisms to adjust to the many and varied influences we encounter in our environment. Ongoing change forms a normal part of our lives. But, of course, the body does not possess adequate compensation mechanisms for all biological effects. Changes that are irreversible and stress the system for long periods of time may constitute a health hazard.

An adverse health effect causes detectable impairment of the health of the exposed individual or of his or her offspring; a biological effect, on the other hand, may or may not result in an adverse health effect.

It is not disputed that electromagnetic fields above certain levels can trigger biological effects. Experiments with healthy volunteers indicate that short-term exposure at the levels present in the environment or in the home do not cause any apparent detrimental effects. Exposures to higher levels that might be harmful are restricted by national and international guidelines. The current debate is centered on whether long-term low level exposure can evoke biological responses and influence people's well-being.

Widespread Concerns for Health

A look at the news headlines of recent years allows some insight into the various areas of public concern. Over the course of the past decade, numerous electromagnetic field sources have become the focus of health concerns, including power lines, microwave ovens, computer and TV screens, security devices, radars, and most recently mobile phones and their base stations.

The International EMF Project

In response to growing public health concerns over possible health effects from exposure to an ever increasing number and diversity of electromagnetic field sources, in 1996 the World Health Organization (WHO) launched a large, multidisciplinary research effort. The International EMF Project brings together current knowledge and available resources of key international and national agencies and scientific institutions.

Conclusions from Scientific Research: In the area of biological effects and medical applications of non-ionizing radiation approximately 25,000 articles have been published over the past 30 years. Despite the feeling of some people that more research needs to be done, scientific knowledge in this area is now more extensive than for most chemicals. Based on a recent in-depth review of the scientific literature, the WHO concluded that current evidence does not confirm the existence of any health consequences from exposure to low level electromagnetic fields. However, some gaps in knowledge about biological effects exist and need further research.

Effects on General Health: Some members of the public have attributed a diffuse collection of symptoms to low levels of exposure to electromagnetic fields at home. Reported symptoms include headaches, anxiety, suicide and depression, nausea, fatigue, and loss of libido. To date, scientific evidence does not support a link between these symptoms and exposure to electromagnetic fields. At least some of these health problems may be caused by noise or other factors in the environment, or by anxiety related to the presence of new technologies.

Effects on Pregnancy Outcome: Many different sources and exposures to electromagnetic fields in the living and working environment, including computer screens, water beds and electric blankets, radiofrequency welding machines, diathermy equipment, and radar, have been evaluated by the WHO and other organizations. The overall weight of evidence shows that exposure to fields at typical environmental levels does not increase the risk of any adverse outcome such as spontaneous abortions, malformations, low birth weight, and congenital diseases. There have been occasional reports of associations between health problems and presumed exposure to electromagnetic fields, such as reports of prematurity and low birth weight in children of workers in the electronics industry, but these have not been regarded by the scientific community as being necessarily caused by the field exposures (as opposed to factors such as exposure to solvents).

Cataracts: General eye irritation and cataracts have sometimes been reported in workers exposed to high levels of radiofrequency and microwave radiation, but animal studies do not support the idea that such forms of eye damage can be produced at levels that are not thermally hazardous. There is no evidence that these effects occur at levels experienced by the general public.

Electromagnetic Fields and Cancer: Despite many studies, the evidence for any effect remains highly controversial. However, it is clear that if electromagnetic fields do have an effect on cancer, then any increase in risk will be extremely small. The results to date contain many inconsistencies, but no large increases in risk have been found for any cancer in children or adults.

A number of epidemiological studies suggest small increases in risk of childhood leukemia with exposure to low frequency magnetic fields in the home. However, scientists have not generally concluded that these results indicate a cause-effect relation between exposure to the fields and disease (as opposed to artifacts in the study or effects unrelated to field exposure). In part, this conclusion has been reached because animal and laboratory studies fail to demonstrate any reproducible effects that are consistent with the hypothesis that fields cause or promote cancer. Large-scale studies are currently underway in several countries and may help resolve these issues.

Electromagnetic Hypersensitivity and Depression: Some individuals report "hypersensitivity" to electric or magnetic fields. They ask whether aches and pains, headaches, depression, lethargy, sleeping disorders, and even convulsions and epileptic seizures could be associated with electromagnetic field exposure.

There is little scientific evidence to support the idea of electromagnetic hypersensitivity. Recent Scandinavian studies found that individuals do not show consistent reactions under properly controlled conditions of electromagnetic field exposure. Nor is there any accepted biological mechanism to explain hypersensitivity. Research on this subject is difficult because many other subjective responses may be involved, apart from direct effects of fields themselves. More studies are continuing on the subject.

The Focus of Current and Future Research: Much effort is currently being directed toward the study of electromagnetic fields in relation to cancer. Studies in search for possible carcinogenic (cancer-producing) effects of power frequency fields is continuing, although at a reduced level compared to that of the late 1990s.

The long-term health effects of mobile telephone use is another topic of much current research. No obvious adverse effect of exposure to low level radiofrequency fields has been discovered. However, given public concerns regarding the safety of cellular telephones, further research aims to determine whether any less obvious effects might occur at very low exposure levels.

Part Five

Foodborne Hazards

Chapter 31

Food Safety

Chapter Contents

Section 31.1

Food Safety Regulations

"A Focus on Hazard Analysis and Critical Control Points," Food Safety Research Information Office, U.S. Department of Agriculture (fsrio.nal.usda.gov), March 2008.

Hazard Analysis and Critical Control Points (HACCP) is a production control system for the food industry. It is a process used to determine the potential danger points in food production and to define a strict management and monitoring system to ensure safe food products for consumers. HACCP is designed to prevent potential microbiological, chemical, and physical hazards, rather than catch them. The Food and Drug Administration (FDA) and the United States Department of Agriculture (USDA) use HACCP programs as an effective approach to food safety and protecting public health.

HACCP began in 1959 when the Pillsbury Corporation cooperated with the U.S. Army and the National Aeronautics Space Association (NASA) to ensure the safety of food in space programs. Originally known as the "Modes of Failure," it was adapted over the next 20 years, and with the help of the National Conference of Food Protection and the National Academy of Science it developed into what is known today as HACCP. Good manufacturing practices (GMPs), standard operating procedures (SOPs), sanitation standard operating procedures (SSOP), and good agricultural practices (GAPs) are also among a number of prerequisite programs that laid the foundation for HACCP.

HACCP Research Areas

- Evaluate the effect of high pressure processing (HPP) on the inactivation of spores of *Clostridium botulinum* types A, B, and E in a model buffer and a food system.
- Organize a committee of HACCP experts from industry, academia, and government and operate in a workshop format to develop a library of generic HACCP plans and models.

- Evaluate the use of biocontrol or biological competition to serve as a secondary barrier against toxin production by *Clostridium botulinum* in extended shelf life refrigerated foods possessing a pH greater than 4.6.
- Study thermal and nonthermal in-shell pasteurization of eggs mathematically and microbiologically to determine the potential for the use of microwave energy in eliminating *Salmonella enteritidis* (SE) in in-shell eggs.
- Develop rapid tests for detecting pathogens is an ongoing and important aspect of food safety in the meat industry. NCBA [National Cattlemen's Beef Association] has sponsored several studies that are assisting companies in development of new diagnostic tests. USDA's Agricultural Research Service is also very active in this area of research.
- Evaluate the genetic makeup of serotypes of organisms such as *E. coli*, *Salmonella*, and *Listeria*; identify where they enter the processing system; and identify which subtypes of the organisms are causing human illness.
- Improve sampling procedures including the development of more sensitive, accurate, and rapid pathogen detection tests for the meat industry to detect microbial contamination that may occur during the meat production process.
- Improve microbial safety of meat and the development of more effective intervention procedures to reduce or control pathogens throughout slaughter and processing.
- Determine new and important CCPs [critical control points] or processing events that require specific contamination-preventative measures to provide unique information regarding the nature of specific pathogens to guide the development of better methods to identify and reduce or eliminate meat contamination.

HACCP and the Food Industry

In addition to human illness, food safety problems can cause economic losses to producers, processors, and consumers, and jeopardize the international competitiveness of the U.S. agricultural industry. According to the U.S. Department of Commerce (DOC), four reasons stated by management to implement a HACCP plan include (1) existing and potential product liability claims, (2) concern over impact on reputation and sales, (3) complying with federal and state statutes, and (4) monitoring the safety of new products and processes.

Juice, meat and poultry, and seafood HACCP are regulated at the federal level with inspectors being responsible for the inspection processes. Meat and poultry HACCP systems are regulated by the USDA, while seafood and juice are regulated by the FDA. The use of HACCP is currently voluntary in other food industries.

Processing plants must develop a HACCP plan for each of their products, and they must identify critical control points during their processes where hazards such as microbial contamination can occur. They must also establish controls to prevent or reduce those hazards and maintain records documenting that the controls are working as intended.

Seven Principles of HACCP

1. *Analyze hazards.* Potential hazards associated with a food and measures to control those hazards are identified. The hazard can be biological, such as a microbe; chemical, such as a toxin; or physical, such as ground glass or metal fragments.

2. *Identify critical control points.* These are points in a food's production—from its raw state through processing and shipping to consumption by the consumer—at which the potential hazard can be controlled or eliminated. Examples are cooking, cooling, packaging, and metal detection.

3. *Establish preventive measures with critical limits for each control point.* For a cooked food, for example, this may include setting the minimum cooking temperature and time required to ensure the elimination of any harmful microbes.

4. *Establish procedures to monitor the critical control points.* Such procedures may include determining how and by whom cooking time and temperature should be monitored.

5. *Establish corrective actions to be taken when monitoring shows that a critical limit has not been met.* For example, reprocessing or disposing of food if the minimum cooking temperature is not met.

6. *Establish procedures to verify that the system is working properly.* For example, testing time- and temperature-recording devices to verify that a cooking unit is working properly.

7. *Establish effective recordkeeping to document the HACCP system.* This may include records of hazards and their control methods, the monitoring of safety requirements, and action taken to correct potential problems. Each of these principles must be science-based such as published microbiological studies on time and temperature factors for controlling foodborne pathogens.

Juice HACCP Regulations

Each year 16,000 to 48,000 Americans experience foodborne illness from fruit and vegetable juices. The FDA's Center for Food Safety and Applied Nutrition (CFSAN) found that most frequently contamination occurs during the growing and harvesting of fruits, but can also occur at any point from harvest to table. In 1998, as a preventative measure to this problem, the FDA released the Final Rule 63 FR 20450 stating that the most effective way to ensure juice safety is to process the products under a system of preventative measures (HACCP). The HACCP juice regulation covers both pasteurized as well as nonpasteurized fruit and vegetable juices. (See Juice—HACCP Final Rule at www.cfsan.fda.gov/~lrd/fr01119a.html.)

The juice HACCP rule applies to both interstate and intrastate commerce. The final rule went into effect for medium and large facilities in January 2002, for small facilities January 2003, and for very small facilities January 2004.

Meat and Poultry HACCP Regulations

The potential threat of *Escherichia coli* O157:H7, *Listeria monocytogenes*, and *Salmonella* in meat and poultry products has created the need to search for new approaches to eliminate pathogen contamination. The Centers for Disease Control (CDC) suggests foodborne microbial pathogens are responsible for nearly five million cases of foodborne illness and more than 4,000 deaths associated with meat and poultry products each year.

In order to address this problem, the USDA Food Safety and Inspection Service (FSIS) determined requirements to reduce the number of foodborne illnesses and pathogens on meat and poultry products in July of 1996. For the first time ever, slaughter plants and plants that produced raw, ground meat and poultry were required to systematically target and reduce harmful bacteria. The final rule went into effect for medium and large facilities in 1998, for small facilities January 1999, and for very small facilities January 2000. (See Meat and Poultry—HACCP Final Rule at www.fsis.usda.gov/OA/fr/haccp_rule.htm.)

The rule consists of the following four elements:

1. All slaughter and processing plants are required to adopt a system of process controls (HACCP) to prevent food safety hazards.
2. Slaughter plants are required to conduct microbial testing for generic *E. coli* to verify that their control systems are working as intended to prevent fecal contamination.
3. Plants must meet pathogen reduction performance standards set by FSIS for their raw products.
4. All plants must adopt and implement a written plan (sanitation standard operating procedures) for meeting its basic sanitation responsibilities.

FSIS has more than 7,400 inspectors in 6,200 slaughter and meat and poultry processing plants to ensure that unsafe and unhealthy animals and birds do not enter the food supply. The inspectors guarantee that sanitation and other requirements are met as well as monitor the volatile levels of chemical residues.

Seafood HACCP Regulations

The FDA has regulated the seafood industry for decades, but in December 1997 it began requiring the use of HACCP programs to further ensure the safety of shellfish and fish (Federal Register 60 FR 65095). Firms in the United States or in foreign countries that engage in handling, storing, preparing, heading, eviscerating, shucking, freezing, changing into different market forms, manufacturing, preserving, packing, labeling, dockside unloading, or holding fish and fishery products are required to comply to the HACCP program. The National Marine Fisheries Service (NMFS) maintains the voluntary fee-for-service inspection program and covers all processors. (See Seafood—HACCP Final Rule at www.cfsan.fda.gov/~comm/haccp4x8.html.)

It is estimated that the implementation of this regulation can prevent anywhere from 20,000 to 60,000 seafood poisonings that occur each year. Since the implementation of the program, inspection frequency has increased from an average of every four years to annually. Unlike many other areas of the food industry, seafood and fish are still primarily harvested from individuals or small businesses, making it more difficult to regulate. Progress is currently being made with improvements in the understanding of seafood safety and upgrades in equipment and facilities.

Beyond the United States, other countries that have adopted seafood HACCP systems and procedures include the following: Canada, Uruguay, Brazil, Chile, Ecuador, Australia, New Zealand, Thailand, Iceland, Argentina, Peru, Ireland, Cuba, Morocco, Norway, Sri Lanka, Vietnam, and Bangladesh.

HACCP Alliances

Three alliances have been developed to provide uniform training and education for the implementation and maintenance of HACCP systems.

- The International HACCP Alliance was developed on March 25, 1994. It is housed within the Department of Animal Science at Texas A&M University to provide a uniform program to assure safer meat and poultry products.
- The Seafood HACCP Alliance is a funded proposal by the National Sea Grant Program to support training and education. The alliance was initiated by the Association of Food and Drug Officials (AFDO) and their regional affiliate of Southern States (AFDOSS) in conjunction with a group of Sea Grant Seafood Specialists who originally assisted the National Fisheries Institute (NFI) with their initial HACCP training programs.
- The Juice HACCP Alliance was organized by the National Center for Food Safety and Technology with the assistance of juice processing experts from government, industry, trade associations, AFDO, and academia to develop a juice HACCP curriculum.

HACCP Research

With industry becoming more consumer driven and the demand for high quality foods that are minimally processed, free of additives and residues, healthy, convenient, and affordable, it is impossible for traditional postharvest processing technologies like canning, fermentation, and drying to satisfy all of these demands simultaneously. Researchers have begun developing new nonthermal processing technologies like irradiation, hydrostatic pressure processing (HPP), and hydrodynamic pressure (HDP) processing. However, HPP and HDP present a unique set of processing potential dangers that must also be addressed.

Today, research is concentrated on evaluating the implementation of HACCP in production and processing facilities. Scientists are surveying the production and processing practices and determining their impact on the incidents and magnitudes of the hazards. The attitudes and perceptions of safety among processors, including risk management and assessment, are also being considered.

New sampling methodologies for different critical control points as well as comparisons of microbial sampling and testing methods to evaluate the HACCP plans are also a large area of study. This knowledge will be integrated into applications usable by the food industry as part of a HACCP program.

Section 31.2

Irradiated Foods

"A Focus on Food Irradiation," Food Safety Research Information Office, U.S. Department of Agriculture (fsrio.nal.usda.gov), December 2005.

Food Irradiation Research Areas

- Radioactive safety for consumers
- Combining beneficial effects of irradiation and other ingredients to improve sensory characteristics
- Effects of vitamin E on meat quality including odor and color after irradiation
- Radiation sensitivity of foodborne pathogens with foods of varying starting temperatures
- Reducing processing costs
- Improving consumer acceptance

FDA-Approved Irradiation in the United States

- Wheat and wheat flour: first approval to rid plants of insects, 1963

- NASA sterilizes meat for astronauts in space, 1972
- Pork products: controlling trichinosis, 1985
- Spices, tea, fruits, vegetables, grains: eliminating insects, 1986
- Fresh and frozen poultry: controlling *Salmonella*, other bacteria, 1990
- Fresh and frozen red meats such as beef, lamb, and pork: pathogen control, 1997
- Fresh shell eggs, 2000
- Animal feed ingredients, including pet treats: reducing risk of *Salmonella* contamination, 2001

What Can Irradiation Do?

At low doses, irradiation delays ripening and sprouting in fruits and vegetables and controls insects and parasites (an alternative to chemicals and fumigation). At medium doses, irradiation extends shelf life, reduces spoilage, and reduces pathogenic organisms. At high doses, irradiation is used for sterilization of meat, poultry, seafood, prepared foods, and disinfection of spices.

Approved Dosages for the United States

- Spices and dry vegetable seasoning, decontaminates and controls insects and microorganisms—30 kGy [kiloGray, radiation unit of measure]
- Dry or dehydrated enzyme preparations, controls insects and microorganisms—10 kGy
- All foods, controls insects—1 kGy
- Fresh foods, delays maturation—1 kGy
- Poultry, controls disease-causing microorganisms—3 kGy
- Red meat (such as beef, lamb, and pork), controls spoilage and disease-causing microorganisms—4.5 kGy (fresh), 7 kGy (frozen)

Uses of Irradiation

Irradiation cannot be used with all food because it can change their acceptability and palatability, usually those with high fat contents.

For example, higher fat dairy products can have undesirable flavor changes. Some fruits, such as peaches and nectarines, may have tissue softening. Oysters and other raw shellfish can be irradiated, but the shelf life and quality decreases because the live oyster inside the shell is damaged or killed by the irradiation.

Currently in the United Sates, strawberries and other fruits in Florida are being irradiated. Tropical fruits from Hawaii's mainland are being irradiated as a replacement to the normal fumigation process. Beef, pork, poultry, and many commercial spices are also being irradiated. Forty countries are permitting food irradiation, including the following: France, the Netherlands, Portugal, Israel, Thailand, Russia, China, and South Africa.

The USDA estimates that the American consumer will receive approximately two dollars in benefits such as reduced spoilage and less illness for each dollar spent on food irradiation. The FDA requires that all food that has been irradiated carry the international symbol of the radura, and the statement "Treated with radiation" or "Treated by Irradiation" on the packaging.

How Food Irradiation Works

The short, high energy waves of radiant energy of the irradiation process transfer into the molecules of the microbe. This energy creates reactive chemicals that damage the cell's DNA. This damage interferes with the cell replication and thus duplication and reproduction of the organism fails.

Depending on the size of the organism, the amount of DNA, and how quickly the organism can repair itself, the sensitivity to the irradiation varies. Larger organisms, such as insects and parasites, are easily eliminated with irradiation because they have a greater amount of DNA that can be affected and damaged. Smaller organisms, such as viruses, are more resistant. Irradiation is measured in units called "Grays" (GY). The killing effect of irradiation on microbes is measured in D-values. One D-value is the amount needed to kill 90% of that organism.

Applications of Food Irradiation

Food irradiation is applied to food products for different purposes, including the following:

- **Controlling foodborne pathogens:** Irradiation is currently used to eliminate pathogens that cause foodborne illnesses, but this process does not protect the food from being recontaminated, and consumers should handle the food in the same manner as nonirradiated products by being aware of storage and handling, refrigeration and cooking time and temperatures, and cross contamination.

- **Preservation:** Irradiation can destroy or inactivate the organisms that cause spoilage and decomposition, thereby extending the shelf life of the food. There are some advantages to irradiation for the purpose of preservation. Unlike canning, the food does not undergo a lot of heat, so the food is much closer to its original fresh state. There is no additional liquid required and there is little loss of its own liquid since the temperature does not rise. Therefore the flavor, texture, and color remain very much like the original food.
- **Sterilization:** As with canned and other heat-sterilized foods, the product can be stored for years at room temperature. This is helpful with military and space flights. It also can be beneficial to immune-compromised patients and hospitals.
- **Controlling sprouting, ripening, and insect damage:** Irradiation is an alternative to chemicals. It can be used with tropical fruits, potatoes, grains, etc. There is no residue left on the food.

Regulators of Food Irradiation

Food irradiation in the United States is primarily regulated by the FDA since it is considered a food additive. Other federal agencies that regulate aspects of food irradiation include the following:

- United States Department of Agriculture (USDA): meat and poultry products
- Nuclear Regulatory Commission (NRC): safety of the processing facility
- Department of Transportation (DOT): safe transport of the radioactive sources

Each new food is approved separately with a guideline specifying a maximum dosage. Packaging materials containing the food processed by irradiation must also undergo approval.

Irradiation Technologies

Currently three different technologies exist for the process of irradiating food products, including the following:

- **The first technology:** Use of radiation given off by a radioactive substance, such as Cobalt 60 or Cesium 137. These particular substances give off photons that produce gamma rays. They do not release neutrons; thus, the food does not become radioactive. The photons can penetrate up to several feet. This is the same technology that has been routinely used to sterilize dental and medical supplies. The photons are constantly released. When the substance is not in use, it is submerged in a pool of water that absorbs the photons safely and completely.

- **Electron beam technology:** No radioactive substance is involved. Electrons are "shot from a gun" toward the substance. Shielding is needed to protect workers from the released electrons. This technology is limited since the electrons can only penetrate up to a little over an inch. The food must be very thin.

- **X-ray technology:** This is the newest technology and is still being developed. A beam of electrons are directed onto a thin plate of gold or other metal, producing a stream of X-rays much stronger than X-ray machines found in hospitals. Like the Cobalt technology, this technology can pass through thick foods, but like the electron beam technology requires protection for the users. A limited number of these machines have been built.

Public Interest

Food irradiation is currently encountering public opposition because many organizations feel there is a danger to the environment and consumer. These concerns include the potential that the food itself may become radioactive or lose its nutritional value, long-term health risks associated with eating the processed food, and environmental risks at the processing facilities.

There is controversy over the production of small amounts of substances called radiolytic products. There is debate over whether the levels produced are harmful and to what degree risk is produced. There is no debate, however, that they are produced when food is irradiated. The public concern also looks ahead into the industry's use of irradiation as a fallback to sterilize "dirty" food.

Currently, 40 countries and a large number of government agencies and medical organizations are advocates of food irradiation as a safe and effective method to reduce the risk of foodborne illness. As identified, research has provided results discounting many of these misconceptions. Ongoing research continues to identify and improve the effectiveness of the irradiation process with the use of other ingredients and established food processes to improve costs, palatability, and safety.

Agencies, such as the CDC, feel that consumer confidence will depend on making food clean first, and then the use of irradiation or pasteurization will make it safe. Food irradiation is a logical next step to reducing the burden of foodborne disease in the United States.

Chapter 32

Food Allergies and Intolerance

What Is Food Allergy?

Food allergy is an abnormal response to a food triggered by the body's immune system. In this chapter, "food allergy" refers to a particular type of response of the immune system in which the body produces what is called an allergic, or IgE, antibody to a food. (IgE, or immunoglobulin E, is a type of protein that works against a specific food.)

Allergic reactions to food can cause serious illness and, in some cases, death. Therefore, if you have a food allergy, it is extremely important for you to work with your health care provider to find out what food or foods cause your allergic reaction.

Sometimes, a reaction to food is not an allergy at all but another type of reaction called "food intolerance."

Food intolerance is more common than food allergy. The immune system does not cause the symptoms of food intolerance, though these symptoms may look and feel like those of a food allergy.

How Do Allergic Reactions Work?

An immediate allergic reaction involves two actions of your immune system:

"Food Allergy," National Institute of Allergy and Infectious Diseases (www3.niaid.nih.gov), January 21, 2009.

- Your immune system produces IgE. This protein is called a food-specific antibody, and it circulates through your blood.
- The food-specific IgE then attaches to basophils and mast cells. Basophils are found in blood. Mast cells are found in body tissues, especially in areas of your body that are typical sites of allergic reactions. Those sites include your nose, throat, lungs, skin, and gastrointestinal (GI) tract.

Generally, your immune system will form IgE against a food if you come from a family in which allergies are common—not necessarily food allergies but perhaps other allergic diseases, such as hay fever or asthma. If you have two allergic parents, you are more likely to develop food allergy than someone with one allergic parent.

If your immune system is inclined to form IgE to certain foods, you must be exposed to the food before you can have an allergic reaction to it.

As this food is digested, it triggers certain cells in your body to produce a food-specific IgE in large amounts. The food-specific IgE is then released and attaches to the surfaces of mast cells and basophils.

- The next time you eat that food, it interacts with food-specific IgE on the surface of the mast cells and basophils and triggers those cells to release chemicals.
- Depending on the tissue in which they are released, these chemicals will cause you to have various symptoms of food allergy.

Food allergens are proteins in the food that enter your bloodstream after the food is digested. From there, they go to target organs, such as your skin or nose, and cause allergic reactions. An allergic reaction to food can take place within a few minutes to an hour. The process of eating and digesting food affects the timing and the location of a reaction.

If you are allergic to a particular food, you may first feel itching in your mouth as you start to eat the food. After the food is digested in your stomach, you may have GI symptoms such as vomiting, diarrhea, or pain. When the food allergens enter and travel through your bloodstream, they may cause your blood pressure to drop. As the allergens reach your skin, they can cause hives or eczema. When the allergens reach your mouth and lungs, they may cause throat tightness and trouble breathing.

Cross-Reactive Food Allergies

If you have a life-threatening reaction to a certain food, your health care provider will show you how to avoid similar foods that might trigger this reaction. For example, if you have a history of allergy to shrimp, allergy testing will usually show that you are not only allergic to shrimp but also to crab, lobster, and crayfish. This is called "cross-reactivity."

Another interesting example of cross-reactivity occurs in people who are highly sensitive to ragweed. During ragweed pollen season, they sometimes find that when they try to eat melons, particularly cantaloupe, they experience itching in their mouths and simply cannot eat the melon. Similarly, people who have severe birch pollen allergy also may react to apple peels. This is called the "oral allergy syndrome."

Common Food Allergies

In adults, the foods that most often cause allergic reactions include the following:

- Shellfish, such as shrimp, crayfish, lobster, and crab
- Peanuts
- Tree nuts, such as walnuts
- Fish
- Eggs

The following are the most common foods that cause problems in children:

- Eggs
- Milk
- Peanuts
- Tree nuts

Peanuts and tree nuts are the leading causes of the potentially deadly food allergy reaction called anaphylaxis.

Adults usually keep their allergies for life, but children sometimes outgrow them. Children are more likely to outgrow allergies to milk, egg, or soy than allergies to peanuts. The foods to which adults or children usually react are those foods they eat often. In Japan, for example, rice allergy is frequent. In Scandinavia, codfish allergy is common.

Food Allergy or Food Intolerance?

If you go to your health care provider and say, "I think I have a food allergy," your provider has to consider other possibilities that may cause symptoms and could be confused with food allergy, such as food intolerance. To find out the difference between food allergy and food intolerance, your provider will go through a list of possible causes for your symptoms. This is called a "differential diagnosis." This type of diagnosis helps confirm that you do indeed have a food allergy rather than a food intolerance or other illness.

Types of Food Intolerance

Food Poisoning: One possible cause of symptoms like those of food allergy is food contaminated with microbes, such as bacteria, and bacterial products, such as toxins. Contaminated meat and dairy products sometimes cause symptoms, including gastrointestinal (GI) discomfort, that resemble a food allergy but are really a type of food poisoning.

Histamine Toxicity: There are substances, such as the powerful chemical histamine, present in certain foods that cause a reaction similar to an allergic reaction. For example, histamine can reach high levels in cheese; some wines; and certain kinds of fish, such as tuna and mackerel.

In fish, histamine is believed to come from contamination by bacteria, particularly in fish that are not refrigerated properly. If you eat one of these foods with a high level of histamine, you could have a reaction that strongly resembles an allergic reaction to food. This reaction is called "histamine toxicity."

Lactose Intolerance: Another cause of food intolerance confused with a food allergy is lactose intolerance or lactase deficiency. This common food intolerance affects at least 1 out of 10 people.

Lactase is an enzyme in the lining of your gut. Lactase breaks down, or digests, lactose, a sugar found in milk and most milk products. Lactose intolerance, or lactase deficiency, happens when there is not enough lactase in your gut to digest lactose. In that case, bacteria in your gut use lactose to form gas, which causes bloating, abdominal pain, and sometimes diarrhea.

Your health care provider can use laboratory tests to find out whether your body can digest lactose.

Food Additives: Another type of food intolerance is a reaction to certain products that are added to food to enhance taste, provide color, or protect against the growth of microbes. Several chemical compounds, such as MSG (monosodium glutamate) and sulfites, are tied to reactions that can be confused with food allergy.

MSG

MSG is a flavor enhancer and, when taken in large amounts, can cause some of the following signs:

- Flushing
- Sensations of warmth
- Headache
- Chest discomfort
- Feelings of detachment

These passing reactions occur rapidly after eating large amounts of food to which MSG has been added.

Sulfites

Sulfites occur naturally in some foods or may be added to increase crispness or prevent mold growth.

Sulfites in high concentrations sometimes pose problems for people with severe asthma. Sulfites can give off a gas called sulfur dioxide. This gas irritates the lungs and can send an asthmatic into severe bronchospasm, a tightening of the lungs.

The Food and Drug Administration (FDA) has banned sulfites as spray-on preservatives in fresh fruits and vegetables. Sulfites are still used in some foods, however, and occur naturally during the fermentation of wine.

Gluten Intolerance: Gluten intolerance is associated with the disease called "gluten-sensitive enteropathy" or "celiac disease." It happens if your immune system responds abnormally to gluten, which is a part of wheat and some other grains. Some researchers include celiac disease as a food allergy. This abnormal immune system response, however, does not involve IgE antibody.

Psychological Causes: Some people may have a food intolerance that has a psychological trigger. If your food intolerance is caused by this type of trigger, a careful psychiatric evaluation may identify an unpleasant event in your life, often during childhood, tied to eating a particular food. Eating that food years later, even as an adult, is associated with a rush of unpleasant sensations.

Other Causes: There are several other conditions, including ulcers and cancers of the GI tract, that cause some of the same symptoms as food allergy. These symptoms include vomiting, diarrhea, and cramping abdominal pain made worse by eating.

Diagnosis

After ruling out food intolerances and other health problems, your health care provider will use several steps to find out if you have an allergy to specific foods.

Detailed History: A detailed history is the most valuable tool for diagnosing food allergy. Your provider will ask you several questions and listen to your history of food reactions to decide if the facts fit a food allergy.

- What was the timing of your reaction?
- Did your reaction come on quickly, usually within an hour after eating the food?
- Did allergy medicines help? Antihistamines should relieve hives, for example.
- Is your reaction always associated with a certain food?
- Did anyone else who ate the same food get sick? For example, if you ate fish contaminated with histamine, everyone who ate the fish should be sick.
- How much did you eat before you had a reaction? The severity of a reaction is sometimes related to the amount of food eaten.
- How was the food prepared? Some people will have a violent allergic reaction only to raw or undercooked fish. Complete cooking of the fish may destroy the allergen, and they can then eat it with no allergic reaction.
- Did you eat other foods at the same time you had the reaction? Some foods may delay digestion and thus delay the start of the allergic reaction.

Diet Diary: Sometimes your health care provider can't make a diagnosis solely on the basis of your history. In that case, you may be asked to record what you eat and whether you have a reaction. This diet diary gives more detail from which you and your provider can see if there is a consistent pattern in your reactions.

Elimination Diet: The next step some health care providers use is an elimination diet. In this step, which is done under your provider's direction, certain foods are removed from your diet. You don't eat a food suspected of causing the allergy, such as eggs. You then substitute another food—in the case of eggs, another source of protein.

Your provider can almost always make a diagnosis if the symptoms go away after you remove the food from your diet. The diagnosis is confirmed if you then eat the food and the symptoms come back. You should do this only when the reactions are not significant and only under direction from your health care provider.

Your provider can't use this technique, however, if your reactions are severe or don't happen often. If you have a severe reaction, you should not eat the food again.

Skin Test: If your history, diet diary, or elimination diet suggests a specific food allergy is likely, your health care provider will then use either the scratch or the prick skin test to confirm the diagnosis.

During a scratch skin test, your health care provider will place an extract of the food on the skin of your lower arm. Your provider will then scratch this portion of your skin with a needle and look for swelling or redness, which would be a sign of a local allergic reaction.

A prick skin test is done by putting a needle just below the surface of your skin of the lower arm. Then, a tiny amount of food extract is placed under the skin.

If the scratch or prick test is positive, it means that there is IgE on the skin's mast cells that is specific to the food being tested. Skin tests are rapid, simple, and relatively safe. You can have a positive skin test to a food allergen, however, without having an allergic reaction to that food. A health care provider diagnoses a food allergy only when someone has a positive skin test to a specific allergen and when the history of reactions suggests an allergy to the same food.

Blood Test: Your health care provider can make a diagnosis by doing a blood test as well. Indeed, if you are extremely allergic and have severe anaphylactic reactions, your provider can't use skin testing because causing an allergic reaction to the skin test could be dangerous. Skin testing also can't be done if you have eczema over a large portion of your body.

Your health care provider may use blood tests such as the RAST (radioallergosorbent test) and newer ones such as the CAP-RAST. Another blood test is called ELISA (enzyme-linked immunosorbent assay). These blood tests measure the presence of food-specific IgE in your blood. The CAP-RAST can measure how much IgE your blood has to a specific food. As with skin testing, positive tests do not necessarily mean you have a food allergy.

Double-Blind Oral Food Challenge: The final method health care providers use to diagnose food allergy is double-blind oral food challenge.

Your health care provider will give you capsules containing individual doses of various foods, some of which are suspected of starting an allergic reaction. Or your provider will mask the suspected food within other foods known not to cause an allergic reaction. You swallow the capsules one at a time or swallow the masked food and are watched to see if a reaction occurs.

In a true double-blind test, your health care provider is also "blinded" (the capsules having been made up by another medical person). In that case your provider does not know which capsule contains the allergen.

The advantage of such a challenge is that if you react only to suspected foods and not to other foods tested, it confirms the diagnosis. The disadvantage is that you cannot be tested this way if you have a history of severe allergic reactions.

In addition, this testing is difficult because it takes a lot of time to perform and many food allergies are difficult to evaluate with this procedure. Consequently, many health care providers do not perform double-blind food challenges.

This type of testing is most commonly used if a health care provider thinks the reaction described is not due to a specific food and wishes to obtain evidence to support this. If your provider finds that your reaction is not due to a specific food, then additional efforts may be used to find the real cause of the reaction.

Controversial and Unproven Diagnostic Methods

Cytotoxicity Testing: One controversial diagnostic technique is cytotoxicity testing, in which a food allergen is added to a blood sample. A technician then examines the sample under the microscope to see if white cells in the blood "die." Scientists have evaluated this technique in several studies and have found it does not effectively diagnose food allergy.

Provocative Challenge: Another controversial approach is called sublingual (placed under the tongue) or subcutaneous (injected under the skin) provocative challenge. In this procedure, diluted food allergen is put under your tongue if you feel that your arthritis, for instance, is due to foods. The technician then asks you if the food allergen has made your arthritis symptoms worse. In clinical studies, researchers have not shown that this procedure can effectively diagnose food allergy.

Sublingual provocative challenge is not the same as a potentially new treatment for food allergy called sublingual immunotherapy, or SLIT. Researchers are currently evaluating this treatment.

Immune Complex Assay: An immune complex assay is sometimes done on people suspected of having food allergies to see if groups, or complexes, of certain antibodies connect to the food allergen in the bloodstream. Some think that these immune groups link with food allergies. The formation of such immune complexes is a normal offshoot of food digestion, however, and everyone, if tested with a sensitive-enough measurement, has them. To date, no one has conclusively shown that this test links with allergies to foods.

IgG Subclass Assay: Another test is the immunoglobulin G (IgG) subclass assay, which looks specifically for certain kinds of IgG antibody. Again, there is no evidence that this diagnoses food allergy.

Treatment

Food allergy is treated by avoiding the foods that trigger the reaction. Once you and your health care provider have identified the food(s) to which you are sensitive, you must remove them from your diet. To do this, you must read the detailed ingredient lists on each food you consider eating.

Many allergy-producing foods such as peanuts, eggs, and milk appear in foods one normally would not associate them with. Peanuts, for example, may be used as a protein source, and eggs are used in some salad dressings.

Because of a new law in the United States, FDA now requires ingredients in a packaged food to appear on its label. You can avoid most of the things to which you are sensitive if you read food labels carefully and avoid restaurant-prepared foods that might have ingredients to which you are allergic.

If you are highly allergic, even the tiniest amounts of a food allergen (for example, a small portion of a peanut kernel) can prompt an allergic reaction.

If you have food allergies, you must be prepared to treat unintentional exposure. Even people who know a lot about what they are sensitive to occasionally make a mistake. To protect yourself if you have had allergic reactions to a food, you should take the following precautions:

- Wear a medical alert bracelet or necklace stating that you have a food allergy and are subject to severe reactions.
- Carry an autoinjector device containing epinephrine (adrenaline), such as an EpiPen or Twinject, that you can get by prescription and give to yourself if you think you are getting a food allergic reaction.
- Seek medical help immediately, even if you have already given yourself epinephrine, by either calling the rescue squad or by getting transported to an emergency room.

Anaphylactic allergic reactions can be fatal even when they start off with mild symptoms such as a tingling in the mouth and throat or gastrointestinal discomfort.

Exercise-Induced Food Allergy

At least one situation may require more than simply eating food with allergens to start a reaction: exercise-induced food allergy. People who have this reaction only experience it after eating a specific food before exercising. Some people get this reaction from many foods, and others get it only after eating a specific food. As exercise increases and body temperature rises, itching and light-headedness start; allergic reactions such as hives may appear and even anaphylaxis may develop.

The management of exercised-induced food allergy is simple—avoid eating for a few hours before exercising.

Childcare Concerns

Schools and day care centers must have plans in place to address any food allergy emergency. Parents and caregivers should take special care with children and learn how to do the following:

- Protect children from foods to which they are allergic
- Manage children if they eat a food to which they are allergic
- Give children epinephrine

Simply washing your hands with soap and water will remove peanut allergens. Also, most household cleaners will remove them from surfaces such as food preparation areas at home, as well as at day care facilities and schools. These easy-to-do measures will help prevent peanut allergy reactions in children and adults.

There are several medicines you can take to relieve food allergy symptoms that are not part of an anaphylactic reaction:

- Antihistamines to relieve GI symptoms, hives, or sneezing and a runny nose
- Bronchodilators to relieve asthma symptoms

It is not easy to determine if a reaction to food is anaphylactic. It is important to develop a plan with a health care provider as to what reactions you should treat with epinephrine first, rather than antihistamines or bronchodilators.

Controversial and Unproven Treatments

One controversial treatment, which sometimes may be used with provocative challenge, includes putting a diluted solution of a particular food under your tongue about a half-hour before you eat the food suspected of causing an allergic reaction. This is an attempt to "neutralize" the subsequent exposure to the food you believe is harmful. The results of carefully conducted clinical research show this procedure does not prevent an allergic reaction.

Allergy Shots: Another unproven treatment involves getting allergy shots (immunotherapy) containing small quantities of the food extracts to which you are allergic. These shots are given regularly for a long period of time with the aim of "desensitizing" you to the food allergen. Researchers have not yet proven that allergy shots reliably relieve food allergies.

Chapter 33

Common Chemical Contaminants in the Food Supply

Chapter Contents

Section 33.1

Persistent Organic Pollutants (POPs)

This section excerpted from "Nowhere to Hide: Persistent Toxic Chemicals in the U.S. Food Supply," by Kristin S. Schafer and Susan E. Kegley of Pesticide Action Network North America, and Sharyle Patton of Commonweal. © 2001 Pesticide Action Network North America (www.panna.org). Reprinted with permission. The complete text of this report including references is available at http://www.panna.org/files/nowhereToHide.pdf. Reviewed by David A. Cooke, MD, FACP, June 2009.

Persistent Toxic Chemicals, the Food Supply, and the Global POPs Treaty

A class of toxic chemicals known as persistent organic pollutants (POPs) are among the most dangerous compounds ever produced. This ubiquitous class of chemicals includes many pesticides, industrial chemicals, and by-products of certain manufacturing processes and waste incineration. The characteristics that make these chemicals unique also make them an urgent global environmental health problem:

- POPs persist in the environment.
- POPs build up in body fat and concentrate at higher levels (bioaccumulate) as they make their way up the food chain.
- POPs travel in global air and water currents.
- POPs are linked with serious health effects in humans and other living organisms.

In just a few decades, POPs have spread throughout the environment to threaten human health and to damage land and water ecosystems all over the world. All living organisms on Earth now carry measurable levels of POPs in their tissues. POPs have been found in sea mammals at levels high enough to qualify their bodies as hazardous waste under U.S. law. Nor are humans immune to contamination. Evidence of POPs contamination in human blood and breast milk has been documented worldwide.

There is strong evidence that exposure to even miniscule amounts of POPs at critical periods of development—particularly in the womb—can cause irreversible damage. The effects of such exposures may take years to develop, sometimes appearing first in the offspring of exposed parents. Some of the human health effects now linked to POPs exposure include cancer, learning disorders, impaired immune function, reproductive problems (e.g., low sperm counts, endometriosis), and diabetes.

Despite their hazards, these chemicals continue to be produced, used, and stored in many countries. Even where national bans or other controls exist, these restrictions are often poorly enforced—and in any case, they cannot protect citizens from exposure to POPs that have migrated from other regions where the chemicals are still in use.

Because they are persistent and continue to be produced and released into the global environment, even POPs already banned in the United States, such as DDT [dichlorodiphenyltrichloroethane] and PCBs [polychlorinated biphenyls], make their way into the U.S. food supply. Once in the air, the water, and the soil, these chemicals resist breaking down. Some have half-lives measured in decades, and they remain in water and soil as well as plants and animals that ultimately, in one form or another, provide food for humans. POPs that were once particles in the sediment of a riverbed, in soil, or in grasses find their way into the fatty tissue and milk of livestock or into the vegetables that pull POPs from the soil in the same way they take in nutrients.

It is no surprise, therefore, that POPs are pervasive in store-bought food as well as in fish and wildlife consumed after being caught in the wild. This presence of POPs in the food supply creates a compelling and urgent need for action to prevent further release and buildup of these dangerous chemicals.

The Global POPs Treaty

Recognizing that the health risks from POPs can neither be managed by individual countries' regulators nor contained by national borders, the United Nations Environment Programme sponsored an international agreement to phase out production, use, and release of POPs. Twelve POPs have been identified as initial phaseout targets under the new treaty. This list includes nine organochlorine pesticides and three industrial chemicals/ byproducts (see Table 33.1). The global POPs treaty is a promising vehicle for addressing POPs accumulation in the U.S. food supply.

The nine pesticides on this initial list have been banned or severely restricted in the United States since the 1970s and 1980s. Most industrialized countries and many developing countries also have banned or restricted the use of these pesticides. It is important to note that while other POPs pesticides are present in the U.S. food supply, the focus of this section is limited to the initial list of chemicals targeted under the POPs treaty. The treaty includes provisions for adding additional POPs chemicals in the future.

Table 33.1. Twelve POPs Targeted for Global Ban

Pesticides		Industrial Toxins and By-Products
Aldrin	Heptachlor	PCBs
Chlordane	Hexachloro-benzene	Furans
Endrin	Mirex	Dioxins
DDT	Toxaphene	
Dieldrin		

PCBs also have been banned in most industrialized countries since the late 1970s. Large quantities, however, remain in storage in many countries, including the United States. PCBs also are still permitted in some closed electrical systems and can be found in old transformers, fluorescent lighting fixtures, and other appliances. Used primarily as coolants and lubricants in electrical transformers and other equipment, this group of chlorinated industrial chemicals is highly toxic to both wildlife and humans. PCBs are stable and persistent, and there is evidence that they have been transported thousands of kilometers in the atmosphere. PCBs are the chemicals that most frequently cause government warnings (advisories) against consumption of fish and wildlife in the United States.

Dioxins and furans are by-products of chlorine-based industrial processes and incineration. Primary sources include the bleaching of paper products, manufacture of chlorinated chemicals, and the burning of hospital, hazardous, and municipal waste. Dioxins are known to be toxic at extremely low levels. The EPA [Environmental Protection Agency] has called one form of dioxin the most potent synthetic carcinogen ever found. Like many POPs, dioxin is also a known endocrine disruptor, mimicking hormones such as estrogen to cause permanent hormonal and metabolic changes in humans and other animals. A recent report documented dioxins in the Arctic environment and linked them to key emissions sources in the United States.

While some POPs have been banned or restricted, they continue to circulate in the global environment at levels of concern. This is due both to the persistence of these chemicals and continued use in some countries. Dioxins continue to be released as by-products of production and waste disposal processes worldwide, adding to the chemical burden of populations around the globe. Rapid ratification and effective implementation of the international treaty is urgently needed to protect present and future generations from POPs-related harm.

How POPs Enter the Food Supply

Worldwide, humans are exposed to persistent toxic chemicals mainly through our food supply. In the United States, POPs enter the human diet in several ways.

Waterways: When released into rivers, lakes, and oceans, POPs collect in sediments. Away from light and oxygen, these pesticides degrade slowly and are ingested with sediments by small invertebrates at the bottom of the food chain. Once inside the organism, POPs accumulate in fatty tissues. Fish that eat pesticide-contaminated invertebrates accumulate more of the chemical with each shrimp or insect they ingest. A large, mature fish is likely to contain much higher pesticide residues because it has eaten more contaminated food over time than a younger fish. The highest concentrations of these persistent, bioaccumulating chemicals are found in those animals at the top of the food chain—humans, predatory birds, seals, and other predatory animals.

Deposition on Land: POPs are deposited on U.S. soil through a well-documented process of transport by air currents and storm systems—sometimes over great distances—and deposition through contact with solid surfaces or through precipitation. For example, dioxin released from an incinerator could be deposited in either a nearby or distant pasture where grazing cattle consume the chemical. The ingested dioxin then contaminates the milk and fatty tissue of the meat consumed by humans. It also can become incorporated in the fatty tissue of nursing calves, including those destined for veal production. By the time the dioxin makes its way into the bodies of consumers, it will have bioaccumulated to much higher levels than originally deposited on the grass.

Banned Pesticides in Soils: Persistent soil residues of POPs pesticides that have been banned for decades provide another primary source of POPs in the food supply. DDT and its breakdown products, as well as dieldrin and other organochlorine chemicals, continue to be taken up by crops grown in soil contaminated by heavy pesticide use in the 1960s and 1970s. These soil-borne POPs residues also are taken up in pastures and crops used as feed for livestock and make their way to consumers through livestock food products.

Pesticides Used to Produce Imported Foods: POPs pesticide residues also are found in produce imported from countries where the pesticides are still in use or were recently banned. There is no clear evidence, however, that imported produce has more POPs residues than fruits and vegetables grown in the United States. In the case of winter squash, for example, dieldrin was found in 35% of the domestically produced samples, and found in only 4.2% of the samples from Mexico. Moreover, the residue levels were significantly higher in the U.S. squash. In the case of carrots, in contrast, DDT was found in 75% of Canadian samples taken, but only found in 6.4% of the U.S.-grown carrots tested. While the data on imported POPs residues collected through USDA's [United States Department of Agriculture] pesticide data program is not comprehensive, the samples collected clearly illustrate that contamination levels depend on a range of variables. U.S. consumers cannot assume that domestically produced fruits and vegetables are less contaminated with POPs than imported produce.

Persistent Toxic Chemicals Pervade the U.S. Food Supply

Overview of Findings

Evaluation of POPs residue data from several government and university sources produced startling results. Residues of five or more persistent toxic chemicals per food product are not unusual. The most commonly found POPs are dieldrin and DDE [dichlorodiphenyl dichloroethylene]. Dieldrin is a highly persistent and very toxic organochlorine pesticide banned since the late 1970s. DDE is a breakdown product of DDT, which has been banned since 1972.

Residues are found in virtually all food categories—baked goods, fruit, vegetables, meat, poultry, and dairy products are all contaminated with POPs that have been banned in the United States. A typical holiday dinner menu of 11 food items can deliver 38 "hits" of POPs exposure, while hypothetical daily meal plans developed for four U.S. regions can each deliver between 63 and 79 POPs exposures per day. By region, the number of exposures found were as follows:

- Northeast: 64 exposures per day
- Midwest: 63 exposures per day
- Southeast: 70 exposures per day
- West: 66 exposures per day

According to FDA's [Food and Drug Administration] Total Diet Study, POPs residues usually occur at less than 100 parts per billion (i.e., 100 pounds of DDT per billion pounds of food). Scientific data indicate, however, that even these low levels of exposure are cause for concern. Moreover, the daily dietary exposure determined from the data on POPs in food products is at or near the safety thresholds established by various federal agencies (see the following full discussion of the health effects of low-level exposure).

For example, both the U.S. Agency for Toxic Substances and Disease Registry (ATSDR) and the EPA have set the level of concern for exposure to the pesticide dieldrin at 0.05 micrograms per kilogram of body weight per day—a total of 3.5 micrograms of dieldrin per day for a 154 pound (70 kg) adult. This amount of dieldrin represents 0.000000005% of an average adult's body weight, similar to a drop of water in an Olympic-size swimming pool (50 meters x 25 meters x 2 meters).

In the case of dioxin, even smaller levels of exposure are cause for concern. Agency standards for "safe" daily intake of dioxin range from EPA's 0.70 picograms a day for a 154 pound adult[1] to the World Health Organization's 70–280 picograms a day—one picogram is one trillionth of a gram.

According to FDA's food residue data, the average daily exposure to dieldrin through food consumption approaches the health-based "safety" thresholds established by ATSDR and EPA for adults, and it can exceed the standards for children. This illustrates that POPs residues are occurring in food at or near levels understood by federal agencies to be cause for concern.

The threat from POPs in food is greater than this, since dieldrin is only one of the chemicals consumers are exposed to through their daily diet. Americans are exposed to an array of persistent toxic chemicals every day through the foods they eat. Health-based thresholds are established for individual chemicals, while actual diets may include PCB residues in a fish filet, dieldrin in a serving of zucchini, and dioxin in an ice cream cone. Bit by bit, these combinations of chemicals, which in many instances cause the same or similar types of negative health effects, accumulate in daily diets at higher levels.

When it comes to protecting children from POPs, "safe" levels of exposure are even lower. The Food Quality Protection Act of 1996 recognized that children are not simply small adults. Following recommendations of an influential National Academy of Sciences study, the law requires EPA to take into consideration the factors that make children uniquely vulnerable to the risks posed by pesticides in the food supply. Children eat disproportionately more of certain foods on a pound-for-pound body weight basis than does an average-weight adult male. For heavily consumed foods, their smaller size means children have a proportionately greater exposure to POPs from those food products. In addition, young children's bodies are engaged in a multitude of developmental processes that are uniquely susceptible to harm from POPs. Proportionately larger exposures and unique susceptibilities combine to make developing children much more vulnerable to POPs than adults.

Top 10 Foods Most Contaminated with Persistent Toxic Chemicals

The foods listed in the following are the 10 foods in FDA's 1999 Total Diet Study found to be most contaminated with residues from POP pesticides and dioxin.

The food products included in the top 10 list are distinguished by their containing residues of at least three, and as many as seven, different POPs at levels higher than those found in other foods. The food items containing three or four POPs have high levels of at least one particularly toxic chemical (e.g., dioxin in meatloaf, chlordane in popcorn). The list reflects contamination from POP pesticides for which FDA has tested and for dioxins, which have been examined by other researchers. Data on the presence of PCBs and furans were not available for this study.

The top 10 POP-contaminated foods, in alphabetical order, are butter, cantaloupe, cucumbers/pickles, meatloaf, peanuts, popcorn, radishes, spinach, summer squash, and winter squash.

1. The EPA's reference dose (RfD) assumes a lifetime of exposure at the level indicated.

Section 33.2

Polychlorinated Biphenyls (PCBs)

"Basic Information: Polychlorinated Biphenyl (PCB)," Environmental Protection Agency (www.epa.gov), December 4, 2008.

PCBs belong to a broad family of man-made organic chemicals known as chlorinated hydrocarbons. PCBs were domestically manufactured from 1929 until their manufacture was banned in 1979. They have a range of toxicity and vary in consistency from thin, light-colored liquids to yellow or black waxy solids. Due to their nonflammability, chemical stability, high boiling point, and electrical insulating properties, PCBs were used in hundreds of industrial and commercial applications including electrical, heat transfer, and hydraulic equipment; as plasticizers in paints, plastics, and rubber products; in pigments, dyes, and carbonless copy paper; and many other industrial applications.

Release and Exposure of PCBs

Prior to the 1979 ban, PCBs entered the environment during their manufacture and use in the United States. Today PCBs can still be released into the environment from poorly maintained hazardous waste sites that contain PCBs, illegal or improper dumping of PCB wastes, leaks or releases from electrical transformers containing PCBs, and disposal of PCB-containing consumer products into municipal or other landfills not designed to handle hazardous waste. PCBs may also be released into the environment by the burning of some wastes in municipal and industrial incinerators.

Once in the environment, PCBs do not readily break down and therefore may remain for long periods of time cycling between air, water, and soil. PCBs can be carried long distances and have been found in snow and sea water in areas far away from where they were released into the environment. As a consequence, PCBs are found all over the world. In general, the lighter the form of PCB, the further it can be transported from the source of contamination.

PCBs can accumulate in the leaves and above-ground parts of plants and food crops. They are also taken up into the bodies of small organisms and fish. As a result, people who ingest fish may be exposed to PCBs that have bioaccumulated in the fish they are ingesting.

Health Effects of PCBs

PCBs have been demonstrated to cause a variety of adverse health effects. PCBs have been shown to cause cancer in animals. PCBs have also been shown to cause a number of serious noncancer health effects in animals, including effects on the immune system, reproductive system, nervous system, endocrine system, and other health effects. Studies in humans provide supportive evidence for potential carcinogenic and noncarcinogenic effects of PCBs. The different health effects of PCBs may be interrelated, as alterations in one system may have significant implications for the other systems of the body. The potential health effects of PCB exposure are discussed in greater detail in the following.

Cancer

EPA uses a weight-of-evidence approach in evaluating the potential carcinogenicity of environmental contaminants. EPA's approach permits evaluation of the complete carcinogenicity database, and allows the results of individual studies to be viewed in the context of all of the other available studies. Studies in animals provide conclusive evidence that PCBs cause cancer. Studies in humans raise further concerns regarding the potential carcinogenicity of PCBs. Taken together, the data strongly suggest that PCBs are probable human carcinogens.

PCBs are one of the most widely studied environmental contaminants, and many studies in animals and human populations have been performed to assess the potential carcinogenicity of PCBs. EPA's first assessment of PCB carcinogenicity was completed in 1987. At that time, data were limited to Aroclor 1260. In 1996, at the direction of Congress, EPA completed a reassessment of PCB carcinogenicity, titled "PCBs: Cancer Dose-Response Assessment and Application to Environmental Mixtures" (www.epa.gov/epawaste/hazard/tsd/pcbs/pubs/pcb.pdf). In addition to Aroclor 1260, new studies provided data on Aroclors 1016, 1242, and 1254. EPA's cancer reassessment reflected the agency's commitment to the use of the best science in evaluating health effects of PCBs. EPA's cancer reassessment was peer reviewed by 15 experts on PCBs, including scientists from government, academia, and industry. The peer reviewers agreed with EPA's conclusion that PCBs are probable human carcinogens.

The cancer reassessment determined that PCBs are probable human carcinogens, based on the following information:

There is clear evidence that PCBs cause cancer in animals. EPA reviewed all of the available literature on the carcinogenicity of PCBs in animals as an important first step in the cancer reassessment. An industry scientist commented that "all significant studies have been reviewed and are fairly represented in the document." The literature presents overwhelming evidence that PCBs cause cancer in animals. An industry-sponsored peer-reviewed rat study, characterized as the "gold standard study" by one peer reviewer, demonstrated that every commercial PCB mixture tested caused cancer. The new studies reviewed in the PCB reassessment allowed EPA to develop more accurate potency estimates than previously available for PCBs. The reassessment provided EPA with sufficient information to develop a range of potency estimates for different PCB mixtures, based on the incidence of liver cancer and in consideration of the mobility of PCBs in the environment.

The reassessment resulted in a slightly decreased cancer potency estimate for Aroclor 1260 relative to the 1987 estimate due to the use of additional dose-response information for PCB mixtures and refinements in risk assessment techniques (e.g., use of a different animal-to-human scaling factor for dose). The reassessment concluded that the types of PCBs likely to be bioaccumulated in fish and bound to sediments are the most carcinogenic PCB mixtures.

In addition to the animal studies, a number of epidemiological studies of workers exposed to PCBs have been performed. Results of human studies raise concerns for the potential carcinogenicity of PCBs. Studies of PCB workers found increases in rare liver cancers and malignant melanoma. The presence of cancer in the same target organ (liver) following exposures to PCBs both in animals and in humans and the finding of liver cancers and malignant melanomas across multiple human studies adds weight to the conclusion that PCBs are probable human carcinogens.

Some of the studies in humans have not demonstrated an association between exposures to PCBs and disease. However, epidemiological studies share common methodological limitations that can affect their ability to discern important health effects (or define them as statistically significant) even when they are present. Often, the number of individuals in a study is too small for an effect to be revealed, or there are difficulties in determining actual exposure levels, or there are multiple confounding factors (factors that tend to co-occur with PCB exposure, including smoking, drinking of alcohol, and exposure to other chemicals in the workplace). Epidemiological studies may not be able to detect small increases in cancer over background unless the cancer rate following contaminant exposure is very high or the exposure produces a very unusual type of cancer. However, studies that do not demonstrate an association between exposure to PCBs and disease should not be characterized as negative studies. These studies are most appropriately viewed as inconclusive. Limited studies that produce inconclusive findings for cancer in humans do not mean that PCBs are safe.

It is very important to note that the composition of PCB mixtures changes following their release into the environment. The types of PCBs that tend to bioaccumulate in fish and other animals and bind to sediments happen to be the most carcinogenic components of PCB mixtures. As a result, people who ingest PCB-contaminated fish or other animal products and contact PCB-contaminated sediment may be exposed to PCB mixtures that are even more toxic than the PCB mixtures contacted by workers and released into the environment.

EPA's peer-reviewed cancer reassessment concluded that PCBs are probable human carcinogens. EPA is not alone in its conclusions regarding PCBs. The International Agency for Research on Cancer has declared PCBs to be probably carcinogenic to humans. The National Toxicology Program has stated that it is reasonable to conclude that PCBs are carcinogenic in humans. The National Institute for Occupational Safety and Health has determined that PCBs are a potential occupational carcinogen.

Noncancer Effects

EPA evaluates all of the available data in determining the potential noncarcinogenic toxicity of environmental contaminants, including PCBs. Extensive study has been conducted in animals, including nonhuman primates using environmentally relevant doses. EPA has found clear evidence that PCBs have significant toxic effects in animals, including effects on the immune system, the reproductive system, the nervous system, and the endocrine system. The body's regulation of all of these systems is complex and interrelated. As a result, it is not surprising that PCBs can exert a multitude of serious adverse health effects. A discussion of the potential noncancer health effects of PCBs is presented here.

Immune Effects: The immune system is critical for fighting infections, and diseases of the immune system have very serious potential implications for the health of humans and animals. The immune effects of PCB exposure have been studied in rhesus monkeys and other animals. It is important to note that the immune systems of rhesus monkeys and humans are very similar. Studies in monkeys and other animals have revealed a number of serious effects on the immune system following exposures to PCBs, including a significant decrease in size of the thymus gland (which is critical to the immune system) in infant monkeys, reductions in the response of the immune system following a challenge with sheep red blood cells (a standard laboratory test that determines the ability of an animal to mount a primary antibody response and develop protective immunity), and decreased resistance to Epstein-Barr virus and other infections in PCB-exposed animals. Individuals with diseases of the immune system may be more susceptible to pneumonia and viral infections. The animal studies were not able to identify a level of PCB exposure that did not cause effects on the immune system.

In humans, a recent study found that individuals infected with Epstein-Barr virus had a greater association of increased exposures to PCBs with increasing risk of non-Hodgkin lymphoma than those who had no Epstein-Barr infection. This finding is consistent with increases in infection with Epstein-Barr virus in animals exposed to PCBs. Since PCBs suppress the immune system and immune system suppression has been demonstrated as a risk factor for non-Hodgkin lymphoma, suppression of the immune system is a possible mechanism for PCB-induced cancer. Immune effects were also noted in humans who experienced exposure to rice oil contaminated with PCBs, dibenzofurans, and dioxins.

Taken together, the studies in animals and humans suggest that PCBs may have serious potential effects on the immune systems of exposed individuals.

Reproductive Effects: Reproductive effects of PCBs have been studied in a variety of animal species, including rhesus monkeys, rats, mice, and mink. Rhesus monkeys are generally regarded as the best laboratory species for predicting adverse reproductive effects in humans. Potentially serious effects on the reproductive system were seen in monkeys and a number of other animal species following exposures to PCB mixtures. Most significantly, PCB exposures were found to reduce the birth weight, conception rates, and live birth rates of monkeys and other species and PCB exposure reduced sperm counts in rats. Effects in monkeys were long lasting and were observed long after the dosing with PCBs occurred.

Studies of reproductive effects have also been carried out in human populations exposed to PCBs. Children born to women who worked with PCBs in factories showed decreased birth weight and a significant decrease in gestational age with increasing exposures to PCBs. Studies in fishing populations believed to have high exposures to PCBs also suggest similar decreases. This same effect was seen in multiple species of animals exposed to PCBs, and suggests that reproductive effects may be important in humans following exposures to PCBs.

Neurological Effects: Proper development of the nervous system is critical for early learning and can have potentially significant implications for the health of individuals throughout their lifetimes. Effects of PCBs on nervous system development have been studied in monkeys and a variety of other animal species. Newborn monkeys exposed to PCBs showed persistent and significant deficits in neurological development, including visual recognition, short-term memory, and learning. Some of these studies were conducted using the types of PCBs most commonly found in human breast milk.

Studies in humans have suggested effects similar to those observed in monkeys exposed to PCBs, including learning deficits and changes in activity associated with exposures to PCBs. The similarity in effects observed in humans and animals provide additional support for the potential neurobehavioral effects of PCBs.

Endocrine Effects: There has been significant discussion and research on the effects of environmental contaminants on the endocrine system ("endocrine disruption"). While the significance of endocrine disruption as a widespread issue in humans and animals is a subject of ongoing study, PCBs have been demonstrated to exert effects on thyroid hormone levels in animals and humans. Thyroid hormone levels are critical for normal growth and development, and alterations in thyroid hormone levels may have significant implications.

It has been shown that PCBs decrease thyroid hormone levels in rodents, and that these decreases have resulted in developmental deficits in the animals, including deficits in hearing. PCB exposures have also been associated with changes in thyroid hormone levels in infants in studies conducted in the Netherlands and Japan. Additional research will be required to determine the significance of these effects in the human population.

Other Noncancer Effects: A variety of other noncancer effects of PCBs have been reported in animals and humans, including dermal and ocular effects in monkeys and humans, and liver toxicity in rodents. Elevations in blood pressure, serum triglyceride, and serum cholesterol have also been reported with increasing serum levels of PCBs in humans.

In summary, PCBs have been demonstrated to cause a variety of serious health effects. PCBs have been shown to cause cancer and a number of serious noncancer health effects in animals, including effects on the immune system, reproductive system, nervous system, and endocrine system. Studies in humans provide supportive evidence for the potential carcinogenicity and noncarcinogenic effects of PCBs. The different health effects of PCBs may be interrelated, as alterations in one system may have significant implications for the other regulatory systems of the body.

Section 33.3

Dioxins (Furan)

This section excerpted from "Questions and Answers about Dioxins," Food and Drug Administration (www.fda.gov), September 2008.

What are dioxins?

"Dioxins" refers to a group of chemical compounds that share certain chemical structures and biological characteristics. Several hundred of these compounds exist and are members of three closely related families: the chlorinated dibenzo-p-dioxins (CDDs), chlorinated dibenzofurans (CDFs), and certain PCBs. Sometimes the term dioxin is also used to refer to the most studied and one of the most toxic dioxins, 2,3,7,8-tetrachlorodibenzo-p-dioxin (TCDD). CDDs and CDFs are not created intentionally, but are produced as a result of human activities. Natural processes also produce CDDs and CDFs. PCBs are manufactured products, but they are no longer produced in the United States.

Dioxins are formed as a result of combustion processes such as commercial or municipal waste incineration and from burning fuels (like wood, coal, or oil). The 2003 draft dioxin reassessment makes the finding that anthropogenic (man-made) emissions dominate current releases in the United States, but acknowledges the need for more data on natural sources. Dioxins can also be formed when household trash is burned and as a result of natural processes such as forest fires. Chlorine bleaching of pulp and paper, certain types of chemical manufacturing and processing, and other industrial processes all can create small quantities of dioxins. Cigarette smoke also contains small amounts of dioxins.

Over the past decade, EPA and industry have worked together to dramatically reduce dioxin emissions. It is important to note that dioxin levels in the United States environment have been declining for the last 30 years due to reductions in man-made sources. However, dioxins break down so slowly that some of the dioxins from past releases will still be in the environment many years from now. Because dioxins are extremely persistent compounds, past releases of dioxins from both man-made and natural sources still exist in the environment. A large part of the current exposures to dioxins in the United States is due to release of man-made dioxins that occurred decades ago. Even if all human-generated dioxins were eliminated, low levels of naturally produced dioxins will remain. EPA is working with other parts of the government to look for ways to further reduce dioxin levels entering the environment and to reduce human exposure to them.

Why are people concerned about dioxins?

Dioxins from natural and anthropogenic (man-made) sources have been widely distributed throughout the environment. Almost every living creature has been exposed to dioxins. Studies have shown that exposure to dioxins at high enough doses may cause a number of adverse health effects. The health effects associated with dioxins depend on a variety of factors including the following: the level of exposure, when someone was exposed, and for how long and how often. Because dioxins are so widespread, we all have some level of dioxins in our bodies.

The most common health effect in people exposed to large amounts of dioxin is chloracne. Chloracne cases have typically been the result of accidents or significant contamination events. Chloracne is a severe skin disease with acne-like lesions that occur mainly on the face and upper body. Other effects of exposure to large amounts of dioxin include skin rashes, skin discoloration, excessive body hair, and possibly mild liver damage.

One of the main concerns over health effects from dioxins is the risk of cancer in adults. Several studies suggest that workers exposed to high levels of dioxins at their workplace over many years have an increased risk of cancer. Animal studies have also shown an increased risk of cancer from long-term exposure to dioxins.

Finally, based on data from animal studies, there is some concern that exposure to low levels of dioxins over long periods (or high-level exposures at sensitive times) might result in reproductive or developmental effects.

What happens to dioxins when they enter the environment?

When released into the air, some dioxins may be transported long distances. Because of this, dioxins are found in most places in the world. When dioxins are released into water, they tend to settle into sediments where they can be further transported or ingested by fish and other aquatic organisms. Dioxins decompose very slowly in the environment and can be deposited on plants and taken up by animals and aquatic organisms. Dioxins may be concentrated in the food chain so that animals have higher concentrations than plants, water, soil, or sediments. Within animals, dioxins tend to accumulate in fat.

Have we made progress in reducing environmental dioxins?

Yes. Dioxin levels in the United States environment have been declining for the last 30 years due to reductions in man-made sources. In fact, as a result of the efforts of EPA, state governments, and industry, known and quantifiable industrial emissions of dioxin in the United States have been reduced by more than 90% from 1987 levels. However, dioxins break down so slowly that some of the dioxins from past releases will still be in the environment many years from now. Dioxins that remain in the environment from past releases are sometimes called "reservoir sources" of dioxins. Because of processes in the natural environment, dioxin levels will never go to zero.

Based on recent measurements in a few states, it appears that levels in our bodies are declining. Federal agencies are continuing to monitor to see if these trends continue. Again, because of background occurrence of dioxin in the environment, the levels will probably never go to zero.

What is meant by "natural background" and "current background" for dioxins?

In addition to man-made sources, natural processes, such as brush and forest fires, produce dioxins. The term "natural background" for dioxins refers to the dioxins that are in the environment because of these natural processes. The natural background level of dioxins cannot be directly measured. The term "current background" refers to the level of dioxin in the environment today. Current background is primarily made up of dioxins from man-made sources.

What are the major sources of dioxins?

The amounts of dioxin released from various sources have changed significantly over time. Historically, commercial or municipal waste incineration, manufacture and use of certain herbicides, and chlorine bleaching of pulp and paper resulted in the major releases of dioxins to air and water. Government regulatory actions along with voluntary industry actions have resulted in dramatic reductions in each of these sources, and they are no longer major contributors of dioxins to the environment in the United States. While the United States has taken action to control this type of emission, some of these sources of dioxin still occur elsewhere in the world. Currently, the uncontrolled burning of residential waste is thought to be the largest sources of dioxins to the environment in the United States.

What is EPA doing to control dioxin releases into the environment?

Over the past few decades, EPA has aggressively looked for ways to reduce and control dioxins in the environment in the United States. Collectively, these actions have resulted in strict controls on all of the known and quantifiable major industrial sources of dioxin releases. As a result of EPA's efforts, along with efforts by state governments and private industry, known and quantifiable industrial emissions in the United States have been reduced by more than 90% from 1987 levels. For example, municipal waste combustors are estimated to have emitted collectively nearly 18 pounds of dioxin toxic equivalents in 1987, but under EPA regulations they are now expected to emit less than 1/2 ounce per year. Similarly, medical waste incinerators emitted about five pounds of dioxin equivalents in 1987, but under EPA regulations they now will be limited to about 1/4 ounce annual emissions. EPA has implemented similarly strict standards for other dioxin sources. Through expanded monitoring and research collaboration with the FDA, the Food Safety and Inspection Service (FSIS), and the Centers for Disease Control and Prevention (CDC), EPA is also making progress in characterizing additional sources.

Should I (or can I) find out what my dioxin levels are?

We do not recommend dioxin testing. Tests for measuring dioxin levels in humans are not routinely available. Laboratories that offer dioxin testing generally do not have the required certification for medical testing. A person's individual dioxin level is not helpful for predicting or screening disease.

How can I reduce my personal dioxin levels?

We all have some levels of dioxins in our bodies. Dioxins have existed in our environment for a long time. Environmental dioxins have declined significantly since 1987 and recent measurements in a few states indicate that levels in our bodies are going down as well. Unfortunately, there are no safe and effective treatments to rid dioxins now in humans. Dioxins metabolize slowly over years. The best way to reduce your personal dioxins level and your potential risks from dioxins is to reduce exposure and intake of dioxins.

Although dioxins are an environmental contaminant, exposure most often occurs through food by consumption of animal fats. Overall, the best strategy for lowering the risk of dioxins while maintaining the benefits of a good diet is to follow the recommendations in the Federal Dietary Guidelines. For most people, following Federal Dietary Guidelines will reduce fat consumption and, consequently, reduce dioxin exposure. The dietary guidelines provide for moderate amounts of fats, which are part of a balanced diet. However, eliminating all fats is not recommended. See the following section for information on preparing and selecting foods.

Should I stop eating particular foods?

No, we do not recommend avoiding particular foods because of dioxins. The EPA's 2003 draft dioxin reassessment indicates that following the science-based advice in the Dietary Guidelines for Americans will also likely help individuals lower their risk of exposure to dioxins. These guidelines include the recommendations to choose meat and dairy products that are lean, low fat, or fat free and to increase consumption of fruits, vegetables, and whole grain products. Meat, milk, and fish are important sources of nutrients for the American public and an appropriate part of a balanced diet. Milk is a major source of calcium, vitamins A and D, and riboflavin; meat is an important source of iron, zinc, and several B vitamins; fish provides beneficial fatty acids as well as certain vitamins and minerals. Each of these foods provides high quality protein in the diet. Lean meat includes meats that are naturally lower in fat, and meat where visible fat has been trimmed. For fish and poultry you can reduce fat by removing the skin. Reducing the amount of butter or lard used in the preparation of foods and cooking methods that reduce fat (such as oven broiling) will also lower the risk of exposure to dioxin. These strategies help lower the intake of saturated fats as well as reduce the risk of exposure to dioxin. Similarly, the 2003 NAS [National Academy of Sciences] report titled "Dioxins and Dioxin-like Compounds in the Food Supply: Strategies to Decrease Exposure" identified options to be considered to reduce dioxin exposure through food-consumption pathways. One of these options was promoting changes in dietary consumption patterns of the general population that more closely conform to recommendations to reduce consumption of animal fats, such as the recommendations of the Dietary Guidelines for Americans. For information on the Federal Dietary Guidelines see www.health.gov/dietaryguidelines/.

You should also pay attention to local fishing advisories for fish that you catch yourself. Fishing advisories may exist that provide recommended consumption rates of particular kinds of fish from particular water bodies where local contamination has occurred. If you do not know whether a water body that you fish in is covered under a fishing advisory, call your local or state health or environmental protection department and ask for their advice. (They are listed in the blue pages of your local telephone directory.) Ask them if there are advisories on the kinds or sizes of fish that should not be eaten from the water body. You can also ask about fishing advisories at local sporting goods or bait shops where fishing licenses are sold.

Can I cook the dioxins out? Or wash them off?

Good food safety practices like washing food and countertops will reduce risk from bacterial infection, but they cannot reduce dioxin levels. Methods that keep fat at a minimum in the food you eat (such as trimming fat and broiling) may help to reduce dioxin exposure.

Does the government monitor food for dioxins?

The government monitors potential dietary sources of dioxins, primarily foods that contain animal fat. The goal of this monitoring is to find any unusually high dioxin levels in foods and then work to determine the dioxin sources for those high levels so that they can be controlled or eliminated before entering the food supply.

What kinds of foods are tested, how often, and in how many locations?

FDA and USDA [United States Department of Agriculture]'s Food Safety and Inspection Service (FSIS) monitoring has been focused on food products in which there is a greater potential to contain dioxins. In the past, it was more difficult to detect or monitor the low levels of dioxins in foods. Recent improvements in dioxin testing methods have allowed the federal government to expand its monitoring efforts. In addition, feed components have emerged as an important target to predict how animal feed may contribute to the dioxin levels in some foods.

FSIS began to monitor dioxins in domestically produced beef, pork, and poultry products with a survey of each of these products being conducted between 1994 and 1996 (163 total samples). A larger survey of these products was conducted in 2002–2003 (510 total samples). Further, FSIS is in the midst of its current survey of over 500 beef, pork, and poultry samples for dioxins (2007–2008).

Since about 1995, FDA dioxin monitoring has involved several hundred samples a year, primarily of fish and dairy products from grocery stores and distribution centers across the country. To date the FDA monitoring of dairy products and fish shows that when detectable levels are found they are generally consistent with EPA estimates for background occurrence of dioxins.

In 1999, FDA began annual monitoring for dioxins as part of FDA's Total Diet Study (TDS). TDS is a yearly program that determines levels of various pesticide residues, contaminants, and nutrients in foods.

In addition to the TDS samples, FDA conducts additional non-TDS (targeted) sampling of food and animal feed in an effort to gather additional information on dioxin. FDA collected approximately 550 food and feed samples in 2001 and approximately 1,050 food and feed samples in 2002 for dioxin analysis. FDA expanded the program to approximately 1,700 food and feed samples in 2003, 2004, and 2005, and collected and analyzed approximately 1,100 food and feed samples in 2006, 2007, and 2008. FDA plans to include additional analytes (nine dioxin-like and nondioxin-like PCBs congeners) in select samples in 2009.

FDA has posted data for dioxin levels in TDS and non-TDS samples and posted exposure estimates using these results. For more information about FDA's posted data see www.cfsan.fda.gov/~lrd/dioxdata.html. For more information about FDA's TDS see http://www.cfsan.fda.gov/~comm/tds-toc.html.

How do dioxin levels now found in food compare to the incidents of dioxin contamination that have been in the news in previous years?

To date the FDA monitoring of dairy products and fish shows that when detectable levels are found they are generally consistent with EPA estimates for background occurrence of dioxins. It is also important to note that known and quantifiable industrial emissions of dioxins in the United States have been reduced significantly since 1987. In addition, recent measurements from a few states show that dioxin levels in our bodies have also been reduced.

There were, however, two incidents involving dioxin in food in past years that received national and international attention. In both incidents, the dioxin levels were higher than background levels typically seen in foods tested by FDA or FSIS. In the first incident in 1997, elevated levels of dioxins were found in some farm-raised fish and poultry products. The levels in fish, poultry, and eggs during this incident were about 10 times higher than background levels. An investigation was quickly launched by FDA, FSIS, and EPA. That investigation discovered that particular clay from one mine in Mississippi used as an additive to animal feed was responsible for the higher dioxin levels. The clay, which appears to have naturally occurring dioxins, was withdrawn from use as an animal feed ingredient. The government is continuing to monitor these foods and will address any situations identified.

In the second incident in 1999, elevated levels of dioxins were discovered in some Belgian animal products, and the source of the dioxins was traced to animal feeds from a particular source. The U.S. government stopped the import of certain foods from a number of European countries until it could be either established that dioxin-contaminated feeds were not fed to the slaughtered animals, or that food derived from the slaughtered animals did not contain elevated dioxins. The levels of dioxins in this incident were a hundred or more times higher than what the current background levels are in similar foods in the United States.

What is the federal government doing to reduce dioxin levels in food?

Relevant federal agencies have taken a number of actions to reduce dioxin levels in food. EPA has taken aggressive actions to reduce dioxin emissions into the environmental by placing strict regulatory controls on all of the major industrial sources of dioxins. The known, quantifiable industrial emissions have been reduced by more the 90% from their levels in the 1980s as a result of EPA's efforts, along with efforts by state government and private industry.

In the long-term, efforts to reduce dioxin in the environment should also reduce dioxin levels in the food supply. Federal agencies have been monitoring the levels in foods and conducting an investigation whenever a particular food has dioxin levels detected over the background levels in that food. If the investigation determines a specific source of the increased dioxins, the FDA and the FSIS take action to remove that source where practicable.

Given that studies have shown that dioxin is in breast milk, should I nurse my infant?

Yes. Studies consistently show that breastfed infants are healthier than formula-fed infants. This statement is even more relevant now than in the past, when the levels of dioxin in breast milk were higher than they are today.

There are overwhelming benefits of breast-feeding both for the mother and her infant. The American Academy of Pediatrics and many other professional organizations have concluded that the benefits of breast-feeding far outweigh the potential effects of dioxin in breast milk. Breast milk is known to be the most complete form of nutrition for infants, with benefits for infant health, growth, immunity, and development. The benefits of breast-feeding for children include fewer cases and less severity of diarrhea, respiratory infections, ear infections, and meningitis, among others. Breast-feeding may also reduce the risk of sudden infant death syndrome and may lower rates of childhood cancer.

In addition to the benefits for children, breast-feeding also has benefits for mothers. Breast-feeding has been shown to reduce postpartum bleeding, promote earlier return to prepregnancy weight, and reduce the risk of breast cancer.

Chapter 34

Contaminants in Fish and Shellfish

Chapter Contents

Section 34.1

Mercury and PCBs

This section includes excerpts from "Methylmercury in Sport Fish: Information for Fish Consumers," © 2003 California Office of Environmental Health Hazard Assessment, and "PCBs in Sport Fish: Information for Consumers," © 2009 California Office of Environmental Health Hazard Assessment. Reprinted with permission. For the complete text of these documents, visit http://www.oehha.ca.gov/fish.html.

Methylmercury in Sport Fish

Methylmercury is a form of mercury that is found in most freshwater and saltwater fish. The Office of Environmental Health Hazard Assessment (OEHHA) has issued health advisories to fishers and their families giving recommendations on how much of the affected fish in these areas can be safely eaten. In these advisories, women of childbearing age and children are encouraged to be especially careful about following the advice because of the greater sensitivity of fetuses and children to methylmercury.

Fish are nutritious and should be a part of a healthy, balanced diet. As with many other kinds of food, however, it is prudent to consume fish in moderation. OEHHA provides advice to the public so that people can continue to eat fish without putting their health at risk.

Where does methylmercury in fish come from?

Methylmercury in fish comes from mercury in the aquatic environment. Mercury, a metal, is widely found in nature in rock and soil, and is washed into surface waters during storms. Mercury evaporates from rock, soil, and water into the air, and then falls back to the earth in rain, often far from where it started. Human activities redistribute mercury and can increase its concentration in the aquatic environment.

Once mercury gets into water, much of it settles to the bottom where bacteria in the mud or sand convert it to the organic form of methylmercury. Fish absorb methylmercury when they eat smaller aquatic organisms. Larger and older fish absorb more methylmercury as they eat other fish. In this way, the amount of methylmercury builds up as it passes through the food chain. Fish eliminate methylmercury slowly, and so it builds up in fish in much greater concentrations than in the surrounding water. Methylmercury generally reaches the highest levels in predatory fish at the top of the aquatic food chain.

How might I be exposed to methylmercury?

Eating fish is the main way that people are exposed to methylmercury. Each person's exposure depends on the amount of methylmercury in the fish that they eat and how much and how often they eat fish.

Women can pass methylmercury to their babies during pregnancy, and this includes methylmercury that has built up in the mother's body even before pregnancy. For this reason, women of childbearing age are encouraged to be especially careful to follow consumption advice, even if they are not pregnant. In addition, nursing mothers can pass methylmercury to their child through breast milk.

You may be exposed to inorganic forms of mercury through dental amalgams (fillings) or accidental spills, such as from a broken thermometer. For most people, these sources of exposure to mercury are minor and of less concern than exposure to methylmercury in fish.

How does methylmercury affect health?

Much of what we know about methylmercury toxicity in humans stems from several mass poisoning events that occurred in Japan during the 1950s and 1960s, and Iraq during the 1970s. In Japan, a chemical factory discharged vast quantities of mercury into several bays near fishing villages. Many people who consumed large amounts of fish from these bays became seriously ill or died over a period of several years. In Iraq, thousands of people were poisoned by eating contaminated bread that was mistakenly made from seed grain treated with methylmercury.

From studying these cases, researchers have determined that the main target of methylmercury toxicity is the central nervous system. At the highest exposure levels experienced in these poisonings, methylmercury toxicity symptoms included such nervous system effects as loss of coordination, blurred vision or blindness, and hearing and speech impairment. Scientists also discovered that the developing nervous systems of fetuses are particularly sensitive to the toxic effects of methylmercury. In the Japanese outbreak, for example, some fetuses developed methylmercury toxicity during pregnancy even when their mothers did not. Symptoms reported in the Japan and Iraq epidemics resulted from methylmercury levels that were much higher than what fish consumers in the U.S. would experience.

Individual cases of adverse health effects from heavy consumption of commercial fish containing moderate to high levels of methylmercury have been reported only rarely. Nervous system symptoms reported in these instances included headaches, fatigue, blurred vision, tremor, and/or some loss of concentration, coordination, or memory. However, because there was no clear link between the severity of symptoms and the amount of mercury to which the person was exposed, it is not possible to say with certainly that these effects were a consequence of methylmercury exposure and not the result of other health problems. The most subtle symptoms in adults known to be clearly associated with methylmercury toxicity are numbness or tingling in the hands and feet or around the mouth.

In recent studies of high fish-eating populations in different parts of the world, researchers have been able to detect more subtle effects of methylmercury toxicity in children whose mothers frequently ate seafood containing low to moderate mercury concentrations during their pregnancy. Several studies found slight decreases in learning ability, language skills, attention, and/or memory in some of these children. These effects were not obvious without using very specialized and sensitive tests. Children may have increased susceptibility to the effects of methylmercury through adolescence, as the nervous system continues to develop during this time.

Methylmercury builds up in the body if exposure continues to occur over time. Exposure to relatively high doses of methylmercury for a long period of time may also cause problems in other organs such as the kidneys and heart.

Is there a way to reduce methylmercury in fish to make them safer to eat?

There is no specific method of cleaning or cooking fish that will significantly reduce the amount of methylmercury in the fish. However, fish should be cleaned and gutted before cooking because some mercury may be present in the liver and other organs of the fish. These organs should not be eaten.

In the case of methylmercury, fish size is important because large fish that prey upon smaller fish can accumulate more of the chemical in their bodies. It is better to eat the smaller fish within the same species, provided that they are legal size.

Is there a medical test to determine exposure to methylmercury?

Mercury in blood and hair can be measured to assess methylmercury exposure. However, this is not routinely done. Special techniques in sample collection, preparation, and analysis are required for these tests to be accurate. Although tests using hair are less invasive, they are also less accurate. It is important to consult with a physician before undertaking medical testing because these tests alone cannot determine the cause of personal symptoms.

How can I reduce the amount of methylmercury in my body?

Methylmercury is eliminated from the body over time provided that the amount of mercury taken in is reduced. Therefore, following the OEHHA consumption advice and eating less of the fish that have higher levels of mercury can reduce your exposure and help to decrease the levels of methylmercury already in your body if you have not followed these recommendations in the past.

What if I eat fish from other sources such as restaurants, stores, or other water bodies that may not have an advisory?

Most commercial fish have relatively low amounts of methylmercury and can be eaten safely in moderate amounts. However, several types of fish such as large, predatory, long-lived fish have high levels of methylmercury, and could cause overly high exposure to methylmercury if eaten often. The U.S. Food and Drug Administration (FDA) is responsible for the safety of commercial seafood. FDA advises that women who are pregnant or could become pregnant, nursing mothers, and young children not eat shark, swordfish, king mackerel, or tilefish.

FDA also advises that women of childbearing age and pregnant women may eat an average of 12 ounces of fish purchased in stores and restaurants each week. However, if 12 ounces of cooked fish from a store or restaurant are eaten in a given week, then fish caught by family or friends should not be eaten the same week. This is important to keep the total level of methylmercury contributed by all fish at a low level in the body. The FDA advice can be found at www.cfsan.fda.gov/~dms/admehg.html.

The United States Environmental Protection Agency (U.S. EPA) has issued the following advice for women and children who eat fish that are caught in freshwater bodies anywhere in the U.S. This advice should be followed for water bodies where OEHHA has not already issued more restrictive guidelines.

"If you are pregnant or could become pregnant, are nursing a baby, or if you are feeding a young child, limit consumption of freshwater fish caught by family and friends to one meal per week. For adults, one meal is six ounces of cooked fish or eight ounces uncooked fish; for a young child, one meal is two ounces cooked fish or three ounces uncooked fish."

For more information on the nationwide advice, check the U.S. EPA website at www.epa.gov/ost/fishadvice/advice.html.

In addition, OEHHA offers the following general advice that can be followed to reduce exposure to methylmercury in fish. Chemical levels can vary from place to place. Therefore, your overall exposure to chemicals is likely to be lower if you fish at a variety of places, rather than at one location that might have high contamination levels. Furthermore, some fish species have higher chemical levels than others in the same location. If possible, eat smaller amounts of several different types of fish rather than a large amount of one type that may be high in contaminants. Smaller fish of a species will usually have lower chemical levels than larger fish in the same location because some of the chemicals may become more concentrated in larger, older fish. It is advisable to eat smaller fish (of legal size) more often than larger fish. Cleaning and cooking fish in a manner that removes fat and organs is an effective way to reduce other contaminants that may be present in fish.

PCBs in Sport Fish

Polychlorinated biphenyls (PCBs) are a large group of structurally related industrial chemicals known individually as congeners. They are oily liquids or solids, clear to light yellow in color, and have no smell or taste. PCBs are common contaminants in fish in many parts of the world. High levels of PCBs in fish may pose a health threat to frequent fish consumers. OEHHA has issued health advisories to fishers and their families with recommendations on how much fish can be eaten safely in areas where PCBs are found.

Where do PCBs come from?

PCBs were manufactured in the United States beginning around 1930 for use as coolants in electrical transformers and capacitors, and as hydraulic fluids, lubricating and cutting oils, and plasticizers. They were banned for most uses by the Toxic Substances Control Act of

1976. Although they are no longer manufactured in significant quantities in the United States, PCBs still occur in the environment as a result of accidental spills and leaks, improper disposal, or runoff from PCB-contaminated soil. Once released to the environment, PCBs cycle freely throughout air, soil, and water and may be transported thousands of miles from their original source.

How might I be exposed to PCBs?

In the environment, PCBs are found primarily in soil, sediment, and fatty tissues of animal origin, including fish, meats, and dairy products. Fish and shellfish usually contain the highest PCB levels of any food source. In general, the highest PCB levels are found in fish at the top of the aquatic food chain, have the highest fat content, or were caught near urban or industrial areas. People may also be exposed to small amounts of PCBs if they use older fluorescent light fixtures or electrical appliances, work with PCB transformers or other PCB-containing devices, breathe the air near hazardous waste sites, or drink water from a PCB-contaminated well. Babies may be exposed to PCBs through the placenta during pregnancy or through breast milk after they are born. PCB exposure has declined since its ban in 1977.

How can PCBs affect health?

People exposed to very high levels of PCBs, as has occurred in the workplace and some accidental poisoning incidents, have shown various adverse health effects, particularly to the skin, eyes, and nervous system. However, simultaneous exposure to other chemicals makes it difficult to tell whether these health effects were caused by PCBs. Because of this, scientists have used experimental studies with animals to determine the likely health effects of PCB exposure. These animal studies show that exposure to high levels of PCBs can harm the liver, the gastrointestinal tract, and the immune, nervous, and reproductive systems. The most sensitive effects of PCB toxicity—those occurring at the lowest experimental doses—have been shown in monkeys. These include distorted growth of fingernails and toenails, eye discharge, and decreased response of the immune system. These effects occurred at experimental doses far higher than would be expected to occur from eating fish. More recent studies have tried to find whether lower levels of PCB exposure (such as those that could occur from frequent consumption of fish containing high levels of PCBs) may subtly affect development of the fetal nervous system during pregnancy. Some studies have suggested that PCBs might cause small decreases in children's I.Q. or affect their memory, especially if exposures occur during pregnancy. Other studies have not confirmed these effects. While human studies have not been consistent, there is enough evidence in humans and animals to justify concern. PCBs have also been found to cause cancer in some laboratory animals. The U.S. EPA considers PCBs to be probable human carcinogens.

Can PCB poisoning occur from eating sport fish in California?

No cases of PCB poisoning have been reported from eating California sport fish. Eating California sport fish is not expected to result in obvious signs of toxicity from exposure to PCBs. Fish consumption advisories are designed to prevent PCBs from building up in your body to levels that could cause subtle adverse effects or increase the risk of cancer.

Is there a way to reduce PCBs in fish to make them safer to eat?

A significant percent of PCBs found in fish can be removed by specific cooking and cleaning techniques. OEHHA recommends that you clean and gut the fish you catch before cooking it because PCBs and some other chemicals tend to concentrate in the organs, particularly in the liver. OEHHA also recommends consuming only the meat or fillet of the fish. For shellfish such as crabs and lobster, do not eat the soft "green stuff" (called "crab butter," mustard, tomalley, liver, or hepatopancreas) in the body section of these shellfish.

PCBs are mainly stored in fat and can be reduced by getting rid of the fat. Trim the fat, remove the skin, and fillet the fish before cooking. Fat is located along the back and the belly, and in the dark meat along the lateral line running along the side of the fish. Skinning fish will remove the thin layer of fat under the skin. Use a cooking method such as baking or grilling that allows the juices to drain away, and then discard the cooking juices. Do not use the fat, skin, organs, juices, or whole fish in soups or stews. These methods may eliminate half or more of the PCBs in fish. OEHHA also recommends fishing in different locations in case the location where you usually fish is highly contaminated. Eating a variety of fish species is likely to reduce your exposure to a species that has high contamination. Eating smaller fish of a species may also reduce your exposure because smaller younger fish tend to contain fewer PCBs than larger older fish.

Section 34.2

Shellfish-Associated Toxins

"Marine Toxins," Centers for Disease Control and Prevention (www.cdc.gov), October 12, 2005.

What are marine toxins?

Marine toxins are naturally occurring chemicals that can contaminate certain seafood. The seafood contaminated with these chemicals frequently looks, smells, and tastes normal. When humans eat such seafood, disease can result.

What sort of diseases do marine toxins cause?

The most common diseases caused by marine toxins in the United States in order of incidence are scombrotoxic fish poisoning, ciguatera poisoning, paralytic shellfish poisoning, neurotoxic shellfish poisoning, and amnesic shellfish poisoning.

Scombrotoxic fish poisoning, also known as scombroid or histamine fish poisoning, is caused by bacterial spoilage of certain finfish such as tuna, mackerel, bonito, and, rarely, other fish. As bacteria break down fish proteins, byproducts such as histamine and other substances that block histamine breakdown build up in fish. Eating spoiled fish that have high levels of these histamines can cause human disease. Symptoms begin within two minutes to two hours after eating the fish. The most common symptoms are rash, diarrhea, flushing, sweating, headache, and vomiting. Burning or swelling of the mouth, abdominal pain, or a metallic taste may also occur. The majority of patients have mild symptoms that resolve within a few hours. Treatment is generally unnecessary, but antihistamines or epinephrine may be needed in certain instances. Symptoms may be more severe in patients taking certain medications that slow the breakdown of histamine by their liver, such as isoniazid and doxycycline.

Ciguatera poisoning or ciguatera is caused by eating contaminated tropical reef fish. Ciguatoxins that cause ciguatera poisoning are actually produced by microscopic sea plants called dinoflagellates. These toxins become progressively concentrated as they move up the food chain from small fish to large fish that eat them, and reach particularly high concentrations in large predatory tropical reef fish. Barracuda are commonly associated with ciguatoxin poisoning, but eating grouper, sea bass, snapper, mullet, and a number of other fish that live in oceans between latitude 35° N and 35° S has caused the disease. These fish are typically caught by sport fishermen on reefs in Hawaii, Guam and other South Pacific islands, the Virgin Islands, and Puerto Rico. Ciguatoxin usually causes symptoms within a few minutes to 3 hours after eating contaminated fish, and occasionally it may take up to six hours. Common nonspecific symptoms include nausea, vomiting, diarrhea, cramps, excessive sweating, headache, and muscle aches. The sensation of burning or "pins-and-needles," weakness, itching, and dizziness can occur. Patients may experience reversal of temperature sensation in their mouth (hot surfaces feeling cold and cold, hot), unusual taste sensations, nightmares, or hallucinations. Ciguatera poisoning is rarely fatal. Symptoms usually clear in one to four weeks.

Paralytic shellfish poisoning is caused by a different dinoflagellate with a different toxin than that causing ciguatera poisoning. These dinoflagellates have a red-brown color, and can grow to such numbers that they cause red streaks to appear in the ocean, called "red tides." This toxin is known to concentrate within certain shellfish that typically live in the colder coastal waters of the Pacific states and New England, though the syndrome has been reported in Central America. Shellfish that have caused this disease include mussels, cockles, clams, scallops, oysters, crabs, and lobsters. Symptoms begin anywhere from 15 minutes to 10 hours after eating the contaminated shellfish, although usually within two hours. Symptoms are generally mild, and begin with numbness or tingling of the face, arms, and legs. This is followed by headache, dizziness, nausea, and muscular incoordination. Patients sometimes describe a floating sensation. In cases of severe poisoning, muscle paralysis and respiratory failure occur, and in these cases death may occur in 2 to 25 hours.

Neurotoxic shellfish poisoning is caused by a third type of dinoflagellate with another toxin that occasionally accumulates in oysters, clams, and mussels from the Gulf of Mexico and the Atlantic coast of the southern states. Symptoms begin one to three hours after eating the contaminated shellfish and include numbness;

tingling in the mouth, arms, and legs; incoordination; and gastrointestinal upset. As in ciguatera poisoning, some patients report temperature reversal. Death is rare. Recovery normally occurs in two to three days.

Amnesic shellfish poisoning is a rare syndrome caused by a toxin made by a microscopic, red-brown, salt-water plant, or diatom, called *Nitzschia pungens*. The toxin produced by these diatoms is concentrated in shellfish such as mussels and causes disease when the contaminated shellfish are eaten. Patients first experience gastrointestinal distress within 24 hours after eating the contaminated shellfish. Other reported symptoms have included dizziness, headache, disorientation, and permanent short-term memory loss. In severe poisoning, seizures, focal weakness or paralysis, and death may occur.

How can these diseases be diagnosed?

Diagnosis of marine toxin poisoning is generally based on symptoms and a history of recently eating a particular kind of seafood. Laboratory testing for the specific toxin in patient samples is generally not necessary because this requires special techniques and equipment available in only specialized laboratories. If suspect, leftover fish or shellfish are available, they can be tested for the presence of the toxin more easily. Identification of the specific toxin is not usually necessary for treating patients because there is no specific treatment.

How can these diseases be treated?

Other than supportive care there are few specific treatments for ciguatera poisoning, paralytic shellfish poisoning, neurotoxic shellfish poisoning, or amnesic shellfish poisoning. Antihistamines and epinephrine, however, may sometimes be useful in treating the symptoms of scombrotoxic fish poisoning. Intravenous mannitol has been suggested for the treatment of severe ciguatera poisoning.

Are there long-term consequences to these diseases?

Ciguatera poisoning has resulted in some neurologic problems persisting for weeks, and in rare cases, even years. Symptoms have sometimes returned after eating contaminated fish a second time. Amnesic shellfish poisoning has resulted in long-term problems with short-term memory. Long-term consequences have not been associated with paralytic shellfish poisoning, neurotoxic shellfish poisoning, and scombrotoxic fish poisoning.

How common are these diseases?

Every year, approximately 30 cases of poisoning by marine toxins are reported in the United States. Because health care providers are not required to report these illnesses and because many milder cases are not diagnosed or reported, the actual number of poisonings may be much greater. Toxic seafood poisonings are more common in the summer than winter because dinoflagellates grow well in warmer seasons. It is estimated from cases with available data that one person dies every four years from toxic seafood poisonings.

What can I do to prevent poisoning by marine toxins?

Follow these general guidelines for safe seafood consumption:

1. Although any person eating fish or shellfish containing toxin or disease-causing bacteria may become ill, persons with weakened immune systems or liver problems should not eat raw seafood because of their higher risk of *Vibrio* infection (see *Vibrio* FAQ at www.cdc.gov/ncidod/DFBMD/diseaseinfo/vibriovulnificus_g.htm).
2. Keep seafood on ice or refrigerated at less than 38° Fahrenheit to prevent spoilage.

Follow this specific advice for avoiding marine toxin poisoning:

1. Keep fresh tuna, mackerel, grouper, and mahi mahi refrigerated to prevent development of histamine. Don't believe that cooking spoiled or toxic seafood will keep you safe. These toxins are not destroyed by cooking.
2. Do not eat barracuda, especially those from the Caribbean.
3. Check with local health officials before collecting shellfish, and look for health department advisories about algal blooms, dinoflagellate growth, or "red tide" conditions that may be posted at fishing supply stores.
4. Do not eat finfish or shellfish sold as bait. Bait products do not need to meet the same food safety regulations as seafood for human consumption.

What is the government doing about these diseases?

Some health departments test shellfish harvested within their jurisdiction to monitor the level of dinoflagellate toxins and asses the risk for contamination. Based on the results of such testing, recreational and commercial seafood harvesting may be prohibited locally during periods of risk. State and federal regulatory agencies monitor reported cases of marine toxin poisoning, and health departments investigate possible outbreaks and devise control measures. The Centers for Disease Control and Prevention (CDC) provides support to investigators as needed.

What else can be done to prevent these diseases?

It is important to notify public health departments about even one person with marine toxin poisoning. Public health departments can then investigate to determine if a restaurant, oyster bed, or fishing area has a problem. This prevents other illnesses. In any food poisoning occurrence, consumers should note foods eaten and freeze any uneaten portions in case they need to be tested. A commercial test has been developed in Hawaii to allow persons to test sport-caught fish for ciguatoxins.

Section 34.3

Imported Shrimp and Your Health

Over the past two decades, Americans have been eating more seafood than ever. Shrimp is the most popular seafood in the United States. In 2005, Americans ate an average of 4.1 pounds of shrimp per person, up from 2.5 pounds in 1995.

The United States increasingly relies on imports—more than 80%—to satisfy consumers' appetites for cheap shrimp. Shrimp imports have increased by 95% in the past 10 years.

The Food and Agriculture Organization of the United Nations estimates that industrial shrimp production accounts for approximately 40% of shrimp worldwide. In 2006, the United States imported 1.3 billion pounds of shrimp, of which Thailand produced more than 30%. Four of the five leading shrimp exporters to the United States are from Asia, the aquaculture epicenter. While the U.S. government does not track whether seafood imports are wild-caught or farm-raised, it is reasonable to conclude that industrially farmed shrimp makes up a growing proportion of U.S. shrimp imports.

Unfortunately, consumers don't know if their shrimp is domestic or imported. In 2005, the U.S. Department of Agriculture developed mandatory country of origin labeling rules, which was intended to inform consumers about where seafood comes from and if it is farm-raised or wild-caught. However, the USDA [U.S. Department of Agriculture] did not create a strong program. "Processed" sea-food is exempt, leaving more than 50% of seafood sold in the United States without labels; 90% of fish sellers, such as wholesale markets and restaurants, are exempt; no enforcement mechanism exists and violators face paltry fines.

Americans are largely unaware of the health concerns associated with imported aquaculture products. The crowded, unsanitary conditions on these industrial shrimp farms breed bacteria, viruses, and parasites, forcing producers to use antibiotics and chemicals illegal in the United States to prevent disease outbreaks. Residues of these chemicals then end up in the shrimp where they can harm the consumers who eat it. Furthermore, transport of seafood imports over long distances presents opportunities for contamination and decomposition due to improper handling and refrigeration.

The U.S. government's Food and Drug Administration has a mandate to oversee the safety of seafood imports by inspecting shipments at the border. In reality, lack of money meant that FDA physically inspected less than 2% of all import shipments in 2006, and laboratory tested only 0.59%—not enough to ensure the safety of America's seafood. Analysis of the seafood shipments FDA refused between 2003 and 2006 found many troubling trends in imported shrimp.

Troubling Trends in Shrimp Imports

Filth was the leading reason that seafood imports were refused. From 2003 to 2006, shrimp accounted for between 26% and 35% of all filth refusals, even though only 22% to 24% of all imports were shrimp.

Salmonella is disproportionately concentrated in shrimp. Refusals for *Salmonella* are most prevalent in shrimp imports. Shrimp imports constituted between 22% and 24% of the weight of all U.S. seafood imports between 2003 and 2006. However, shrimp was responsible for more than double that percentage of all *Salmonella* refusals, ranging from a high of 56.1% in 2005 to a low of 42.9% in 2006.

Approximately 60% of the *Salmonella* refusals of shrimp were processed shrimp, products that are not subject to country of origin labeling. As a result, Americans purchase these products without knowledge of whether or not they were imported. *Salmonella* contamination is particularly troublesome with ready-to-eat shrimp products, which consumers do not cook before eating.

Heavy Use of Antibiotics and Chemicals in Shrimp

Industrial shrimp producers use antibiotics and chemicals during production to prevent disease and parasites. Nitrofurans and chloramphenicol are substances widely used in shrimp production. In 2004 and 2006, about 20% of all drug refusals were for shrimp imports. However, in 2003 and 2005, shrimp were responsible for 84% and 65% of all refusals for drug residues, respectively. Since refusals of drug residues fluctuate widely, a consistent and thorough inspection program is necessary.

These troubling trends in shrimp imports are a serious concern for American consumers, given that they eat shrimp more than any other seafood. FDA must increase physical inspection of imported seafood. Congress must appropriate the money to make this happen, and USDA must expand country of origin labeling to include processed seafood products so consumers are aware of where their seafood originates. Together, these measures would better ensure the safety of America's seafood.

What Can You Do?

- Choose wild-caught, sustainably produced, domestic shrimp over imported shrimp. Consumers should ask grocery stores and restaurants where their shrimp comes from and how it was produced.
- Tell FDA to increase inspection of imported shrimp.
- Ask Congress to increase funding and oversight for FDA's seafood import inspection program.
- Tell USDA to expand country of origin labeling so that it includes processed seafood and expands to every store and restaurant.

Editor's Note: The information in this section represents the opinion of the copyright holder and is presented as one viewpoint on a complex subject.

Section 34.4

How the U.S. Food and Drug Administration Regulates Imported Seafood

"How FDA Regulates Seafood: FDA Detains Imports of Farm-Raised Chinese Seafood," Food and Drug Administration (www.fda.gov), June 28, 2007.

On June 28, 2007, FDA announced a broader import control of farm-raised catfish, basa, shrimp, dace (related to carp), and eel from China. FDA will start to detain these products at the border until the shipments are proven to be free of residues from drugs that are not approved in the United States for use in farm-raised aquatic animals. The agency took this action to protect American consumers from unsafe residues detected in these products. There have been no reports of illnesses to date.

FDA is taking this strong step now because of continuing evidence that certain Chinese aquaculture products imported into the United States contain illegal substances. Aquaculture, also known as fish farming, involves raising fish in enclosed areas to be sold for food. Almost half of all imported seafood is from aquaculture, according to the U.S. Department of Commerce.

During targeted sampling, from October 2006 through May 2007, FDA repeatedly found that farm-raised seafood from China was contaminated with antimicrobial agents that are not approved for use in the United States. More specifically, the antimicrobials nitrofuran, malachite green, gentian violet, and fluoroquinolones were detected. Nitrofurans, malachite green, and gentian violet have been shown to cause cancer with long-term exposure in lab animals. The use of fluoroquinolones in food animals may increase antibiotic resistance, making it harder for this class of drugs to fight certain infections in people.

"Consumers should know that this is not an immediate public health hazard," says Robert Brackett, PhD, director of FDA's Center for Food Safety and Applied Nutrition. "The levels of contaminants that have been found are very low, and FDA is not advising consumers to destroy or return farm-raised seafood that they may have already purchased and have in their homes. The agency also is not seeking a recall of products already in the marketplace."

FDA is taking this action as a precautionary measure to prevent problems that may occur from long-term exposure to harmful residues. The agency is also concerned about the possible development of antibiotic resistance. "This action serves to keep contaminated products from entering the country so that they don't reach American consumers," Brackett says.

Here's a look at how FDA works to protect consumers from unsafe seafood.

How do drug residues end up in fish?

Some fish are given drugs to treat bacterial and parasitic diseases that cause major mortalities in fish. FDA's Center for Veterinary Medicine (CVM) regulates drugs given to animals. CVM conducts research to improve the drug approval process and expand the number of safe drugs available for fish production. CVM also develops methods to detect unapproved chemicals in fish tissues so that harmful drug residues don't wind up in the fish on your plate.

Is imported seafood required to meet the same standards as domestic seafood?

Yes. Imported foods must be pure, wholesome, safe to eat, and produced under sanitary conditions. FDA requires imported seafood to be free of harmful residues. Importers must comply with regulations under the Federal Food, Drug, and Cosmetic Act and the Fair Packaging and Labeling Act. In addition, seafood must be processed in accordance with FDA's Hazard Analysis and Critical Control Point (HACCP) regulations. A 1997 regulation, "Procedures for the Safe and Sanitary Processing and Importing of Fish and Fishery Products," requires seafood processors to identify food safety hazards and apply preventive measures to control hazards that could cause foodborne illness.

What other specific FDA regulatory programs focus on seafood?

- **National Shellfish Sanitation Program:** Administered by FDA, this program provides for the sanitary harvest and production of fresh and frozen molluscan shellfish (oysters, clams, and mussels). FDA conducts reviews of foreign and domestic molluscan shellfish safety programs.

- **Salmon Control Plan:** This is a voluntary, cooperative program among industry, FDA, and the Grocery Manufacturers Association/Food Products Association. It's designed to provide control over processing and plant sanitation, and to address concerns in the salmon canning industry.
- **Low-Acid Canned Food (LACF) Program:** To ensure safety from harmful bacteria or their toxins, especially the deadly *Clostridium botulinum* (*C. botulinum*), in canned foods, regulations were established to ensure that commercial canning establishments apply proper processing controls, such as heating the canned food at the proper temperature for a sufficient time to destroy the toxin-forming bacteria. Products such as canned tuna and salmon are examples of LACF seafood products.

How does FDA know when there is a safety concern associated with seafood?

FDA, in collaboration with state regulatory counterparts, conducts in-plant inspections that focus on product safety, plant/food hygiene, economic fraud, and other compliance concerns. FDA also receives notice of every seafood entry coming from a foreign country and selects entries from which to collect and analyze samples. FDA laboratories analyze samples for the presence of various safety hazards and contaminants, such as pathogens, chemical contaminants, unapproved food additives and drugs, pesticides, and toxins. Through close collaboration with CDC and state and foreign regulatory partners, FDA also learns of seafood safety concerns that arise through reports of illness potentially associated with seafood products.

What steps does FDA take when problems with seafood are detected?

For imported seafood, FDA has the authority to detain the food at the border to keep it from entering the country. This happens when FDA's analysis of such products indicate that they are not in compliance with the laws and regulations enforced by FDA. FDA can subsequently refuse entries of detained products if evidence of compliance is not provided by the importer or the importer does not correct the problem.

FDA has developed a number of import alerts that address problems found in seafood products in the past. An import alert identifies products that are suspected of violating the law so that FDA field personnel and U.S. Customs and Border Protection staff can stop these entries at the border prior to distribution in the United States. Usually, these import alerts will describe the products or firms that are subject to detention without physical examination. When products are detained without physical examination, the burden for demonstrating compliance of the product falls on the importer. Such compliance must be demonstrated before the product can enter U.S. commerce.

FDA can recommend criminal prosecution or injunction of responsible domestic firms and individuals, as well as seizure of contaminated products in commercial distribution within the United States. FDA also works with domestic seafood processors to initiate voluntary recalls of contaminated products that may pose a safety concern to consumers.

What kind of research on seafood safety does FDA do?

FDA conducts research to better understand the nature and severity posed by various safety hazards, and other defects which may affect quality and economic integrity and to develop methods to minimize these risks. There are FDA laboratories specializing in seafood research on the Atlantic, Gulf, and Pacific coasts to address regional problems related to toxins and contaminants. FDA also has a facility in Laurel, Maryland, for conducting state-of-the-art research on drugs used in aquaculture.

What is the consumer's role in seafood safety?

As with any food, consumers should take precautions to reduce the risk of foodborne illness associated with seafood. This includes properly selecting, preparing, and storing seafood. For example, consumers should only buy food from reputable sources and buy fresh seafood that is refrigerated or properly iced. Also, most seafood should be cooked to an internal temperature of 145° F. Some people are at greater risk for foodborne illness and should not eat raw or partially cooked fish or shellfish. This includes pregnant women, young children, older adults, and people with compromised immune systems.

Chapter 35

Antibiotics and Hormones in Dairy and Meat

Section 35.1

Antibiotics

"Use of antimicrobials outside human medicine and resultant antimicrobial resistance in humans," Fact Sheet Number 268, January 2002, http://www.who.int/mediacentre/factsheets/fs268/en/index.html. © 2002 World Health Organization. Reprinted with permission. *Health Reference Series* Medical Advisor's note added by David A. Cooke, MD, FACP, June 2009.

Antimicrobials are natural or synthetic drugs which inhibit or kill bacteria. This capability makes them unique for the control of deadly infectious diseases caused by a large variety of pathogenic bacteria.

Today, more than 15 different classes of antimicrobials are known. They differ in chemical structure and mechanism of action. Specific antimicrobials are necessary for the treatment of specific pathogens.

Following their 20th-century triumph in human medicine, antimicrobials have also been used increasingly for the treatment of bacterial disease in animals, fish, and plants. In addition, they became an important element of intense animal husbandry because of their observed growth-enhancing effect, when added in subtherapeutic doses to animal feed. Antimicrobials are also used in industry, e.g., to eliminate bacterial growth on the inside of oil pipelines.

The Antimicrobial Resistance Problem

- The widespread use of antimicrobials outside human medicine is of serious concern given the alarming emergence in humans of bacteria, which have acquired, through this use, resistance to antimicrobials.
- Most of the rising antimicrobial resistance problem in human medicine is due to the overuse and misuse of antimicrobials by doctors, other health personnel, and patients.
- However, some of the newly emerging resistant bacteria in animals are transmitted to humans; mainly via meat and other food of animal origin or through direct contact with farm animals. The best-known examples are the foodborne pathogenic

bacteria *Salmonella* and *Campylobacter* and the commensal (harmless in healthy persons and animals) bacteria *Enterococcus*. Research has shown that resistance of these bacteria to classic treatment in humans is often a consequence of the use of certain antimicrobials in agriculture.

- Further study is required to investigate other possible ways of transmission of antimicrobial resistant bacteria to humans. For example, the impact on human health of the widespread distribution of nonmetabolized antimicrobials through manure and other effluents from farm animals into the environment is still unknown.

Antimicrobial Use in Food Animals

- In addition to being administered to sick food animals individually to treat them, antimicrobials are used for mass treatment against infectious diseases or continuously in feed at very low doses (parts per million) for growth promotion, particularly in pig and poultry production. Use of antimicrobials for these purposes has become an important part of intense animal husbandry.
- Some growth promoters belong to groups of antimicrobials (e.g., glycopeptides and streptogramins), which are essential drugs in human medicine for the treatment of serious, potentially life-threatening, bacterial diseases, such as *Staphylococcus* or *Enterococcus* infections.

Scale of Antimicrobial Use outside Human Medicine

- The amount of antimicrobials used in food animals is not known precisely. National statistics on the amount and pattern of use of antimicrobials in human medicine or elsewhere exist in only a few countries.
- It is estimated that about half of the total amount of antimicrobials produced globally is used in food animals.
- In Europe, all classes of antimicrobials licensed for disease therapy in humans are also registered for use in animals, a situation comparable with other regions in the world where comprehensive registration data are much more difficult to obtain.
- A recent review in Europe has shown that an average amount of 100 milligrams of antimicrobials is used in animals for the production of one kilogram of meat for human consumption.

- The increase in meat production in many developing countries is mainly due to intensified farming, which is often coupled with increased antimicrobial usage for both disease therapy and growth promotion.

Factors Contributing to Overuse of Antimicrobials in Food Animals

- Education on antimicrobial resistance and prudent antimicrobial use is lacking amongst dispensers and prescribers of antimicrobials. In many countries, antimicrobials are dispensed by inadequately trained individuals. One study reported that more than 90% of all veterinary drugs used in animals in the United States in 1987 were administered without professional veterinary consultation. In addition, inappropriate doses and combinations of drugs are frequently used in animals. Furthermore, administering antimicrobials to animal flocks and herds in their feed causes problems of inaccurate dosing and inevitable treatment of all animals irrespective of health status.
- Empiric treatment (based on clinical investigations, rather than isolation and typing of the causative pathogen) predominates because of the widespread lack of diagnostic services (particularly in developing countries). In many countries, submission of clinical specimens and samples from sick animals is uncommon due to costs involved, time restrictions, and the limited number of laboratories.
- In many countries, including several developed countries, antimicrobials are available over-the-counter and may be purchased without prescription.
- Inefficient regulatory mechanisms or poor enforcement of regulations, with lack of quality assurance and marketing of substandard drugs, are important contributory factors. Discrepancies between regulatory requirements and prescribing/dispensing realities are often wider in veterinary medicine than in human medicine.
- Antimicrobial growth promoters are not considered as drugs and are licensed, if at all, as feed additives.
- As in human medicine, pharmaceutical industry marketing of antimicrobials influences prescribing behavior and use patterns of veterinarians and farmers. Unlike in human medicine, there

are currently few countries with industry codes or government rules that oversee advertising practices for antimicrobials for nonhuman use.

- There is a significant increase in intensive animal production, particularly in countries with economies in transition, where the aforementioned general factors are present: improper prescription and dispensing; lack of licensing and enforcement; poor drug quality, veterinary education, and food safety; etc.

Examples of the Consequences of the Overuse of Antimicrobials in Food Animals

- Studies in several countries, including the United Kingdom and United States, have demonstrated the association between the use of antimicrobials in food animals and antimicrobial resistance. Shortly after the licensing and use of fluoroquinolone, a powerful new class of antimicrobials, in poultry, fluoroquinolone-resistant *Salmonella* and *Campylobacter* isolations from animals, and shortly afterward such isolations from humans, became more common. Community and family outbreaks, as well as individual cases, of salmonellosis and campylobacteriosis resistant to treatment with fluoroquinolones have since been reported from several countries. The U.S. Food and Drug Administration (FDA) believes that each year the health of at least 5,000 Americans is affected by use of these drugs in chickens. (WHO Fact Sheets on "*Campylobacter*" and "Multidrug Resistant *Salmonella typhimurium*" can be found at the following URLs: www.who.int/entity/mediacentre/factsheets/fs255/en/index.html and www.who.int/entity/mediacentre/factsheets/fs139/en/index.html respectively.)

- With the emergence of vancomycin-resistant strains of *Enterococcus* bacteria in many hospitals around the world, the question arose if the use of vancomycin in agriculture could have compounded the worsening problem. Indeed, vancomycin-resistant *enterococci* were isolated in animals, food, and nontreated volunteers in countries where vancomycin is also used as a growth promoter in animals.

- Because of the health threat from vancomycin-resistant *enterococci*, Denmark banned use of vancomycin as an animal growth promoter in 1995 and all European countries followed suit in

1997. After the ban, prevalence of resistant *Enterococcus* in animals and food, particularly in poultry meat, fell sharply.

Antimicrobial Use in Aquaculture

- Various antimicrobials are licensed and used in fish and shrimp production, particularly in Asia. Unfortunately, little information is available on the type and amount of antimicrobials used in aquaculture, making assessment of emerging public health risks more difficult.
- There is an urgent need to review the current usage patterns of antimicrobials in aquaculture to identify looming hazards in food safety and infectious disease control in humans. (This also applies to other uses of antimicrobials, including for plant protection and in industry.)
- Because of lessons learned from antimicrobial use in species living on land, some countries have been looking for non-antimicrobial alternatives for some time. Norway, for instance, has been able to diminish antimicrobial use in aquaculture by more than 90% in a very short period of time after changing certain production practices and increasing use of vaccines.

Containment of Antimicrobial Resistance

1. The World Health Organization (WHO) is developing a Global Strategy for the Containment of Antimicrobial Resistance. This strategy targets all areas where antimicrobials are used in the community, hospitals, and agriculture.
2. As part of this strategy, WHO, jointly with other organizations such as the United Nations Food and Agriculture Organization (FAO) and the Office International des Epizooties (OIE), developed global principles (recommendations) for antimicrobial use in agriculture. The overall aim of this activity is to minimize the potential negative public health impact of the use of antimicrobial agents in animals used for human food, whilst at the same time providing for their safe and effective use in veterinary medicine. The global principles may be consulted on the Internet at the following address: www.who.int/emc/diseases/zoo/who_global_principles/index.htm.
3. Few countries have active surveillance for antimicrobial resistance in bacteria from food animals and food of animal

origin. Existing programs rarely involve all relevant zoonotic and commensal microorganisms and do not test for all the antimicrobials that may be relevant from a public health perspective. Furthermore, methods used are not sufficiently standardized to enable comparison of data between different surveillance programs focused on animals or humans. Consequently, there is an absence of adequate data to evaluate the consequences of antimicrobial use in animals and to monitor the effect of different interventions applied to reduce antimicrobial resistance in bacteria from animals.

4. Through a concerted effort with partners from national agencies and research institutions, WHO is enhancing foodborne disease surveillance and antimicrobial resistance testing of foodborne bacteria. The laboratory strengthening focuses on salmonellosis and antimicrobial resistance surveillance in foodborne *Salmonella* and includes the following activities:

   - Development of the Global Salm-Surv (www.who.int/salmsurv), a web-based, up-to-date databank on national and regional laboratories
   - Establishment of a network of electronically linked national and regional reference laboratories; currently, more than 260 scientists, microbiologists, epidemiologists, and others from 109 institutions in 101 countries are participating
   - Conducting external quality assurance programs; by the end of 2000, 80 national reference laboratories will have completed evaluation of their *Salmonella* typing and antimicrobial susceptibility testing
   - Establishment of international centers of excellence for surveillance and containment of antimicrobial resistance resulting from antimicrobial use in agriculture

5. Containment of antimicrobial resistance will require national and local efforts to reduce use of antimicrobials. Through legislation, some countries have recently taken steps to reduce the problem of antimicrobial resistance in food animals. The European Union banned all antimicrobial animal growth promoters which are also used in human medicine in 1997. Already in 1986, Sweden banned the use of all animal growth promoters, even those which are not used in human medicine. Denmark voluntarily suspended the use of all animal growth

promoters in 1999 and Switzerland did the same in 2000. Studies in Denmark have shown that voluntary suspension resulted in an overall reduction of antimicrobial use in Danish livestock of more than 60% with no significant economic impact or negative change in animal health status and food safety.

6. WHO encourages countries to use all opportunities to reduce, to the extent possible, the use of antimicrobials outside human medicine. This will minimize the risk of the emergence of antimicrobial resistance in bacteria, which can be transmitted to humans from animals or the environment. The overall aim is to ensure that infectious disease in humans can be controlled more efficiently.

Health Reference Series Medical Advisor's note: Since the original publication of this article, the European Union has banned all feeding of antibiotics to livestock for promoting growth. This was in reaction to concerns about promotion of antibiotic resistance. Antibiotics are still frequently used in animal feed in the United States, but restrictions on this are under discussion due to an increasing number of highly resistant bacterial strains that are suspected to be due to use in livestock.

Section 35.2

Recombinant Bovine Growth Hormone (rBGH)

What is rBGH?

Recombinant Bovine Growth Hormone (rBGH or rBST) is a genetically engineered hormone injected into cows to increase milk production by 8–17%. The Monsanto Corporation manufactures the product, which is sold under the trade name Posilac.

Background

In 1993, the FDA approved rBGH, even though many scientists and government leaders were critical of the hormone, the inadequate research on its risks, and the approval process. Twelve years after it was approved in the U.S., significant health concerns regarding rBGH remain. The European Union, as well as Japan, Canada, and Australia, have banned rBGH. Codex Alimentarius, the U.N. [United Nations] body that sets food safety standards, has refused to approve the safety of rBGH three times.

Health Effects

Recombinant bovine growth hormone causes harm to cows and may pose harm to humans.

Cancer Risk

Injections of rBGH increase another powerful hormone, called IGF-1, in the cow and the cow's milk. Numerous studies indicate that IGF-1 survives digestion. Too much IGF-1 in humans is linked with increased rates of colon, breast, and prostate cancer. "Definitive studies demonstrating the lack of absorption of rBST or IGF-1 upon oral administration were neither conducted nor requested," Health Canada concluded. "Simply not enough is known about how IGF-1 functions to properly evaluate the potential health impacts."

While it's not clear that rBGH given to cows significantly increases IGF-1 in humans, why take the chance simply so dairies can produce more milk from fewer cows?

Mastitis and Antibiotic Resistance

Use of rBGH on dairy cows increases the rate of mastitis, a bacterial udder infection, by 25%. Mastitis leads to increased use of antibiotics, including important ones used to treat humans, like penicillin. The overuse of antibiotics is already a serious problem in the livestock industry—giving rise to new strains of "superbugs" that are becoming more resistant to antibiotics and are strongly linked to hard-to-treat illnesses in people.

In 1992, the U.S. General Accounting Office [GAO] recommended that the FDA not approve rBGH until the mastitis problem was further studied. "Concern exists now about whether antibiotic levels in milk are already too high," the GAO wrote. "There has been no examination of whether rBGH use will increase antibiotic levels in milk or beef beyond that which currently exist and, if so, to what degree those levels are acceptable." RBGH also increases birth defects, pus in milk, and clinical lameness in cows.

Possible Allergic Reactions

In one study, rats that were fed rBGH, including one given a relatively low dose, developed antibodies to rBGH. This effect, if validated, "would suggest the possibility of occasional hypersensitivity reactions in those consuming food products from rBST-treated cattle." The FDA brushed aside these disturbing results and did not fully investigate these results.

A Tool for Factory Farms

In the United States, about 15% of the dairy herds use recombinant bovine growth hormone; overall, approximately 22% of dairy cows in the U.S. are injected with the hormone. For the most part, this hormone is a tool for dairy factory farms to eke out even more milk per cow. The hormone is used in 54% of large herds (500 animals or more), 32% of medium herds, and only 8% of small herds.

Consumer Backlash

Consumers are seeking dairy products produced without rBGH, and companies are responding. Most recently, the Tillamook County Creamery Association, a 150–dairy farmer cooperative, voted to ban rBGH in their cheese production due to consumer requests. Ben & Jerry's ice cream brand is also rBGH-free. The company explains this decision by saying, "We think its use is a step in the wrong direction toward a synthetic, chemically-intensive, factory-produced food supply."

Several years ago, Oakhurst Dairy in Maine was sued for advertising their products as rBGH-free; they were eventually required to state that the FDA has not found any significant difference between products with and without the hormone on their products. Nevertheless, almost all dairy products sold in Maine are rBGH-free, in response to consumer rejection of the product. And organic food, which cannot be produced with growth hormones, is a skyrocketing market, growing almost 20% annually over the last decade. Organic dairy products constituted $1.3 billion in sales in 2003.

What You Can Do

Purchase dairy products that are labeled "rBGH-free," "rBST-free," or "organic." Also, tell your supermarket, favorite dairy brand, and school district that you want dairy products that were not made with rBGH.

Editor's Note: The information in this section represents the opinion of the copyright holder and is presented as one viewpoint on a complex subject.

Chapter 36

Food Additives

Acesulfame-K

- Artificial sweetener: Baked goods, chewing gum, gelatin desserts, diet soda, Sunette

This artificial sweetener, manufactured by Hoechst, a giant German chemical company, is widely used around the world. It is about 200 times sweeter than sugar. In the United States, for several years acesulfame-K (the *K* is the chemical symbol for potassium) was permitted only in such foods as sugar-free baked goods, chewing gum, and gelatin desserts. In July 1998, the FDA [Food and Drug Administration] allowed this chemical to be used in soft drinks, thereby greatly increasing consumer exposure. It is often used together with sucralose.

The safety tests of acesulfame-K were conducted in the 1970s and were of mediocre quality. Key rat tests were afflicted by disease in the animal colonies; a mouse study was several months too brief and did not expose animals during gestation. Two rat studies suggest that the additive might cause cancer. It was for those reasons that in 1996 the Center for Science in the Public Interest [CSPI] urged the FDA to require better testing before permitting acesulfame-K in soft drinks.

Excerpted from "Food Additives," http://www.cspinet.org/reports/chemcuisine.htm.

In addition, large doses of acetoacetamide, a breakdown product, have been shown to affect the thyroid in rats, rabbits, and dogs. Hopefully, the small amounts in food are not harmful.

Artificial Colorings

Most artificial colorings are synthetic chemicals that do not occur in nature. Because colorings are used almost solely in foods of low nutritional value (candy, soda pop, gelatin desserts, etc.), you should simply avoid all artificially colored foods. In addition to problems mentioned in the following, colorings cause hyperactivity in some sensitive children. The use of coloring usually indicates that fruit or other natural ingredient has not been used.

Artificial Colorings: Blue 1

- Beverages, candy, baked goods

Inadequately tested; suggestions of a small cancer risk.

Artificial Colorings: Blue 2

- Pet food, beverages, candy

The largest study suggested, but did not prove, that this dye caused brain tumors in male mice. The FDA concluded that there is "reasonable certainty of no harm."

Artificial Colorings: Green 3

- Candy, beverages

A 1981 industry-sponsored study gave hints of bladder cancer, but FDA reanalyzed the data using other statistical tests and concluded that the dye was safe. Fortunately, this possibly carcinogenic dye is rarely used.

Artificial Colorings: Red 3

- Cherries in fruit cocktail, candy, baked goods

The evidence that this dye caused thyroid tumors in rats is "convincing," according to a 1983 review committee report requested by

FDA. FDA's recommendation that the dye be banned was overruled by pressure from elsewhere in the Reagan Administration.

Artificial Colorings: Yellow 6

- Beverages, sausage, baked goods, candy, gelatin

Industry-sponsored animal tests indicated that this dye, the third most widely used, causes tumors of the adrenal gland and kidney. In addition, small amounts of several carcinogens contaminate Yellow 6. However, the FDA reviewed those data and found reasons to conclude that Yellow 6 does not pose a significant cancer risk to humans. Yellow 6 may also cause occasional allergic reactions.

Aspartame

- Artificial sweetener: "Diet" foods, including soft drinks, drink mixes, gelatin desserts, low-calorie frozen desserts, packets

Aspartame (Equal, NutraSweet), a chemical combination of two amino acids and methanol, was initially thought to be the perfect artificial sweetener, but it might cause cancer or neurological problems such as dizziness or hallucinations.

A 1970s study suggested that aspartame caused brain tumors in rats. However, the FDA persuaded an independent review panel to reverse its conclusion that aspartame was unsafe. The California Environmental Protection Agency and others have urged that independent scientists conduct new animal studies to resolve the cancer question. In 2005, researchers at the Ramazzini Foundation in Bologna, Italy, conducted the first such study. It indicated that rats first exposed to aspartame at eight weeks of age caused lymphomas and leukemias in females. However, the European Food Safety Authority reviewed the study and concluded that the tumors probably occurred just by chance.

In 2007, the same Italian researchers published a follow-up study that began exposing rats to aspartame in utero. This study found that aspartame caused leukemias/lymphomas and mammary (breast) cancer. It is likely that the new studies found problems that earlier company-sponsored studies did not because the Italian researchers monitored the rats for three years instead of two.

In a 2006 study, U.S. National Cancer Institute researchers studied a large number of adults 50 to 69 years of age over a five-year period. There was no evidence that aspartame posed any risk. However, the study was limited in three major regards: It did not involve truly elderly people (the rat studies monitored the rats until they died a natural death), the subjects had not consumed aspartame as children, and it was not a controlled study (the subjects provided only a rough estimate of their aspartame consumption, and people who consumed aspartame might have had other dietary or lifestyle differences that obscured the chemical's effects).

The bottom line is that lifelong consumption of aspartame probably increases the risk of cancer. People—especially young children—should not consume foods and beverages sweetened with aspartame, should switch to products sweetened with sucralose (Splenda), or should avoid all artificially sweetened foods. Two other artificial sweeteners, saccharin and acesulfame-K, have also been linked to a risk of cancer.

Butylated Hydroxyanisole (BHA)

- Antioxidant: Cereals, chewing gum, potato chips, vegetable oil

BHA retards rancidity in fats, oils, and oil-containing foods. While some studies indicate it is safe, other studies demonstrate that it causes cancer in rats, mice, and hamsters. Those cancers are controversial because they occur in the forestomach, an organ that humans do not have. However, a chemical that causes cancer in at least one organ in three different species indicates that it might be carcinogenic in humans. That is why the U.S. Department of Health and Human Services considers BHA to be "reasonably anticipated to be a human carcinogen." Nevertheless, the FDA still permits BHA to be used in foods. This synthetic chemical can be replaced by safer chemicals (e.g., vitamin E), safer processes (e.g., packing foods under nitrogen instead of air), or can simply be left out (many brands of oily foods, such as potato chips, don't use any antioxidant).

Cyclamate

- Artificial sweetener: Diet foods

This controversial high-potency sweetener was used in the United States in diet foods until 1970, at which time it was banned. Animal studies indicated that it causes cancer. Now, based on animal studies, it (or a by-product) is believed not to cause cancer directly, but to increase the potency of other carcinogens and to harm the testes.

Olestra (Olean)

- Fat substitute: Lay's Light Chips, Pringles Light Chips

Olestra is Procter & Gamble's synthetic fat that is not absorbed as it passes through the digestive system, so it has no calories. Procter & Gamble suggests that replacing regular fat with olestra will help people lose weight and lower the risk of heart disease.

Olestra can cause diarrhea and loose stools, abdominal cramps, flatulence, and other adverse effects. Those symptoms are sometimes severe. Afflicted consumers can file reports with the Center for Science in the Public Interest [at www.cspinet.org/olestraform/index.htm].

Even more importantly, olestra reduces the body's ability to absorb fat-soluble carotenoids (such as alpha and beta-carotene, lycopene, lutein, and canthaxanthin) from fruits and vegetables. Those nutrients are thought by many experts to reduce the risk of cancer and heart disease. Olestra enables manufacturers to offer greasy-feeling low-fat snacks, but consumers would be much better off with baked snacks, which are perfectly safe and just as low in calories. Products made with olestra should not be called "fat free," because they contain substantial amounts of indigestible fat.

Partially Hydrogenated Vegetable Oil, Hydrogenated Vegetable Oil (Trans Fat)

- Fat, oil, shortening: Stick margarine, crackers, fried restaurant foods, baked goods, icing, microwave popcorn

Vegetable oil, usually a liquid, can be made into a semisolid shortening by reacting it with hydrogen. Partial hydrogenation reduces the levels of polyunsaturated oils—and also creates trans fats, which promote heart disease. A committee of the FDA concluded in 2004 that on a gram-for-gram basis, trans fat is even more harmful than saturated fat. Ideally, food manufacturers would replace hydrogenated shortening with less-harmful ingredients. The Institute of Medicine has advised consumers to consume as little trans fat as possible, ideally less than about two grams a day (that much might come from naturally occurring trans fat in beef and dairy products). Harvard School of Public Health researchers estimate that trans fat had been causing about 50,000 premature heart attack deaths annually, making partially hydrogenated oil one of the most harmful ingredients in the food supply.

Beginning in 2006, nutrition facts labels have had to list the amount of trans fat in a serving. That spurred many companies, including Frito-Lay, Kraft, ConAgra, and others, to replace most or all of the partially hydrogenated oil in almost all their products. Usually the substitutes are healthier and the total of saturated plus trans fat is no higher than it was. Foods labeled "0 g trans fat" are permitted to contain 0.5 g per serving, while "no trans fat" means none at all. Consumers need to read labels carefully: foods labeled "0 g trans" or "no trans" may still have large amounts of saturated fat.

Restaurants, which do not provide nutrition information, have been slower to change, but the pace of change has picked up. They use partially hydrogenated oil for frying chicken, potatoes, and fish, as well as in biscuits and other baked goods. McDonald's, Wendy's, KFC, Taco Bell, Ruby Tuesday, and Red Lobster are some of the large chains that have largely eliminated trans fat or soon will. Most large chains and many smaller independent restaurants continue to fry in partially hydrogenated oil and their french fries, fried chicken, fried fish, and pot pies contain substantial amounts of trans fat. Fortunately, the use of partially hydrogenated oil dropped by 50% from around 2000 to 2007.

In Denmark, the government has virtually banned partially hydrogenated oil. In 2004, the Center for Science in the Public Interest petitioned the FDA to immediately require restaurants to disclose when they use partially hydrogenated oil and to begin the process of eliminating partially hydrogenated oil from the entire food supply. While the FDA rejected the idea of requiring restaurants to disclose the presence of trans fat, New York City, Philadelphia, Boston, and other jurisdictions have set tight limits on the trans-fat content of restaurant foods. Meanwhile, the FDA is continuing to consider CSPI's petition to revoke the legal status of partially hydrogenated oil (the FDA considers that oil to be "generally recognized as safe," even though it and everyone else considers it to be "generally recognized as dangerous").

Fully hydrogenated vegetable oil does not have any trans fat, but it also does not have any polyunsaturated oils. It is sometimes mixed (physically or chemically) with polyunsaturated liquid soybean oil to create trans-free shortening. When it is chemically combined with liquid oil, the ingredient is called inter-esterified vegetable oil. Meanwhile, oil processors are trying to improve the hydrogenation process so that less trans fat forms.

Potassium Bromate

- Flour improver: White flour, bread, and rolls

This additive has long been used to increase the volume of bread and to produce bread with a fine crumb (the not-crust part of bread) structure. Most bromate rapidly breaks down to form innocuous bromide. However, bromate itself causes cancer in animals. The tiny amounts of bromate that may remain in bread pose a small risk to consumers. Bromate has been banned virtually worldwide except in Japan and the United States. It is rarely used in California because a cancer warning might be required on the label. In 1999, the Center for Science in the Public Interest petitioned the FDA to ban bromate. Since then, numerous millers and bakers have stopped using bromate.

Propyl Gallate

- Antioxidant preservative: Vegetable oil, meat products, potato sticks, chicken soup base, chewing gum

Propyl gallate retards the spoilage of fats and oils and is often used with BHA and BHT [butylated hydroxytoluene], because of the synergistic effects these preservatives have. The best studies on rats and mice were peppered with suggestions (but not proof) that this preservative might cause cancer.

Saccharin

- Artificial sweetener: Diet, no-sugar-added products, soft drinks, sweetener packets

Saccharin (Sweet 'N Low) is 350 times sweeter than sugar and is used in diet foods or as a tabletop sugar substitute. Many studies on animals have shown that saccharin can cause cancer of the urinary bladder. In other rodent studies, saccharin has caused cancer of the uterus, ovaries, skin, blood vessels, and other organs. Other studies have shown that saccharin increases the potency of other cancer-causing chemicals. And the best epidemiology study (done by the National Cancer Institute) found that the use of artificial sweeteners (saccharin and cyclamate) was associated with a higher incidence of bladder cancer.

In 1977, the FDA proposed that saccharin be banned, because of studies that it causes cancer in animals. However, Congress intervened and permitted it to be used, provided that foods bear a warning notice. It has been replaced in many products by aspartame (NutraSweet). In 1997, the diet-food industry began pressuring the U.S. and Canadian governments and the World Health

Organization to take saccharin off their lists of cancer-causing chemicals. The industry acknowledges that saccharin causes bladder cancer in male rats, but argues that those tumors are caused by a mechanism that would not occur in humans. Many public health experts respond by stating that, even if that still-unproved mechanism were correct in male rats, saccharin could cause cancer by additional mechanisms and that, in some studies, saccharin has caused bladder cancer in mice and in female rats and other cancers in both rats and mice.

In May 2000, the U.S. Department of Health and Human Services removed saccharin from its list of cancer-causing chemicals. Later that year, Congress passed a law removing the warning notice that likely will result in increased use in soft drinks and other foods and in a slightly greater incidence of cancer.

Sodium Nitrite, Sodium Nitrate

- Preservative, coloring, flavoring: Bacon, ham, frankfurters, luncheon meats, smoked fish, corned beef

Meat processors love sodium nitrite because it stabilizes the red color in cured meat (without nitrite, hot dogs and bacon would look gray) and gives a characteristic flavor. Sodium nitrate is used in dry cured meat, because it slowly breaks down into nitrite. Adding nitrite to food can lead to the formation of small amounts of potent cancer-causing chemicals (nitrosamines), particularly in fried bacon. Nitrite, which also occurs in saliva and forms from nitrate in several vegetables, can undergo the same chemical reaction in the stomach. Companies now add ascorbic acid or erythorbic acid to bacon to inhibit nitrosamine formation, a measure that has greatly reduced the problem. While nitrite and nitrate cause only a small risk, they are still worth avoiding.

Several studies have linked consumption of cured meat and nitrite by children, pregnant women, and adults with various types of cancer. Although those studies have not yet proven that eating nitrite in bacon, sausage, and ham causes cancer in humans, pregnant women would be prudent to avoid those products.

The meat industry justifies its use of nitrite and nitrate by claiming that it prevents the growth of bacteria that cause botulism poisoning. That's true, but freezing and refrigeration could also do that, and the U.S. Department of Agriculture has developed a safe method using lactic-acid-producing bacteria. The use of nitrite and nitrate has decreased greatly over the decades, because of refrigeration and restrictions on the amounts used. The meat industry could do the public's health a favor by cutting back even further. Because nitrite is used primarily in fatty, salty foods, consumers have important nutritional reasons for avoiding nitrite-preserved foods.

Editor's Note: The information in this chapter represents the opinion of the copyright holder and is presented as one viewpoint on a complex subject.

Chapter 37

Foodborne Illnesses

Chapter Contents

Section 37.1

Introduction to Foodborne Illnesses

"Foodborne Illness," Centers for Disease Control and Prevention (www.cdc.gov), October 5, 2005.

What is foodborne disease?

Foodborne disease is caused by consuming contaminated foods or beverages. Many different disease-causing microbes, or pathogens, can contaminate foods, so there are many different foodborne infections. In addition, poisonous chemicals or other harmful substances can cause foodborne diseases if they are present in food.

More than 250 different foodborne diseases have been described. Most of these diseases are infections, caused by a variety of bacteria, viruses, and parasites that can be foodborne. Other diseases are poisonings caused by harmful toxins or chemicals that have contaminated the food—for example, poisonous mushrooms. These different diseases have many different symptoms, so there is no one "syndrome" that is foodborne illness. However, the microbe or toxin enters the body through the gastrointestinal tract, and often causes the first symptoms there, so nausea, vomiting, abdominal cramps, and diarrhea are common symptoms in many foodborne diseases.

Many microbes can spread in more than one way, so we cannot always know that a disease is foodborne. The distinction matters, because public health authorities need to know how a particular disease is spreading to take the appropriate steps to stop it. For example, *Escherichia coli* O157:H7 infections can spread through contaminated food, contaminated drinking water, contaminated swimming water, and from toddler to toddler at a day care center. Depending on which means of spread caused a case, the measures to stop other cases from occurring could range from removing contaminated food from stores, chlorinating a swimming pool, or closing a child day care center.

What are the most common foodborne diseases?

The most commonly recognized foodborne infections are those caused by the bacteria *Campylobacter*, *Salmonella*, and *E. coli* O157:H7, and by a group of viruses called Calicivirus, also known as the Norwalk and Norwalk-like viruses.

Campylobacter is a bacterial pathogen that causes fever, diarrhea, and abdominal cramps. It is the most commonly identified bacterial cause of diarrheal illness in the world. These bacteria live in the intestines of healthy birds, and most raw poultry meat has *Campylobacter* on it. Eating undercooked chicken, or other food that has been contaminated with juices dripping from raw chicken, is the most frequent source of this infection.

Salmonella is also a bacterium that is widespread in the intestines of birds, reptiles, and mammals. It can spread to humans via a variety of different foods of animal origin. The illness it causes, salmonellosis, typically includes fever, diarrhea, and abdominal cramps. In persons with poor underlying health or weakened immune systems, it can invade the bloodstream and cause life-threatening infections.

E. coli O157:H7 is a bacterial pathogen that has a reservoir in cattle and other similar animals. Human illness typically follows consumption of food or water that has been contaminated with microscopic amounts of cow feces. The illness it causes is often a severe and bloody diarrhea and painful abdominal cramps, without much fever. In 3% to 5% of cases, a complication called hemolytic uremic syndrome (HUS) can occur several weeks after the initial symptoms. This severe complication includes temporary anemia, profuse bleeding, and kidney failure.

Calicivirus, or Norwalk-like virus, is an extremely common cause of foodborne illness, though it is rarely diagnosed because the laboratory test is not widely available. It causes an acute gastrointestinal illness, usually with more vomiting than diarrhea, that resolves within two days. Unlike many foodborne pathogens that have animal reservoirs, it is believed that Norwalk-like viruses spread primarily from one infected person to another. Infected kitchen workers can contaminate a salad or sandwich as they prepare it if they have the virus on their hands. Infected fishermen have contaminated oysters as they harvested them.

Some common diseases are occasionally foodborne, even though they are usually transmitted by other routes. These include infections caused by *Shigella*, hepatitis A, and the parasites *Giardia lamblia* and *Cryptosporidia*. Even strep throats have been transmitted occasionally through food.

In addition to disease caused by direct infection, some foodborne diseases are caused by the presence of a toxin in the food that was produced by a microbe in the food. For example, the bacterium *Staphylococcus aureus* can grow in some foods and produce a toxin that causes intense vomiting. The rare but deadly disease botulism occurs when the bacterium *Clostridium botulinum* grows and produces a powerful paralytic toxin in foods. These toxins can produce illness even if the microbes that produced them are no longer there.

Other toxins and poisonous chemicals can cause foodborne illness. People can become ill if a pesticide is inadvertently added to a food, or if naturally poisonous substances are used to prepare a meal. Every year, people become ill after mistaking poisonous mushrooms for safe species, or after eating poisonous reef fishes.

Are the types of foodborne diseases changing?

The spectrum of foodborne diseases is constantly changing. A century ago, typhoid fever, tuberculosis, and cholera were common foodborne diseases. Improvements in food safety, such as pasteurization of milk, safe canning, and disinfection of water supplies, have conquered those diseases. Today other foodborne infections have taken their place, including some that have only recently been discovered. For example, in 1996, the parasite *Cyclospora* suddenly appeared as a cause of diarrheal illness related to Guatemalan raspberries. These berries had just started to be grown commercially in Guatemala, and somehow became contaminated in the field there with this unusual parasite. In 1998, a new strain of the bacterium *Vibrio parahaemolyticus* contaminated oyster beds in Galveston Bay and caused an epidemic of diarrheal illness in persons eating the oysters raw. The affected oyster beds were near the shipping lanes, which suggested that the bacterium arrived in the ballast water of freighters and tankers coming into the harbor from distant ports. Newly recognized microbes emerge as public health problems for several reasons: microbes can easily spread around the world, new microbes can evolve, the environment and ecology are changing, food production practices and consumption habits change, and because better laboratory tests can now identify microbes that were previously unrecognized.

In the last 15 years, several important diseases of unknown cause have turned out to be complications of foodborne infections. For example, we now know that Guillain-Barré syndrome can be caused by *Campylobacter* infection, and that the most common cause of acute kidney failure in children, hemolytic uremic syndrome, is caused by infection with *E. coli* O157:H7 and related bacteria. In the future, other diseases whose origins are currently unknown may turn out be related to foodborne infections.

What happens in the body after the microbes that produce illness are swallowed?

After they are swallowed, there is a delay, called the incubation period, before the symptoms of illness begin. This delay may range from hours to days, depending on the organism and on how many of them were swallowed. During the incubation period, the microbes pass through the stomach into the intestine, attach to the cells lining the intestinal walls, and begin to multiply there. Some types of microbes stay in the intestine, some produce a toxin that is absorbed into the bloodstream, and some can directly invade the deeper body tissues. The symptoms produced depend greatly on the type of microbe. Numerous organisms cause similar symptoms, especially diarrhea, abdominal cramps, and nausea. There is so much overlap that it is rarely possible to say which microbe is likely to be causing a given illness unless laboratory tests are done to identify the microbe, or unless the illness is part of a recognized outbreak.

How are foodborne diseases diagnosed?

The infection is usually diagnosed by specific laboratory tests that identify the causative organism. Bacteria such as *Campylobacter*, *Salmonella*, and *E. coli* O157 are found by culturing stool samples in the laboratory and identifying the bacteria that grow on the agar or other culture medium. Parasites can be identified by examining stools under the microscope. Viruses are more difficult to identify, as they are too small to see under a light microscope and are difficult to culture. Viruses are usually identified by testing stool samples for genetic markers that indicate a specific virus is present.

Many foodborne infections are not identified by routine laboratory procedures and require specialized, experimental, and/or expensive tests that are not generally available. If the diagnosis is to be made, the patient has to seek medical attention, the physician must decide to order diagnostic tests, and the laboratory must use the appropriate procedures. Because many ill persons do not seek attention, and of those that do, many are not tested, many cases of foodborne illness go undiagnosed. For example, CDC [Centers for Disease Control and Prevention] estimates that 38 cases of salmonellosis actually occur for every case that is actually diagnosed and reported to public health authorities.

How are foodborne diseases treated?

There are many different kinds of foodborne diseases and they may require different treatments, depending on the symptoms they cause.

Illnesses that are primarily diarrhea or vomiting can lead to dehydration if the person loses more body fluids and salts (electrolytes) than they take in. Replacing the lost fluids and electrolytes and keeping up with fluid intake are important. If diarrhea is severe, oral rehydration solution such as Ceralyte*, Pedialyte* or Oralyte* should be drunk to replace the fluid losses and prevent dehydration. Sports drinks such as Gatorade* do not replace the losses correctly and should not be used for the treatment of diarrheal illness. Preparations of bismuth subsalicylate (e.g., Pepto-Bismol*) can reduce the duration and severity of simple diarrhea. If diarrhea and cramps occur, without bloody stools or fever, taking an antidiarrheal medication may provide symptomatic relief, but these medications should be avoided if there is high fever or blood in the stools because they may make the illness worse.

*CDC does not endorse commercial products or services.

When should I consult my doctor about a diarrheal illness?

A health care provider should be consulted for a diarrheal illness that is accompanied by any of the following symptoms:

- High fever (temperature over 101.5° F, measured orally)
- Blood in the stools
- Prolonged vomiting that prevents keeping liquids down (which can lead to dehydration)
- Signs of dehydration, including a decrease in urination, a dry mouth and throat, and feeling dizzy when standing up
- Diarrheal illness that lasts more than three days

Do not be surprised if your doctor does not prescribe an antibiotic. Many diarrheal illnesses are caused by viruses and will improve in two or three days without antibiotic therapy. In fact, antibiotics have no effect on viruses, and using an antibiotic to treat a viral infection could cause more harm than good. It is often not necessary to take an antibiotic even in the case of a mild bacterial infection. Other treatments can help the symptoms, and careful hand washing can prevent the spread of infection to other people. Overuse of antibiotics is the principal reason many bacteria are becoming resistant. Resistant bacteria are no longer killed by the antibiotic. This means that it is important to use antibiotics only when they are really needed. Partial treatment can also cause bacteria to become resistant. If an antibiotic is prescribed, it is important to take all of the medication as prescribed, and not stop early just because the symptoms seem to be improving.

How many cases of foodborne disease are there in the United States?

An estimated 76 million cases of foodborne disease occur each year in the United States. The great majority of these cases are mild and cause symptoms for only a day or two. Some cases are more serious, and CDC estimates that there are 325,000 hospitalizations and 5,000 deaths related to foodborne diseases each year. The most severe cases tend to occur in the very old, the very young, those who have an illness already that reduces their immune system function, and in healthy people exposed to a very high dose of an organism.

How do public health departments track foodborne diseases?

Routine monitoring of important diseases by public health departments is called disease surveillance. Each state decides which diseases are to be under surveillance in that state. In most states, diagnosed cases of salmonellosis, *E. coli* O157:H7, and other serious infections are routinely reported to the health department. The county reports them to the state health department, which reports them to CDC. Tens of thousands of cases of these "notifiable conditions" are reported every year. For example, nearly 35,000 cases of *Salmonella* infection were reported to CDC in 1998. However, most foodborne infections go undiagnosed and unreported, either because the ill person does not see a doctor or the doctor does not make a specific diagnosis. Also, infections with some microbes are not reportable in the first place.

To get more information about infections that might be diagnosed but not reported, CDC developed a special surveillance system called FoodNet. FoodNet provides the best available information about specific foodborne infections in the United States, and summarizes them in an annual report.

In addition to tracking the number of reported cases of individual infections, states also collect information about foodborne outbreaks and report a summary of that information to CDC. About 400–500 foodborne outbreaks investigated by local and state health departments are reported each year. This includes information about many diseases that are not notifiable and thus are not under individual surveillance, so it provides some useful general information about foodborne diseases.

What are foodborne disease outbreaks and why do they occur?

An outbreak of foodborne illness occurs when a group of people consume the same contaminated food and two or more of them come down with the same illness. It may be a group that ate a meal together somewhere, or it may be a group of people who do not know each other at all, but who all happened to buy and eat the same contaminated item from a grocery store or restaurant. For an outbreak to occur, something must have happened to contaminate a batch of food that was eaten by a group of people. Often, a combination of events contributes to the outbreak. A contaminated food may be left out at room temperature for many hours, allowing the bacteria to multiply to high numbers, and then be insufficiently cooked to kill the bacteria.

Many outbreaks are local in nature. They are recognized when a group of people realize that they all became ill after a common meal, and someone calls the local health department. This classic local outbreak might follow a catered meal at a reception, a potluck supper, or eating a meal at an understaffed restaurant on a particularly busy day. However, outbreaks are increasingly being recognized that are more widespread, that affect persons in many different places, and that are spread out over several weeks. For example, a recent outbreak of salmonellosis was traced to persons eating a breakfast cereal produced at a factory in Minnesota and marketed under several different brand names in many different states. No one county or state had very many cases and the cases did not know each other. The outbreak was recognized because it was caused by an unusual strain of *Salmonella*, and because state public health laboratories that type *Salmonella* strains noticed a sudden increase in this one rare strain. In another recent outbreak, a particular peanut snack food caused the same illness in Israel, Europe, and North America. Again, this was recognized as an increase in infections caused by a rare strain of *Salmonella*.

The vast majority of reported cases of foodborne illness are not part of recognized outbreaks, but occurs as individual or "sporadic" cases. It may be that many of these cases are actually part of unrecognized widespread or diffuse outbreaks. Detecting and investigating such widespread outbreaks is a major challenge to our public health system. This is the reason that new and more sophisticated laboratory methods are being used at CDC and in state public health department laboratories.

Why do public health officials investigate outbreaks?

A foodborne outbreak is an indication that something needs to be improved in our food safety system. Public health scientists investigate outbreaks to control them, and also to learn how similar outbreaks can be prevented in the future. Just as when a fire breaks out in a large building or when an airliner crashes, two activities are critical when an outbreak occurs. First, emergency action is needed to keep the immediate danger from spreading, and second, a detailed objective scientific investigation is needed to learn what went wrong, so that future similar events can be prevented. Much of what we know about foodborne disease and its prevention comes from detailed investigation of outbreaks. This is often how a new pathogen is identified, and this is how the critical information linking a pathogen to a specific food and animal reservoir is first gathered. The full investigation can require a team with multiple talents, including the epidemiologist, microbiologist, food sanitarian, food scientist, veterinarian, and factory process engineer.

How are outbreaks of foodborne disease detected?

The initial clue that an outbreak is occurring can come in various ways. It may be when a person realizes that several other people who were all together at an event have become ill and he or she calls the local health department. It may be when a physician realizes she has seen more than the usual number of patients with the same illness. It may be when a county health department gets an unusually large number of reports of illness. The hardest outbreaks to detect are those that are spread over a large geographic area, with only a few cases in each state. These outbreaks can be detected by combining surveillance reports at the regional or national level and looking for increases in infections of a specific type. This is why state public health laboratories determine the serotype of *Salmonella* bacteria isolated from people. New "DNA fingerprinting" technologies can make detecting outbreaks easier too. For example, the new molecular subtyping network, PulseNet, allows state laboratories and CDC to compare strains of *E. coli* O157:H7 and an increasing number of other pathogens from all across the United States to detect widespread outbreaks.

After an apparent cluster of cases is detected, it is important to determine whether these cases represent a real increase above the expected number of cases and whether they really might be related. Sometimes a cluster of reported cases is caused by something other than an actual outbreak of illness. For example, if the person responsible for reporting has just returned from a vacation and is clearing up a backlog of cases by reporting them all at once, the sudden surge of reports is just a false cluster.

How is a foodborne disease outbreak investigated?

Once an outbreak is strongly suspected, an investigation begins. A search is made for more cases among persons who may have been exposed. The symptoms and time of onset and location of possible cases are determined, and a "case definition" is developed that describes these typical cases. The outbreak is systematically described by time, place, and person. A graph is drawn of the number of people who fell ill on each successive day to show pictorially when it occurred. A map of where the ill people live, work, or eat may be helpful to show where it occurred. Calculating the distribution of cases by age and sex shows who is affected. If the causative microbe is not known, samples of stool or blood are collected from ill people and sent to the public health laboratory to make the diagnosis.

To identify the food or other source of the outbreak, the investigators first interview a few persons with the most typical cases about exposures they may have had in the few days before they got sick. In this way, certain potential exposures may be excluded while others that are mentioned repeatedly emerge as possibilities. Combined with other information, such as the likely sources for the specific microbe involved, these hypotheses are then tested in a formal epidemiologic investigation. The investigators conduct systematic interviews about a list of possible exposures with the ill persons and with a comparable group of people who are not ill. By comparing how often an exposure is reported by ill people and by well people, investigators can measure the association of the exposure with illness. Using probability statistics, similar to those used to describe coin flips, the probability of no association is directly calculated.

For example, imagine that an outbreak has occurred after a catered event. Initial investigation suggested that hollandaise sauce was eaten by at least some of the attendees, so it is on the list of possible hypotheses. Now, we interview 20 persons who attended the affair, 10 of whom became ill and 10 who remained well. Each ill or well person is interviewed about whether or not they ate the hollandaise sauce, as well as various other food items. If half the people ate the sauce, but the sauce was not associated with the illness, then we would expect each person to have a 50/50 chance of reporting that they ate it, regardless of whether they were ill or not. Suppose, however, that we find that all 10 ill people but none of the well persons reported eating hollandaise sauce at the event. This would be very unlikely to occur by chance alone if eating the hollandaise sauce were not somehow related to the risk of illness. In fact, it would be about as unlikely as getting heads 10 times in a row by flipping a coin (that is 50% multiplied by itself 10 times over, or a chance of just under 1 in 1,000). So the epidemiologist concludes that eating the hollandaise sauce was very likely to be associated with the risk of illness. Note that the investigator can draw this conclusion even though there is no hollandaise sauce left to test in a laboratory. The association is even stronger if she can show that those who ate second helpings of hollandaise were even more likely to become ill, or that persons who ate leftover hollandaise sauce that went home in doggie bags also became ill.

Once a food item is statistically implicated in this manner, further investigation into its ingredients and preparation, and microbiologic culture of leftover ingredients or the food itself (if available), may provide additional information about the nature of contamination. Perhaps the hollandaise sauce was made using raw eggs. The source of the raw eggs can be determined, and it may even be possible to trace them back to the farm and show that chickens on the farm are carrying the same strain of *Salmonella* in their ovaries. If so, the eggs from that farm can be pasteurized to prevent them from causing other outbreaks.

Some might think that the best investigation method would be just to culture all the leftover foods in the kitchen and conclude that the one that is positive is the one that caused the outbreak. The trouble is that this can be misleading, because it happens after the fact. What if the hollandaise sauce is all gone, but the spoon that was in the sauce got placed in potato salad that was not served at the function? Now, cultures of the potato salad yield a pathogen, and the unwary tester might call that the source of the outbreak, even though the potato salad had nothing to do with it. This means that laboratory testing without epidemiologic investigation can lead to the wrong conclusion.

Even without isolating microbes from food, a well-conducted epidemiologic investigation can guide immediate efforts to control the outbreak. A strong and consistent statistical association between illness and a particular food item that explains the distribution of the outbreak in time, place, and person should be acted upon immediately to stop further illness from occurring.

An outbreak ends when the critical exposure stops. This may happen because all the contaminated food is eaten or recalled, because a restaurant is closed or a food processor shuts down or changes its procedures, or because an infected food handler is no longer infectious or is no longer working with food. An investigation that clarifies the nature and mechanism of contamination can provide critical information even if the outbreak is over. Understanding the contamination event well enough to prevent it can guide the decision to resume usual operations and lead to more general prevention measures that reduce the risk of similar outbreaks happening elsewhere.

How does food become contaminated?

We live in a microbial world, and there are many opportunities for food to become contaminated as it is produced and prepared. Many foodborne microbes are present in healthy animals (usually in their intestines) raised for food. Meat and poultry carcasses can become contaminated during slaughter by contact with small amounts of intestinal contents. Similarly, fresh fruits and vegetables can be contaminated if they are washed or irrigated with water that is contaminated with animal manure or human sewage. Some types of *Salmonella* can infect a hen's ovary so that the internal contents of a normal-looking egg can be contaminated with *Salmonella* even before the shell is formed. Oysters and other filter-feeding shellfish can concentrate *Vibrio* bacteria that are naturally present in sea water, or other microbes that are present in human sewage dumped into the sea.

Later in food processing, other foodborne microbes can be introduced from infected humans who handle the food, or by cross-contamination from some other raw agricultural product. For example, *Shigella* bacteria, hepatitis A virus, and Norwalk virus can be introduced by the unwashed hands of food handlers who are themselves infected. In the kitchen, microbes can be transferred from one food to another food by using the same knife, cutting board, or other utensil to prepare both without washing the surface or utensil in between. A food that is fully cooked can become recontaminated if it touches other raw foods or drippings from raw foods that contain pathogens.

The way that food is handled after it is contaminated can also make a difference in whether or not an outbreak occurs. Many bacterial microbes need to multiply to a larger number before enough are present in food to cause disease. Given warm moist conditions and an ample supply of nutrients, one bacterium that reproduces by dividing itself every half hour can produce 17 million progeny in 12 hours. As a result, lightly contaminated food left out overnight can be highly infectious by the next day. If the food were refrigerated promptly, the bacteria would not multiply at all. In general, refrigeration or freezing prevents virtually all bacteria from growing but generally preserves them in a state of suspended animation. This general rule has a few surprising exceptions. Two foodborne bacteria, *Listeria monocytogenes* and *Yersinia enterocolitica*, can actually grow at refrigerator temperatures. High salt, high sugar, or high acid levels keep bacteria from growing, which is why salted meats, jam, and pickled vegetables are traditional preserved foods.

Microbes are killed by heat. If food is heated to an internal temperature above 160° F, or 78° C, for even a few seconds this is sufficient to kill parasites, viruses, or bacteria, except for the *Clostridium* bacteria, which produce a heat-resistant form called a spore. *Clostridium* spores are killed only at temperatures above boiling. This is why canned foods must be cooked to a high temperature under pressure as part of the canning process.

The toxins produced by bacteria vary in their sensitivity to heat. The staphylococcal toxin that causes vomiting is not inactivated even if it is boiled. Fortunately, the potent toxin that causes botulism is completely inactivated by boiling.

What foods are most associated with foodborne illness?

Raw foods of animal origin are the most likely to be contaminated; that is, raw meat and poultry, raw eggs, unpasteurized milk, and raw shellfish. Because filter-feeding shellfish strain microbes from the sea over many months, they are particularly likely to be contaminated if there are any pathogens in the seawater. Foods that mingle the products of many individual animals, such as bulk raw milk, pooled raw eggs, or ground beef, are particularly hazardous because a pathogen present in any one of the animals may contaminate the whole batch. A single hamburger may contain meat from hundreds of animals. A single restaurant omelet may contain eggs from hundreds of chickens. A glass of raw milk may contain milk from hundreds of cows. A broiler chicken carcass can be exposed to the drippings and juices of many thousands of other birds that went through the same cold water tank after slaughter.

Fruits and vegetables consumed raw are a particular concern. Washing can decrease but not eliminate contamination, so the consumers can do little to protect themselves. Recently, a number of outbreaks have been traced to fresh fruits and vegetables that were processed under less than sanitary conditions. These outbreaks show that the quality of the water used for washing and chilling the produce after it is harvested is critical. Using water that is not clean can contaminate many boxes of produce. Fresh manure used to fertilize vegetables can also contaminate them. Alfalfa sprouts and other raw sprouts pose a particular challenge, as the conditions under which they are sprouted are ideal for growing microbes as well as sprouts, and because they are eaten without further cooking. That means that a few bacteria present on the seeds can grow to high numbers of pathogens on the sprouts. Unpasteurized fruit juice can also be contaminated if there are pathogens in or on the fruit that is used to make it.

What can consumers do to protect themselves from foodborne illness?

A few simple precautions can reduce the risk of foodborne diseases:

Cook meat, poultry, and eggs thoroughly. Using a thermometer to measure the internal temperature of meat is a good way to be sure that it is cooked sufficiently to kill bacteria. For example, ground beef should be cooked to an internal temperature of 160° F. Eggs should be cooked until the yolk is firm.

Separate: Don't cross-contaminate one food with another. Avoid cross-contaminating foods by washing hands, utensils, and cutting boards after they have been in contact with raw meat or poultry and before they touch another food. Put cooked meat on a clean platter, rather back on one that held the raw meat.

Chill: Refrigerate leftovers promptly. Bacteria can grow quickly at room temperature, so refrigerate leftover foods if they are not going to be eaten within four hours. Large volumes of food will cool more quickly if they are divided into several shallow containers for refrigeration.

Clean: Wash produce. Rinse fresh fruits and vegetables in running tap water to remove visible dirt and grime. Remove and discard the outermost leaves of a head of lettuce or cabbage. Because bacteria can grow well on the cut surface of fruit or vegetable, be careful not to contaminate these foods while slicing them up on the cutting board, and avoid leaving cut produce at room temperature for many hours. Don't be a source of foodborne illness yourself. Wash your hands with soap and water before preparing food. Avoid preparing food for others if you yourself have a diarrheal illness. Changing a baby's diaper while preparing food is a bad idea that can easily spread illness.

Report: Report suspected foodborne illnesses to your local health department. The local public health department is an important part of the food safety system. Often calls from concerned citizens are how outbreaks are first detected. If a public health official contacts you to find our more about an illness you had, your cooperation is important. In public health investigations, it can be as important to talk to healthy people as to ill people. Your cooperation may be needed even if you are not ill.

Are some people more likely to contract a foodborne illness? If so, are there special precautions they should take?

Some persons at particularly high risk should take more precautions.

Pregnant women, the elderly, and those with weakened immune systems are at higher risk for severe infections such as *Listeria* and should be particularly careful not to consume undercooked animal products. They should avoid soft French-style cheeses, pates, uncooked hot dogs, and sliced deli meats, which have been sources of *Listeria* infections. Persons at high risk should also avoid alfalfa sprouts and unpasteurized juices.

A bottle-fed infant is at higher risk for severe infections with *Salmonella* or other bacteria that can grow in a bottle of warm formula if it is left at room temperature for many hours. Particular care is needed to be sure the baby's bottle is cleaned and disinfected and that leftover milk formula or juice is not held in the bottle for many hours.

Persons with liver disease are susceptible to infections with a rare but dangerous microbe called *Vibrio vulnificus*, found in oysters. They should avoid eating raw oysters.

What can consumers do when they eat in restaurants?

You can protect yourself first by choosing which restaurant to patronize. Restaurants are inspected by the local health department to make sure they are clean and have adequate kitchen facilities. Find out how restaurants did on their most recent inspections, and use that score to help guide your choice. In many jurisdictions, the latest inspection score is posted in the restaurant. Some restaurants have specifically trained their staff in principles of food safety. This is also good to know in deciding which restaurant to patronize.

You can also protect yourself from foodborne disease when ordering specific foods, just as you would at home. When ordering a hamburger, ask for it to be cooked to a temperature of 160° F and send it back if it is still pink in the middle. Before you order something that is made with many eggs pooled together, such as scrambled eggs, omelets, or french toast, ask the waiter whether it was made with pasteurized egg, and choose something else if it was not.

There is only so much the consumer can do. How can food be made safer in the first place?

Making food safe in the first place is a major effort, involving the farm and fishery, the production plant or factory, and many other points from the farm to the table. Many different groups in public health, industry, regulatory agencies, and academia have roles to play in making the food supply less contaminated. Consumers can promote general food safety with their dollars by purchasing foods that have been processed for safety. For example, milk pasteurization was a major advance in food safety that was developed 100 years ago. Buying pasteurized milk rather than raw unpasteurized milk still prevents an enormous number of foodborne diseases every day. Now juice pasteurization is a recent important step forward that prevents *E. coli* O157:H7 infections and many other diseases. Consumers can look for and buy pasteurized fruit juices and ciders. In the future, meat and other foods will be available that have been treated for safety with irradiation. These new technologies are likely to be as important a step forward as the pasteurization of milk.

Foodborne diseases are largely preventable, though there is no simple one-step prevention measure like a vaccine. Instead, measures are needed to prevent or limit contamination all the way from farm to table. A variety of good agricultural and manufacturing practices can reduce the spread of microbes among animals and prevent the contamination of foods. Careful review of the whole food production process can identify the principal hazards and the control points where contamination can be prevented, limited, or eliminated. A formal method for evaluating the control of risk in foods that exists is called the Hazard Analysis Critical Control Point, or HACCP, system. This was first developed by NASA [National Aeronautics and Space

Administration] to make sure that the food eaten by astronauts was safe. HACCP safety principles are now being applied to an increasing spectrum of foods, including meat, poultry, and seafood.

For some particularly risky foods, even the most careful hygiene and sanitation are insufficient to prevent contamination, and a definitive microbe-killing step must be included in the process. For example, early in the century, large botulism outbreaks occurred when canned foods were cooked insufficiently to kill the botulism spores. After research was done to find out exactly how much heat was needed to kill the spores, the canning industry and the government regulators went to great lengths to be sure every can was sufficiently cooked. As a result, botulism related to commercial canned foods has disappeared in this country. Similarly, the introduction of careful pasteurization of milk eliminated a large number of milk-borne diseases. This occurred after sanitation in dairies had already reached a high level. In the future, other foods can be made much safer by new pasteurizing technologies, such as in-shell pasteurization of eggs and irradiation of ground beef. Just as with milk, these new technologies should be implemented in addition to good sanitation, not as a replacement for it.

In the end, it is up to the consumer to demand a safe food supply; up to industry to produce it; up to researchers to develop better ways of doing so; and up to government to see that it happens, to make sure it works, and to identify problems still in need of solutions.

Section 37.2

Bovine Spongiform Encephalopathy (Mad Cow Disease)

"A Focus on Bovine Spongiform Encephalopathy," Food Safety Research Information Office, U.S. Department of Agriculture (fsrio.nal.usda.gov), November 2007.

Bovine spongiform encephalopathy (BSE), commonly known as "mad cow disease," is a fatal neurodegenerative disease in cattle that causes a spongy degeneration in the brain and spinal cord. BSE has a long incubation period, about four years, usually affecting adult cattle at a peak-age onset of four to five years, all breeds being equally susceptible. Postmortem pathological tests of the brain tissue are the only existing methods to confirm BSE.

Mad cow disease is believed to be linked to the variant Creutzfeldt-Jakob disease (vCJD), a fatal transmissible spongiform encephalopathy (TSE) disease found in humans. The relationship of the infective BSE agent and vCJD in humans is not completely understood and no direct correlation has been confirmed; however, a strong association exists between humans infected with vCJD and exposure to BSE-infected products. Understanding the TSE agent's ability to cross species barriers and developing more sensitive antemortem diagnostic tests are two current areas of research.

BSE was first identified in the United Kingdom (UK) in 1987. Between 1988 and 2002 more than 182,000 cases were found, accounting for 98% of the cases found worldwide. Epidemiological studies have found that BSE is a feed-borne infection transmitted to animals through BSE-infected meat-and-bone meal in animal feed. The exact origin of BSE in cattle is not known, but it is possible that it came from either scrapie in sheep, a transmissible spongiform encephalopathy in another mammalian species, or a spontaneous mutation in cattle. Risk analysis studies on BSE transmission have initiated research to determine the following: risk materials and infectivity levels, infectious dose, route of infection, strain of the agent, genotype of the animals at risk, and the nature and size of species barriers.

Transmissible Spongiform Encephalopathies

BSE is one disease from a family of related but distinct, neurodegenerative diseases called transmissible spongiform encephalopathies. TSEs are characterized by the long incubation period (with respect to the life expectancy of the host species) and by the existence of many different strains of infectious agents. Strains of TSE differ in their lesion profile, incubation period, pathogenicity, resistance to chemical and heat inactivation, and distribution in the infected organism. TSE agents are similar to conventional viruses in that they can compete for replication in a single host. This means that slow-growing strains interfere with infection/replication of more rapid growing strains. Unlike traditional viruses, TSEs are resistant to most virus-inactivating treatments and do not provoke a systemic inflammatory response or antigenicity.

The following is a list of different types of TSEs that have been identified in animals and humans:

- Chronic wasting disease (CWD) in elk and deer
- Transmissible mink encephalopathy (TME) in ranch-reared mink
- Feline spongiform encephalopathy (FSE) in cats and captive exotic felids
- Scrapie in sheep, goats, and moufflon*
- Kuru, Gerstmann-Straussler-Scheinker disease, fatal familial insomnia, Creutzfeldt-Jakob disease (CJD), and new variant Creutzfeldt-Jakob disease, all found in humans

*The oldest TSE is scrapie.

Variant Creutzfeldt-Jakob Disease (vCJD)

Two types of CJDs are known to exist:

- Classical CJD
- New variant form, vCJD

The vCJD was first diagnosed in 1996 in the UK by the National CJD Surveillance Unit. According to May 2007 statistical data, the total number of deaths in the United Kingdom from definite or probable vCJD cases is 160.

Patients range in age from 12 to 74 years old and live an average of one year after showing clinical symptoms. The incubation period is believed to be 10 to 15 years, but could be longer.

vCJD is linked to eating BSE-contaminated beef products but the potential for transmission between people is not understood and extensive research is currently being conducted in order to understand the transmission, detection, and treatment.

Specified Risk Materials

Specified risk materials (SRM) is the general term designated for infective tissues that transmit the disease. The BSE infective agent has been found to concentrate in specific tissues of BSE-infected cattle and these tissues are all part of the central nervous system, as BSE has not been shown to infect muscle. The World Organization for Animal Health (OIE) has established recommendations and guidelines for SRM removal based on the level of risk. In both the United States and Canada, considered low risk countries, SRMs are defined as: skull, brain, trigeminal ganglia (nerves attached to brain and close to the skull exterior), eyes, spinal cord, distal ileum, and the dorsal root ganglia (nerves attached to the spinal cord and close to the vertebral column) of cattle aged 30 months or older. In the United States, tonsils are removed from cattle of all ages. SRMs must be removed at slaughter and disposed as inedible material. The dorsal root ganglia must be removed during the deboning process, and, in animals older than 30 months, the vertebral column (excluding the vertebrae of the tail, the transverse processes of the lumbar and thoracic vertebrae, and the wings of the sacrum) is removed to be certain the dorsal root ganglia is extracted in its entirety.

In the United Kingdom, and other countries classified as moderate to high risk, the OIE code recommends SRM removal as follows: tonsils and intestines in cattle at all ages; and, brains, eyes, spinal cord, skull, and vertebral column from animals over 12 months of age.

The removal of SRMs is believed by many experts to be the single most important action in protecting the public health.

BSE Surveillance

An active BSE surveillance program has existed in the United States since May 1990, in order to safeguard the American cattle population. The U.S. surveillance program is an interagency effort coordinated by the USDA [U.S. Department of Agriculture] Animal and

Plant Health Inspection Service (APHIS) and includes both active and passive surveillance. It is designed to prevent infection and transmission of foreign animal diseases like BSE, or any TSE, from infecting U.S. cattle. In addition, measures are in place to quickly detect and respond to an outbreak. The BSE surveillance program was enhanced when the first BSE outbreak occurred in the United States in 2003.

Surveillance tests are not food safety tests and can only be used for the purpose of statistical analysis. Current detection methodology is limited and OIE suggest that the likelihood of detecting BSE in cattle varies depending on the characteristics of the subpopulation. The closer the animal is to exhibiting clinical BSE symptoms, the better the likelihood of detection. Currently, positive cases have been detected three months prior to clinical signs; however, given that the incubation period is about four years long, much time exists when infected cattle are tested and false negatives result. According to European data, it is 100 times more likely that BSE will be detected in cattle exhibiting clinical signs of BSE, than in downers on farms; and it is 5,000 to 10,000 more times than in healthy, 30-month-old cattle at slaughter. Another estimate is that the current test methodology has a false negative test rate of 92%, meaning in a population of 100 clinically normal BSE-infected adult cattle, 92 would test negative even though infected.

The U.S. surveillance strategy is to regionally represent the distribution of adult cattle across the nation. The regions are based on the movement of cattle going to slaughter. Each region has different surveillance goals and is treated as an individual country. A scientific approach allows for uniform surveillance across the nation while representing regional differences. Nationally, 12,500 samples are tested in order to detect one BSE-infected cattle per million. This approach is widely accepted around the world. The United States has an adult cattle population of 45 million, so if it is assumed that one per million is BSE infected, then 45 U.S. cattle would be infected. However, in the accuracy of random sampling of adult animals, three million cattle would need to be tested in order to obtain a 95% confidence level.

The United States has an active targeted surveillance plan rather than a random sampling strategy in order to establish a more efficient and effective survey. APHIS focuses on the higher risk population of cattle that are not going to slaughter. BSE-infected cattle have never been detected under the age of 20 months, and 88% of the U.S. slaughter population is under this age. The higher risk population is those most likely to have been exposed to the BSE, and it is in this population where the disease will more likely be detected. European surveillance testing has defined nonambulatory cattle as high risk. A survey conducted by the American Association of Bovine Practitioners estimated that 195,000 nonambulatory cattle exist in the United States. If it is assumed that 45 BSE-infected cattle can potentially be detected in a high-risk population of 195,000, the level of disease that is detected is 0.023%. According to a statistical analysis formulation by Cannon and Roe, a sample size of 12,500 is necessary to detect BSE at a prevalence of 0.023%. The national sample size of 12,500 established to detect one BSE-infected cattle per million is based upon scientific risk analysis methods. In addition, the OIE has established international surveillance standards for the number of samples to be tested each year within a country. In the last five years, the United States has exceeded the OIE recommendation of 433 samples per year.

Feed Ban

The European Union (EU) introduced a ban on ruminant feedstuffs containing protein derived from mammalian tissues in 1994 as part of their BSE eradication program. Originally, feed-borne contamination as a vehicle of disease transmission was just scientific opinion, but now epidemiological evidence, as well as the effect of feed bans, proves this to be true. During the slaughter process prior to the 1994 ban, ruminant tissues were rendered and processed for use in feedstuffs in the form of meat-and-bone meal (MBM).

MBM is defined as processed mammalian tissue used directly or indirectly for animal feed. The 1994 ban concerned animal proteins of ruminant origin being fed to ruminants, so ruminant protein continued to be fed to nonruminants. The continuation of BSE after the 1994 feed ban was blamed on unintentional cross-contamination during feed production since most of the feed mill facilities produced both ruminant and nonruminant feedstuffs. In 2000, the Scientific Steering Committee (SSC) of the EU recognized that the cross-contamination of mammalian MBM with all animal feedstuffs was unavoidable due to mixed-species feed mills and the lack of test methods to distinguish animal proteins of ruminant origin. In January 2001, EU legislation imposed a total ban, which specified that processed proteins derived from all mammals, birds, and fish be prohibited for all farmed animals intended for the production of food.

The SSC had various opinions on the total ban and provided four crucial conditions that, if followed and cross-contamination avoided or detected, would greatly reduce the risk of BSE transmission through recycled animal tissues in feed for nonruminant farmed animals. The four conditions are as follows: raw material fit for human consumption; SRMs and fallen stock removed; pressure-cooking standards (133° C, 20 minutes, 3 bar) followed; and control of the MBM ban to ruminants implemented effectively. In 2002, the EC [European Commission] issued an animal by-product regulation. Only materials from animals fit for human consumption following veterinarian inspection are allowed to be used in animal feed production. This regulation excludes fallen livestock and other condemned materials from the feed chain and it banned intraspecies recycling.

EC legislation made developing rapid control methods for distinguishing and identifying animal proteins of different species a necessity in order to enforce the bans implemented. Currently, different methods are being considered for the identification of animal protein in feed; however, feed microscopy is the official analysis method of the EU. In January 2001, an EC project called STRATFEED was initiated in order to test several of these analytical techniques: classical microscopy; polymerase chain reaction (PCR); near infrared microscopy (NIRM); and near infrared spectroscopy (NIRS). The enzyme-linked immunoabsorbent assay (ELISA) is also an available test, but is not part of the STRATFEED project.

Section 37.3

Campylobacter

"Campylobacter," Centers for Disease Control and Prevention (www.cdc.gov), May 21, 2008.

What is campylobacteriosis?

Campylobacteriosis is an infectious disease caused by bacteria of the genus *Campylobacter*. Most people who become ill with campylobacteriosis get diarrhea, cramping, abdominal pain, and fever within two to five days after exposure to the organism. The diarrhea may be bloody and can be accompanied by nausea and vomiting. The illness typically lasts one week. Some infected persons do not have any symptoms. In persons with compromised immune systems, *Campylobacter* occasionally spreads to the bloodstream and causes a serious life-threatening infection.

How common is Campylobacter?

Campylobacter is one of the most common causes of diarrheal illness in the United States. The vast majority of cases occur as isolated, sporadic events, not as part of recognized outbreaks. Active surveillance through FoodNet indicates that about 13 cases are diagnosed each year for each 100,000 persons in the population. Many more cases go undiagnosed or unreported, and campylobacteriosis is estimated to affect over 2.4 million persons every year, or 0.8% of the population. Campylobacteriosis occurs much more frequently in the summer months than in the winter. The organism is isolated from infants and young adults more frequently than from persons in other age groups and from males more frequently than females. Although *Campylobacter* does not commonly cause death, it has been estimated that approximately 124 persons with *Campylobacter* infections die each year.

What sort of germ is Campylobacter?

Campylobacter organisms are spiral-shaped bacteria that can cause disease in humans and animals. Most human illness is caused by one species, called *Campylobacter jejuni*, but human illness can also be caused by other species. *Campylobacter jejuni* grows best at the body temperature of a bird, and seems to be well adapted to birds, who carry it without becoming ill. These bacteria are fragile. They cannot tolerate drying and can be killed by oxygen. They grow only in places with less oxygen than the amount in the atmosphere. Freezing reduces the number of *Campylobacter* bacteria on raw meat.

How is the infection diagnosed?

Many different kinds of infections can cause diarrhea and bloody diarrhea. *Campylobacter* infection is diagnosed when a culture of a stool specimen yields the organism.

How can campylobacteriosis be treated?

Almost all persons infected with *Campylobacter* recover without any specific treatment. Patients should drink extra fluids as long as the diarrhea lasts. In more severe cases, antibiotics such as erythromycin or a fluoroquinolone can be used, and can shorten the duration of symptoms if given early in the illness. Your doctor will decide whether antibiotics are necessary.

Are there long-term consequences?

Most people who get campylobacteriosis recover completely within 2 to 5 days, although sometimes recovery can take up to 10 days. Rarely, *Campylobacter* infection results in long-term consequences. Some people develop arthritis. Others may develop a rare disease called Guillain-Barré syndrome, which affects the nerves of the body beginning several weeks after the diarrheal illness. This occurs when a person's immune system is "triggered" to attack the body's own nerves resulting in paralysis that lasts several weeks and usually requires intensive care. It is estimated that approximately 1 in every 1,000 reported *Campylobacter* illnesses leads to Guillain-Barré syndrome. As many as 40% of Guillain-Barré syndrome cases in this country may be triggered by campylobacteriosis.

How do people get infected with this germ?

Campylobacteriosis usually occurs in single, sporadic cases, but it can also occur in outbreaks, when a number of people become ill at one time. Most cases of campylobacteriosis are associated with eating raw or undercooked poultry meat or from cross-contamination of other foods by these items. Infants may get the infection by contact with poultry packages in shopping carts. Outbreaks of *Campylobacter* are usually associated with unpasteurized milk or contaminated water. Animals can also be infected, and some people have acquired their infection from contact with the stool of an ill dog or cat. The organism is not usually spread from one person to another, but this can happen if the infected person is producing a large volume of diarrhea.

A very small number of *Campylobacter* organisms (fewer than 500) can cause illness in humans. Even one drop of juice from raw chicken meat can infect a person. One way to become infected is to cut poultry meat on a cutting board, and then use the unwashed cutting board or utensil to prepare vegetables or other raw or lightly cooked foods. The *Campylobacter* organisms from the raw meat can thus spread to the other foods.

How does food or water get contaminated with Campylobacter*?*

Many chicken flocks are infected with *Campylobacter* but show no signs of illness. *Campylobacter* can be easily spread from bird to bird through a common water source or through contact with infected feces. When an infected bird is slaughtered, *Campylobacter* organisms can be transferred from the intestines to the meat. In 2005, *Campylobacter* was present on 47% of raw chicken breasts tested through the FDA-NARMS [Food and Drug Administration National Antimicrobial Resistance Monitoring System] Retail Food program. *Campylobacter* is also present in the giblets, especially the liver.

Unpasteurized milk can become contaminated if the cow has an infection with *Campylobacter* in her udder or the milk is contaminated with manure. Surface water and mountain streams can become contaminated from infected feces from cows or wild birds. This infection is common in the developing world, and travelers to foreign countries are also at risk for becoming infected with *Campylobacter*.

What can be done to prevent Campylobacter *infection?*

Some simple food handling practices can help prevent *Campylobacter* infections.

- Cook all poultry products thoroughly. Make sure that the meat is cooked throughout (no longer pink) and any juices run clear.

All poultry should be cooked to reach a minimum internal temperature of 165° F.

- If you are served undercooked poultry in a restaurant, send it back for further cooking.
- Wash hands with soap before preparing food.
- Wash hands with soap after handling raw foods of animal origin and before touching anything else.
- Prevent cross-contamination in the kitchen by using separate cutting boards for foods of animal origin and other foods and by carefully cleaning all cutting boards, countertops, and utensils with soap and hot water after preparing raw food of animal origin.
- Avoid consuming unpasteurized milk and untreated surface water.
- Make sure that persons with diarrhea, especially children, wash their hands carefully and frequently with soap to reduce the risk of spreading the infection.
- Wash hands with soap after contact with pet feces.

Physicians who diagnose campylobacteriosis and clinical laboratories that identify this organism should report their findings to the local health department. If many cases occur at the same time, it may mean that many people were exposed to a common contaminated food item or water source that might still be available to infect more people. When outbreaks occur, community education efforts can be directed toward proper food handling techniques and toward avoiding consumption of raw (not pasteurized) milk.

Section 37.4

Escherichia Coli

"Questions & Answers: Sickness Caused by *E. coli*," Centers for Disease Control and Prevention (www.cdc.gov), December 10, 2006.

What is E. coli*?*

E. coli is a common kind of bacteria that lives in the intestines of animals and people. There are many strains of *E. coli*. Most are harmless. However, one dangerous strain is called *E. coli* O157:H7. It produces a powerful poison. You can become very sick if it gets into your food or water.

In 1999 it was estimated that about 73,000 people in the United States got sick each year from *E. coli*. About 60 died. It's believed that the number of illnesses and deaths has been dropping since then.

How is E. coli *O157:H7 spread?*

Outbreaks often are caused by food that has gotten the bacteria, *E. coli*, in it. Bacteria can get accidentally mixed into ground beef before packaging. Eating undercooked meat can spread the bacteria, even though the meat looks and smells normal. *E. coli* can also live on cows' udders. It may get into milk that is not pasteurized.

Raw vegetables, sprouts, and fruits that have been grown or washed in dirty water can carry *E. coli* O157:H7. It can get into drinking water, lakes, or swimming pools that have sewage in them. It is also spread by people who have not washed their hands after going to the toilet.

E. coli can be spread to playmates by toddlers who are not toilet trained or by adults who do not wash their hands carefully after changing diapers. Children can pass the bacteria in their stool to another person for two weeks after they have gotten well from an *E. coli* O157:H7 illness. Older children and adults rarely carry the bacteria without symptoms.

What are the signs of **E. coli** *O157:H7 sickness?*

Bloody diarrhea and stomach pain are the most common signs of *E. coli* O157:H7 sickness. People usually do not have a fever, or may have only a slight fever.

Some people, especially children under five and the elderly, can become very sick from *E. coli* O157:H7. The infection damages their red blood cells and their kidneys. This only happens to about 1 out of 50 people, but it is very serious. Without hospital care, they can die. See a doctor right away if you think you may have gotten sick from *E. coli* O157:H7.

How will my doctor know if **E. coli** *O157:H7 made me sick?*

Your doctor will test to see if your sickness was caused by *E. coli* by sending a stool sample to a lab. The lab will test for the bacteria.

Anyone who suddenly has diarrhea with blood in it should call or see a doctor.

How is **E. coli** *O157:H7 treated?*

Your doctor will tell you what is best. Taking medicine on your own may not help you get better, and it could make things worse. Do not take antibiotics or diarrhea medicine like Imodium® unless your doctor tells you to.

Will **E. coli** *O157:H7 infection cause problems for me later?*

People who have only diarrhea and stomach ache usually get completely well in 5–10 days. They do not have problems later.

For those people who get very sick and have kidney failure, about one out of three may have kidney problems later. In rare cases, people have other problems like high blood pressure, blindness, or are paralyzed. Talk to your doctor if you have questions about this.

What is the U.S. government doing to keep food safe from **E. coli** *O157:H7?*

New laws have helped keep food from being contaminated with *E. coli* O157:H7. They keep meat safer during slaughter and grinding, and vegetables safer when they are grown, picked, and washed. But there is still a chance that *E. coli* O157:H7 could reach your food, so you should take the precautions listed here.

What can I do to stay safe from E. coli *O157:H7?*

- During an outbreak: Carefully follow instructions provided by public health officials on what foods to avoid in order to protect yourself and your family from infection.
- Cook all ground beef thoroughly. During an outbreak of *E. coli* O157:H7, vegetables should be boiled for at least one minute before serving.
- Cook ground beef to 160° F. Test the meat by putting a food thermometer in the thickest part of the meat. Do not eat ground beef that is still pink in the middle.
- If a restaurant serves you an undercooked hamburger, send it back for more cooking. Ask for a new bun and a clean plate, too.
- Don't spread bacteria in your kitchen. Keep raw meat away from other foods. Wash your hands, cutting board, counter, dishes, and knives and forks with hot soapy water after they touch raw meat, spinach, greens, or sprouts.
- Never put cooked hamburgers or meat on the plate they were on before cooking. Wash the meat thermometer after use.
- Drink only pasteurized milk, juice, or cider. Frozen juice or juice sold in boxes and glass jars at room temperature has been pasteurized, although it may not say so on the label.
- Drink water from safe sources like municipal water that has been treated with chlorine, wells that have been tested, or bottled water.
- Do not swallow lake or pool water while you are swimming.

Section 37.5

Salmonella

"Salmonellosis," Centers for Disease Control and Prevention (www.cdc.gov), May 21, 2008.

What is salmonellosis?

Salmonellosis is an infection with bacteria called *Salmonella*. Most persons infected with *Salmonella* develop diarrhea, fever, and abdominal cramps 12 to 72 hours after infection. The illness usually lasts four to seven days, and most persons recover without treatment. However, in some persons, the diarrhea may be so severe that the patient needs to be hospitalized. In these patients, the *Salmonella* infection may spread from the intestines to the blood stream and then to other body sites and can cause death unless the person is treated promptly with antibiotics. The elderly, infants, and those with impaired immune systems are more likely to have a severe illness.

What sort of germ is Salmonella*?*

Salmonella is actually a group of bacteria that can cause diarrheal illness in humans. They are microscopic living creatures that pass from the feces of people or animals to other people or other animals. There are many different kinds of *Salmonella* bacteria. *Salmonella* serotype *Typhimurium* and *Salmonella* serotype *Enteritidis* are the most common in the United States. *Salmonella* germs have been known to cause illness for over 100 years. They were discovered by an American scientist named Salmon, for whom they are named.

How can Salmonella *infections be diagnosed?*

Many different kinds of illnesses can cause diarrhea, fever, or abdominal cramps. Determining that *Salmonella* is the cause of the illness depends on laboratory tests that identify *Salmonella* in the stool of an infected person. Once *Salmonella* has been identified, further testing can determine its specific type.

How can Salmonella *infections be treated?*

Salmonella infections usually resolve in five to seven days and often do not require treatment other than oral fluids. Persons with severe diarrhea may require rehydration with intravenous fluids. Antibiotics, such as ampicillin, trimethoprim-sulfamethoxazole, or ciprofloxacin, are not usually necessary unless the infection spreads from the intestines. Some *Salmonella* bacteria have become resistant to antibiotics, largely as a result of the use of antibiotics to promote the growth of food animals.

Are there long-term consequences to a Salmonella *infection?*

Persons with diarrhea usually recover completely, although it may be several months before their bowel habits are entirely normal. A small number of persons with *Salmonella* develop pain in their joints, irritation of the eyes, and painful urination. This is called Reiter's syndrome. It can last for months or years, and can lead to chronic arthritis, which is difficult to treat. Antibiotic treatment does not make a difference in whether or not the person develops arthritis.

How do people catch Salmonella?

Salmonella live in the intestinal tracts of humans and other animals, including birds. *Salmonella* are usually transmitted to humans by eating foods contaminated with animal feces. Contaminated foods usually look and smell normal. Contaminated foods are often of animal origin, such as beef, poultry, milk, or eggs, but any food, including vegetables, may become contaminated. Thorough cooking kills *Salmonella*. Food may also become contaminated by the hands of an infected food handler who did not wash hands with soap after using the bathroom.

Salmonella may also be found in the feces of some pets, especially those with diarrhea, and people can become infected if they do not wash their hands after contact with pets or pet feces. Reptiles, such as turtles, lizards, and snakes, are particularly likely to harbor *Salmonella*. Many chicks and young birds carry *Salmonella* in their feces. People should always wash their hands immediately after handling a reptile or bird, even if the animal is healthy. Adults should also assure that children wash their hands after handling a reptile or bird, or after touching its environment.

What can a person do to prevent this illness?

There is no vaccine to prevent salmonellosis. Because foods of animal origin may be contaminated with *Salmonella*, people should not eat raw or undercooked eggs, poultry, or meat. Raw eggs may be unrecognized in some foods, such as homemade hollandaise sauce, Caesar and other homemade salad dressings, tiramisu, homemade ice cream, homemade mayonnaise, cookie dough, and frostings. Poultry and meat, including hamburgers, should be well-cooked, not pink in the middle. Persons also should not consume raw or unpasteurized milk or other dairy products. Produce should be thoroughly washed.

Cross-contamination of foods should be avoided. Uncooked meats should be kept separate from produce, cooked foods, and ready-to-eat foods. Hands, cutting boards, counters, knives, and other utensils should be washed thoroughly after touching uncooked foods. Hands should be washed before handling food, and between handling different food items.

People who have salmonellosis should not prepare food or pour water for others until their diarrhea has resolved. Many health departments require that restaurant workers with *Salmonella* infection have a stool test showing that they are no longer carrying the *Salmonella* bacterium before they return to work.

People should wash their hands after contact with animal feces. Because reptiles are particularly likely to have *Salmonella*, and it can contaminate their skin, everyone should immediately wash their hands after handling reptiles. Reptiles (including turtles) are not appropriate pets for small children and should not be in the same house as an infant. *Salmonella* carried in the intestines of chicks and ducklings contaminates their environment and the entire surface of the animal. Children can be exposed to the bacteria by simply holding, cuddling, or kissing the birds. Children should not handle baby chicks or other young birds. Everyone should immediately wash their hands after touching birds, including baby chicks and ducklings, or their environment.

How common is salmonellosis?

Every year, approximately 40,000 cases of salmonellosis are reported in the United States. Because many milder cases are not diagnosed or reported, the actual number of infections may be thirty or more times greater. Salmonellosis is more common in the summer than winter.

Children are the most likely to get salmonellosis. The rate of diagnosed infections in children less than five years old is about five times higher than the rate in all other persons. Young children, the elderly, and the immunocompromised are the most likely to have severe infections. It is estimated that approximately 400 persons die each year with acute salmonellosis.

What else can be done to prevent salmonellosis?

It is important for the public health department to know about cases of salmonellosis. It is important for clinical laboratories to send isolates of *Salmonella* to the city, county, or state public health laboratories so the specific type can be determined and compared with other *Salmonella* in the community. If many cases occur at the same time, it may mean that a restaurant, food, or water supply has a problem that needs correction by the public health department.

Some prevention steps occur every day without you thinking about it. Pasteurization of milk and treatment of municipal water supplies are highly effective prevention measures that have been in place for decades. In the 1970s, small pet turtles were a common source of salmonellosis in the United States, so in 1975, the sale of small turtles was banned in this country. However, in 2008, they were still being sold, and cases of *Salmonella* associated with pet turtles have been reported. Improvements in farm animal hygiene, in slaughter plant practices, and in vegetable and fruit harvesting and packing operations may help prevent salmonellosis caused by contaminated foods. Better education of food industry workers in basic food safety and restaurant inspection procedures may prevent cross-contamination and other food handling errors that can lead to outbreaks. Wider use of pasteurized egg in restaurants, hospitals, and nursing homes is an important prevention measure. In the future, irradiation or other treatments may greatly reduce contamination of raw meat.

What is the government doing about salmonellosis?

The CDC monitors the frequency of *Salmonella* infections in the country and assists the local and state health departments in investigating outbreaks and devising control measures. CDC also monitors the different types of *Salmonella* that are reported annually by public health laboratories of state and local health departments. FDA inspects imported foods, oversees inspection of milk pasteurization plants, promotes better food preparation techniques in restaurants and food processing plants, and regulates the sale of turtles. The FDA also regulates the use of specific antibiotics as growth promotants in food animals. The U.S. Department of Agriculture monitors the health of food animals, inspects egg pasteurization plants, and is responsible for the quality of slaughtered and processed meat. The U.S. Environmental Protection Agency regulates and monitors the safety of drinking water supplies.

How can I learn more about this and other public health problems?

You can discuss any medical concerns you may have with your doctor or other heath care provider. Your local city or county health department can provide more information about this and other public health problems that are occurring in your area. General information about the public health of the nation is published every week in the *Morbidity and Mortality Weekly Report (MMWR)* by the CDC in Atlanta, Georgia. Every spring, the *MMWR* publishes a report of the incidence of *Salmonella* and other infections during the previous year in FoodNet sentinel surveillance sites. Epidemiologists in your local and state health departments are tracking many important public health problems, investigating special problems that arise, and helping to prevent them from occurring in the first place, and from spreading when they occur.

What can I do to prevent salmonellosis?

- Cook poultry, ground beef, and eggs thoroughly. Do not eat or drink foods containing raw eggs, or raw (unpasteurized) milk.
- If you are served undercooked meat, poultry, or eggs in a restaurant, don't hesitate to send it back to the kitchen for further cooking.
- Wash hands, kitchen work surfaces, and utensils with soap and water immediately after they have been in contact with raw meat or poultry.
- Be particularly careful with foods prepared for infants, the elderly, and the immunocompromised.
- Wash hands with soap after handling reptiles, birds, or baby chicks, and after contact with pet feces.
- Avoid direct or even indirect contact between reptiles (turtles, iguanas, other lizards, snakes) and infants or immunocompromised persons.

- Don't work with raw poultry or meat and an infant (e.g., feed, change diaper) at the same time.
- Mother's milk is the safest food for young infants. Breastfeeding prevents salmonellosis and many other health problems.

Section 37.6

Listeria

"Listeriosis," Centers for Disease Control and Prevention (www.cdc.gov), March 27, 2008.

What is listeriosis?

Listeriosis, a serious infection caused by eating food contaminated with the bacterium *Listeria monocytogenes*, has recently been recognized as an important public health problem in the United States. The disease affects primarily persons of advanced age, pregnant women, newborns, and adults with weakened immune systems. However, persons without these risk factors can also rarely be affected. The risk may be reduced by following a few simple recommendations.

What are the symptoms of listeriosis?

A person with listeriosis has fever, muscle aches, and sometimes gastrointestinal symptoms such as nausea or diarrhea. If infection spreads to the nervous system, symptoms such as headache, stiff neck, confusion, loss of balance, or convulsions can occur.

Infected pregnant women may experience only a mild, flulike illness; however, infections during pregnancy can lead to miscarriage or stillbirth, premature delivery, or infection of the newborn.

How great is the risk for listeriosis?

In the United States, an estimated 2,500 persons become seriously ill with listeriosis each year. Of these, 500 die. At increased risk are the following:

- Pregnant women (they are about 20 times more likely than other healthy adults to get listeriosis; about one-third of listeriosis cases happen during pregnancy)
- Newborns (newborns rather than the pregnant women themselves suffer the serious effects of infection in pregnancy)
- Persons with weakened immune systems
- Persons with cancer, diabetes, or kidney disease
- Persons with AIDS (they are almost 300 times more likely to get listeriosis than people with normal immune systems)
- Persons who take glucocorticosteroid medications
- The elderly

Healthy adults and children occasionally get infected with *Listeria*, but they rarely become seriously ill.

How does Listeria *get into food?*

Listeria monocytogenes is found in soil and water. Vegetables can become contaminated from the soil or from manure used as fertilizer.

Animals can carry the bacterium without appearing ill and can contaminate foods of animal origin such as meats and dairy products. The bacterium has been found in a variety of raw foods, such as uncooked meats and vegetables, as well as in processed foods that become contaminated after processing, such as soft cheeses and cold cuts at the deli counter. Unpasteurized (raw) milk or foods made from unpasteurized milk may contain the bacterium.

Listeria is killed by pasteurization and cooking; however, in certain ready-to-eat foods such as hot dogs and deli meats, contamination may occur after cooking but before packaging.

How do you get listeriosis?

You get listeriosis by eating food contaminated with *Listeria*. Babies can be born with listeriosis if their mothers eat contaminated food during pregnancy. Although healthy persons may consume contaminated foods without becoming ill, those at increased risk for infection can probably get listeriosis after eating food contaminated with even a few bacteria. Persons at risk can prevent *Listeria* infection by avoiding certain high-risk foods and by handling food properly.

Can listeriosis be prevented?

The general guidelines recommended for the prevention of listeriosis are similar to those used to help prevent other foodborne illnesses, such as salmonellosis. In addition, there are specific recommendations for persons at high risk for listeriosis.

How can you reduce your risk for listeriosis?

General recommendations include the following procedures:

- Thoroughly cook raw food from animal sources, such as beef, pork, or poultry.
- Wash raw vegetables thoroughly before eating.
- Keep uncooked meats separate from vegetables and from cooked foods and ready-to-eat foods.
- Avoid unpasteurized (raw) milk or foods made from unpasteurized milk.
- Wash hands, knives, and cutting boards after handling uncooked foods.
- Consume perishable and ready-to-eat foods as soon as possible.

The following are recommendations for persons at high risk, such as pregnant women and persons with weakened immune systems, in addition to the recommendations listed above:

- Do not eat hot dogs, luncheon meats, or deli meats, unless they are reheated until steaming hot.
- Avoid getting fluid from hot dog packages on other foods, utensils, and food preparation surfaces, and wash hands after handling hot dogs, luncheon meats, and deli meats.
- Do not eat soft cheeses such as feta, Brie, and Camembert, blue-veined cheeses, or Mexican-style cheeses such as queso blanco, queso fresco, and Panela, unless they have labels that clearly state they are made from pasteurized milk.
- Do not eat refrigerated pâtés or meat spreads. Canned or shelf-stable pâtés and meat spreads may be eaten.
- Do not eat refrigerated smoked seafood, unless it is contained in a cooked dish, such as a casserole. Refrigerated smoked seafood,

such as salmon, trout, whitefish, cod, tuna, or mackerel, is most often labeled as "nova-style," "lox," "kippered," "smoked," or "jerky." The fish is found in the refrigerator section or sold at deli counters of grocery stores and delicatessens. Canned or shelf-stable smoked seafood may be eaten.

How do you know if you have listeriosis?

There is no routine screening test for listeriosis during pregnancy, as there is for rubella and some other congenital infections. If you have symptoms such as fever or stiff neck, consult your doctor. A blood or spinal fluid test (to cultivate the bacteria) will show if you have listeriosis. During pregnancy, a blood test is the most reliable way to find out if your symptoms are due to listeriosis.

What should you do if you've eaten a food recalled because of **Listeria** *contamination?*

The risk of an individual person developing *Listeria* infection after consumption of a contaminated product is very small. If you have eaten a contaminated product and do not have any symptoms, we do not recommend that you have any tests or treatment, even if you are in a high-risk group. However, if you are in a high-risk group, have eaten the contaminated product, and within two months become ill with fever or signs of serious illness, you should contact your physician and inform him or her about this exposure.

Can listeriosis be treated?

When infection occurs during pregnancy, antibiotics given promptly to the pregnant woman can often prevent infection of the fetus or newborn.

Babies with listeriosis receive the same antibiotics as adults, although a combination of antibiotics is often used until physicians are certain of the diagnosis. Even with prompt treatment, some infections result in death. This is particularly likely in the elderly and in persons with other serious medical problems.

Section 37.7

Shigella

"Shigellosis," Centers for Disease Control and Prevention (www.cdc.gov), March 27, 2008.

What is shigellosis?

Shigellosis is an infectious disease caused by a group of bacteria called *Shigella*. Most people who are infected with *Shigella* develop diarrhea, fever, and stomach cramps starting a day or two after they are exposed to the bacteria. The diarrhea is often bloody. Shigellosis usually resolves in five to seven days. Persons with shigellosis in the United States rarely require hospitalization. A severe infection with high fever may be associated with seizures in children less than two years old. Some persons who are infected may have no symptoms at all, but may still pass the *Shigella* bacteria to others.

What sort of germ is Shigella*?*

The *Shigella* germ is actually a family of bacteria that can cause diarrhea in humans. They are microscopic living creatures that pass from person to person. *Shigella* were discovered over 100 years ago by a Japanese scientist named Shiga, for whom they are named. There are several different kinds of *Shigella* bacteria: *Shigella sonnei*, also known as "group D" *Shigella*, accounts for over two-thirds of shigellosis in the United States. *Shigella flexneri*, or "group B" *Shigella*, accounts for almost all the rest. Other types of *Shigella* are rare in this country, though they continue to be important causes of disease in the developing world. One type found in the developing world, *Shigella dysenteriae* type 1, can cause deadly epidemics.

How can Shigella *infections be diagnosed?*

Many different kinds of germs can cause diarrhea, so establishing the cause will help guide treatment. Determining that *Shigella* is the cause of the illness depends on laboratory tests that identify *Shigella* in the stools of an infected person. The laboratory can also do special tests to determine which antibiotics, if any, would be best to treat the infection.

How can Shigella *infections be treated?*

Persons with mild infections usually recover quickly without antibiotic treatment. However, appropriate antibiotic treatment kills *Shigella* bacteria, and may shorten the illness by a few days. The antibiotics commonly used for treatment are ampicillin, trimethoprim/sulfamethoxazole (also known as Bactrim* or Septra*), ceftriaxone (Rocephin*), or, among adults, ciprofloxacin. Some *Shigella* bacteria have become resistant to antibiotics. This means some antibiotics might not be effective for treatment. Using antibiotics to treat shigellosis can sometimes make the germs more resistant. Therefore, when many persons in a community are affected by shigellosis, antibiotics are sometimes used to treat only the most severe cases. Antidiarrheal agents such as loperamide (Imodium*) or diphenoxylate with atropine (Lomotil*) can make the illness worse and should be avoided.

Are there long-term consequences of a Shigella *infection?*

Persons with diarrhea usually recover completely, although it may be several months before their bowel habits are entirely normal. About 2% of persons who are infected with one type of *Shigella*, *Shigella flexneri*, later develop pains in their joints, irritation of the eyes, and painful urination. This is called post-infectious arthritis. It can last for months or years, and can lead to chronic arthritis. Post-infectious arthritis is caused by a reaction to *Shigella* infection that happens only in people who are genetically predisposed to it.

Once someone has had shigellosis, they are not likely to get infected with that specific type again for at least several years. However, they can still get infected with other types of *Shigella*.

How do people catch Shigella?

The *Shigella* bacteria pass from one infected person to the next. *Shigella* are present in the diarrheal stools of infected persons while they are sick and for up to a week or two afterwards. Most *Shigella* infections are the result of the bacterium passing from stools or soiled fingers of one person to the mouth of another person. This happens when basic hygiene and hand-washing habits are inadequate and can happen during certain types of sexual activity. It is particularly likely to occur among toddlers who are not fully toilet trained. Family members and playmates of such children are at high risk of becoming infected.

Shigella infections may be acquired from eating contaminated food. Contaminated food usually looks and smells normal. Food may become contaminated by infected food handlers who forget to wash their hands with soap after using the bathroom. Vegetables can become contaminated if they are harvested from a field with sewage in it. Flies can breed in infected feces and then contaminate food. Water may become contaminated with *Shigella* bacteria if sewage runs into it or if someone with shigellosis swims in or plays with it (especially in splash tables, untreated wading pools, or shallow play fountains used by day care centers). *Shigella* infections can then be acquired by drinking, swimming in, or playing with the contaminated water. Outbreaks of shigellosis have also occurred among men who have sex with men.

What can a person do to prevent this illness?

Currently, there is no vaccine to prevent shigellosis. However, the spread of *Shigella* from an infected person to other persons can be stopped by frequent and careful hand washing with soap. Frequent and careful hand washing is important among all age groups. Hand washing among children should be frequent and supervised by an adult in day care centers and homes with children who have not been fully toilet trained.

If a child in diapers has shigellosis, everyone who changes the child's diapers should be sure the diapers are disposed of properly in a closed-lid garbage can, and should wash his or her hands and the child's hands carefully with soap and warm water immediately after changing the diapers. After use, the diaper-changing area should be wiped down with a disinfectant such as diluted household bleach, Lysol*, or bactericidal wipes. When possible, young children with a *Shigella* infection who are still in diapers should not be in contact with uninfected children.

Basic food safety precautions and disinfection of drinking water prevents shigellosis from food and water. However, people with shigellosis should not prepare food or drinks for others until they have been shown to no longer be carrying the *Shigella* bacterium, or if they have had no diarrhea for at least two days. At swimming beaches, having enough bathrooms and hand-washing stations with soap near the swimming area helps keep the water from becoming contaminated. Day care centers should not provide water play areas.

Simple precautions taken while traveling to the developing world can prevent shigellosis. Drink only treated or boiled water, and eat only cooked hot foods or fruits you peel yourself. The same precautions prevent other types of traveler's diarrhea.

How common is shigellosis?

Every year, about 14,000 cases of shigellosis are reported in the United States. Because many milder cases are not diagnosed or reported, the actual number of infections may be 20 times greater. Shigellosis is particularly common and causes recurrent problems in settings where hygiene is poor and can sometimes sweep through entire communities. It is more common in summer than winter. Children, especially toddlers aged two to four, are the most likely to get shigellosis. Many cases are related to the spread of illness in child care settings, and many are the result of the spread of the illness in families with small children.

In the developing world, shigellosis is far more common and is present in most communities most of the time.

What else can be done to prevent shigellosis?

It is important for the public health department to know about cases of shigellosis. It is important for clinical laboratories to send isolates of *Shigella* to the city, county, or state public health laboratory so the specific type can be determined. If many cases occur at the same time, it may mean that a restaurant, food, or water supply has a problem that needs correction by the public health department. If a number of cases occur in a day care center, the public health department may need to coordinate efforts to improve hand washing among the staff, children, and their families. When a community-wide outbreak occurs, a community-wide approach to promote hand washing and basic hygiene among children can stop the outbreak. Improvements in worker hygiene during vegetable and fruit picking and packing may prevent shigellosis caused by contaminated produce.

Some prevention measures in place in most communities help to prevent shigellosis. Making municipal water supplies safe and treating sewage are highly effective prevention measures that have been in place for many years.

Some tips for preventing the spread of shigellosis include the following:

- Wash hands with soap carefully and frequently, especially after going to the bathroom, after changing diapers, and before preparing foods or beverages.
- Dispose of soiled diapers properly.
- Disinfect diaper-changing areas after using them.
- Keep children with diarrhea out of child care settings.
- Supervise hand washing of toddlers and small children after they use the toilet.
- Do not prepare food for others while ill with diarrhea.
- Avoid swallowing water from ponds, lakes, or untreated pools.

*CDC does not endorse commercial products or services.

Section 37.8

Botulism

"Botulism," Centers for Disease Control and Prevention (www.cdc.gov), May 21, 2008.

What is botulism?

Botulism is a rare but serious paralytic illness caused by a nerve toxin that is produced by the bacterium *Clostridium botulinum*. There are three main kinds of botulism. Foodborne botulism is caused by eating foods that contain the botulism toxin. Wound botulism is caused by toxin produced from a wound infected with *Clostridium botulinum*. Infant botulism is caused by consuming the spores of the *botulinum* bacteria, which then grow in the intestines and release toxin. All forms of botulism can be fatal and are considered medical emergencies. Foodborne botulism can be especially dangerous because many people can be poisoned by eating a contaminated food.

How common is botulism?

In the United States, an average of 145 cases are reported each year. Of these, approximately 15% are foodborne, 65% are infant botulism, and 20% are wound. Adult intestinal colonization and iatrogenic botulism also occur, but rarely. Outbreaks of foodborne botulism involving two or more persons occur most years and are usually caused by eating contaminated home-canned foods. The number of cases of foodborne and infant botulism has changed little in recent years, but wound botulism has increased because of the use of black-tar heroin, especially in California.

What are the symptoms of botulism?

The classic symptoms of botulism include double vision, blurred vision, drooping eyelids, slurred speech, difficulty swallowing, dry mouth, and muscle weakness. Infants with botulism appear lethargic, feed poorly, are constipated, and have a weak cry and poor muscle tone. These are all symptoms of the muscle paralysis caused by the bacterial toxin. If untreated, these symptoms may progress to cause paralysis of the arms, legs, trunk, and respiratory muscles. In foodborne botulism, symptoms generally begin 18 to 36 hours after eating a contaminated food, but they can occur as early as 6 hours or as late as 10 days.

How is botulism diagnosed?

Physicians may consider the diagnosis if the patient's history and physical examination suggest botulism. However, these clues are usually not enough to allow a diagnosis of botulism. Other diseases such as Guillain-Barré syndrome, stroke, and myasthenia gravis can appear similar to botulism, and special tests may be needed to exclude these other conditions. These tests may include a brain scan, spinal fluid examination, nerve conduction test (electromyography, or EMG), and a Tensilon test for myasthenia gravis. The most direct way to confirm the diagnosis is to demonstrate the *botulinum* toxin in the patient's serum or stool by injecting serum or stool into mice and looking for signs of botulism. The bacteria can also be isolated from the stool of persons with foodborne and infant botulism. These tests can be performed at some state health department laboratories and at CDC.

How can botulism be treated?

The respiratory failure and paralysis that occur with severe botulism may require a patient to be on a breathing machine (ventilator) for weeks, plus intensive medical and nursing care. After several weeks, the paralysis slowly improves. If diagnosed early, foodborne and wound botulism can be treated with an equine antitoxin that blocks the action of toxin circulating in the blood. This can prevent patients from worsening, but recovery still takes many weeks. Physicians may try to remove contaminated food still in the gut by inducing vomiting or by using enemas. Wounds should be treated, usually surgically, to remove the source of the toxin-producing bacteria followed by administration of appropriate antibiotics. Good supportive care in a hospital is the mainstay of therapy for all forms of botulism. A human-derived antitoxin is used to treat cases of infant botulism and is available from the California Department of Public Health.

Are there complications from botulism?

Botulism can result in death due to respiratory failure. However, in the past 50 years the proportion of patients with botulism who die has fallen from about 50% to 3–5%. A patient with severe botulism may require a breathing machine as well as intensive medical and nursing care for several months. Patients who survive an episode of botulism poisoning may have fatigue and shortness of breath for years and long-term therapy may be needed to aid recovery.

How can botulism be prevented?

Botulism can be prevented. Foodborne botulism has often been from home-canned foods with low acid content, such as asparagus, green beans, beets, and corn. However, outbreaks of botulism can come from more unusual sources such as chopped garlic in oil, chili peppers, tomatoes, carrot juice, improperly handled baked potatoes wrapped in aluminum foil, and home-canned or fermented fish. Persons who do home canning should follow strict hygienic procedures to reduce contamination of foods. Oils infused with garlic or herbs should be refrigerated. Potatoes that have been baked while wrapped in aluminum foil should be kept hot until served or refrigerated. Because the botulism toxin is destroyed by high temperatures, persons who eat home-canned foods should consider boiling the food for 10 minutes before eating it to ensure safety. Instructions on safe home canning can be obtained from county extension services or from the U.S. Department of Agriculture. Because honey can contain spores of *Clostridium botulinum* and this has been a source of infection for infants, children less than 12 months old should not be fed honey. Honey is safe for persons one year of age and older. Wound botulism can be prevented by promptly seeking medical care for infected wounds and by not using injectable street drugs.

Section 37.9

Staphylococcus

"Staphylococcal Food Poisoning," Centers for Disease Control and Prevention (www.cdc.gov), March 29, 2006.

What is Staphylococcus?

Staphylococcus aureus is a common bacterium found on the skin and in the noses of up to 25% of healthy people and animals. *Staphylococcus aureus* is important because it has the ability to make seven different toxins that are frequently responsible for food poisoning.

What is staphylococcal food poisoning?

Staphylococcal food poisoning is a gastrointestinal illness. It is caused by eating foods contaminated with toxins produced by *Staphylococcus aureus*. The most common way for food to be contaminated with *Staphylococcus* is through contact with food workers who carry the bacteria or through contaminated milk and cheeses. *Staphylococcus* is salt tolerant and can grow in salty foods like ham. As the germ multiplies in food, it produces toxins that can cause illness. Staphylococcal toxins are resistant to heat and cannot be destroyed by cooking. Foods at highest risk of contamination with *Staphylococcus aureus* and subsequent toxin production are those that are made by hand and require no cooking. Some examples of foods that have caused staphylococcal food poisoning are sliced meat, puddings, some pastries, and sandwiches.

What are the symptoms of staphylococcal food poisoning?

Staphylococcal toxins are fast acting, sometimes causing illness in as little as 30 minutes. Symptoms usually develop within one to six hours after eating contaminated food. Patients typically experience several of the following: nausea, vomiting, stomach cramps, and diarrhea. The illness is usually mild and most patients recover after one to three days. In a small minority of patients the illness may be more severe.

How do I know if I have staphylococcal food poisoning?

Toxin-producing *Staphylococcus aureus* can be identified in stool or vomit, and toxin can be detected in food items. Diagnosis of staphylococcal food poisoning in an individual is generally based only on the signs and symptoms of the patient. Testing for the toxin-producing bacteria or the toxin is not usually done in individual patients. Testing is usually reserved for outbreaks involving several persons. If you think you may have food poisoning, contact your physician.

How should a patient with suspected staphylococcal food poisoning be treated?

For most patients, staphylococcal food poisoning will cause a brief illness. The best treatments for these patients are rest, plenty of fluids, and medicines to calm their stomachs. Highly susceptible patients, such as the young and the elderly, are more likely to have severe illness requiring intravenous therapy and care in a hospital.

Antibiotics are not useful in treating this illness. The toxin is not affected by antibiotics.

Is a sick patient infectious?

Patients with this illness are not contagious. Toxins are not transmitted from one person to another.

How can staphylococcal food poisoning be prevented?

It is important to prevent the contamination of food with *Staphylococcus* before the toxin can be produced.

- Wash hands and under fingernails vigorously with soap and water before handling and preparing food.
- Do not prepare food if you have a nose or eye infection.
- Do not prepare or serve food for others if you have wounds or skin infections on your hands or wrists.
- Keep kitchens and food-serving areas clean and sanitized.
- If food is to be stored longer than two hours, keep hot foods hot (over 140° F) and cold foods cold (40° F or under).
- Store cooked food in a wide, shallow container and refrigerate as soon as possible.

Could staphylococcal toxins be used in a bioterrorist attack?

Staphylococcal toxins could be used as a biological agent either by contamination of food/water or by aerosolization and inhalation. Breathing in low doses of staphylococcal enterotoxin B may cause fever, cough, difficulty breathing, headache, and some vomiting and nausea. High doses of the toxin have a much more serious effect.

Chapter 38

Foodborne Viruses

Chapter Contents

Section 38.1

Hepatitis A

"Hepatitis A: FAQs for the Public," Centers for Disease Control and Prevention (www.cdc.gov), June 23, 2008.

What is hepatitis A?

Hepatitis A is a contagious liver disease that results from infection with the hepatitis A virus. It can range in severity from a mild illness lasting a few weeks to a severe illness lasting several months. Hepatitis A is usually spread when a person ingests fecal matter—even in microscopic amounts—from contact with objects, food, or drinks contaminated by the feces, or stool, of an infected person.

How common is hepatitis A in the United States?

In the United States, there were an estimated 32,000 new hepatitis A virus infections in 2006. (However, the official number of reported hepatitis A cases is much lower since many people who are infected never have symptoms and are never reported to public health officials.)

Is hepatitis A decreasing in the United States?

Yes. Rates of hepatitis A in the United States are the lowest they have been in 40 years. The hepatitis A vaccine was introduced in 1995, and health professionals now routinely vaccinate all children, travelers to certain countries, and persons at risk for the disease. Many experts believe hepatitis A vaccination has dramatically affected rates of the disease in the United States.

How is hepatitis A spread?

Hepatitis A is usually spread when the hepatitis A virus is taken in by mouth from contact with objects, food, or drinks contaminated by the feces (or stool) of an infected person. A person can get hepatitis A through the following:

- Person-to-person contact
  - When an infected person does not wash his or her hands properly after going to the bathroom and touches other objects or food
  - When a parent or caregiver does not properly wash his or her hands after changing diapers or cleaning up the stool of an infected person
  - When someone engages in certain sexual activities, such as oral-anal contact with an infected person
- Contaminated food or water

Hepatitis A can be spread by eating or drinking food or water contaminated with the virus. This is more likely to occur in countries where hepatitis A is common and in areas where there are poor sanitary conditions or poor personal hygiene. The food and drinks most likely to be contaminated are fruits, vegetables, shellfish, ice, and water. In the United States, chlorination of water kills hepatitis A virus that enters the water supply.

I think I have been exposed to hepatitis A. What should I do?

If you have any questions about potential exposure to hepatitis A, call your health professional or your local or state health department.

If you were recently exposed to hepatitis A virus and have not been vaccinated against hepatitis A, you might benefit from an injection of either immune globulin or hepatitis A vaccine. However, the vaccine or immune globulin must be given within the first two weeks after exposure to be effective. A health professional can decide what is best on the basis of your age and overall health.

What should I do if I ate at a restaurant that had an outbreak of hepatitis A?

Talk to your health professional or a local health department official for guidance. Outbreaks usually result from one of two sources of contamination: an infected food handler or an infected food source. Your health department will investigate the cause of the outbreak.

Keep in mind that most people do not get sick when someone at a restaurant has hepatitis A. However, if an infected food handler is infectious and has poor hygiene, the risk goes up for patrons of that restaurant. In such cases, health officials might try to identify patrons and provide hepatitis A vaccine or immune globulin if they can find them within two weeks of exposure.

On rare occasions, the source of the infection can be traced to contaminated food. Foods can become contaminated at any point along the process: growing, harvesting, processing, handling, and even after cooking. In these cases, health officials will try to determine the source of the contamination and the best ways to minimize health threats to the public.

If I have had hepatitis A in the past, can I get it again?

No. Once you recover from hepatitis A, you develop antibodies that protect you from the virus for life. An antibody is a substance found in the blood that the body produces in response to a virus. Antibodies protect the body from disease by attaching to the virus and destroying it.

Does hepatitis A cause symptoms?

Not always. Some people get hepatitis A and have no symptoms of the disease. Adults are more likely to have symptoms than children.

What are the symptoms of hepatitis A?

Some people with hepatitis A do not have any symptoms. If you do have symptoms, they may include the following:

- Fever
- Fatigue
- Loss of appetite
- Nausea
- Vomiting
- Abdominal pain
- Dark urine
- Clay-colored bowel movements
- Joint pain
- Jaundice (a yellowing of the skin or eyes)

How soon after exposure to hepatitis A will symptoms appear?

If symptoms occur, they usually appear anywhere from two to six weeks after exposure. Symptoms usually develop over a period of several days.

How long do hepatitis A symptoms last?

Symptoms usually last less than two months, although some people can be ill for as long as six months.

Can a person spread hepatitis A without having symptoms?

Yes. Many people, especially children, have no symptoms. In addition, a person can transmit the virus to others up to two weeks before symptoms appear.

How serious is hepatitis A?

Almost all people who get hepatitis A recover completely and do not have any lasting liver damage, although they may feel sick for months. Hepatitis A can sometimes cause liver failure and death, although this is rare and occurs more commonly in persons 50 years of age or older and persons with other liver diseases, such as hepatitis B or C.

How will I know if I have hepatitis A?

A doctor can determine if you have hepatitis A by discussing your symptoms and taking a blood sample.

How is hepatitis A treated?

There are no special treatments for hepatitis A. Most people with hepatitis A will feel sick for a few months before they begin to feel better. A few people will need to be hospitalized. During this time, doctors usually recommend rest, adequate nutrition, and fluids. People with hepatitis A should check with a health professional before taking any prescription pills, supplements, or over-the-counter medications, which can potentially damage the liver. Alcohol should be avoided.

Can hepatitis A be prevented?

Yes. The best way to prevent hepatitis A is through vaccination with the hepatitis A vaccine. Vaccination is recommended for all children, for travelers to certain countries, and for people at high risk for infection with the virus. Frequent hand washing with soap and warm water after using the bathroom, changing a diaper, or before preparing food can help prevent the spread of hepatitis A.

Why is the hepatitis A vaccine recommended before traveling?

Traveling to places where hepatitis A virus is common puts a person at high risk for hepatitis A. The risk exists even for travelers to urban areas, those who stay in luxury hotels, and those who report that they have good hygiene and are careful about what they eat and drink. Travelers can minimize their risk by avoiding potentially contaminated water or food, such as drinking beverages (with or without ice) of unknown purity, eating uncooked shellfish, and eating uncooked fruits or vegetables that are not peeled or prepared by the traveler personally. Risk for infection increases with duration of travel and is highest for those who live in or visit rural areas, trek in backcountry areas, or frequently eat or drink in settings with poor sanitation. Since a simple, safe vaccine exists, experts recommend that travelers to certain countries be vaccinated.

Section 38.2

Noroviruses

"Noroviruses: Q and A," Centers for Disease Control and Prevention (www.cdc.gov), February 2009.

What are noroviruses?

Noroviruses are a group of viruses that cause the "stomach flu," or gastroenteritis, in people. The term norovirus was recently approved as the official name for this group of viruses. Several other names have been used for noroviruses, including the following:

- Norwalk-like viruses (NLVs)
- Caliciviruses (because they belong to the virus family *Caliciviridae*)
- Small round structured viruses

Viruses are very different from bacteria and parasites, some of which can cause illnesses similar to norovirus infection. Like all viral infections, noroviruses are not affected by treatment with antibiotics, and cannot grow outside of a person's body.

What are the symptoms of illness caused by noroviruses?

The symptoms of norovirus illness usually include nausea, vomiting, diarrhea, and some stomach cramping. Sometimes people additionally have a low-grade fever, chills, headache, muscle aches, and a general sense of tiredness. The illness often begins suddenly, and the infected person may feel very sick. In most people the illness is self-limiting with symptoms lasting for about one or two days. In general, children experience more vomiting than adults.

What is the name of the illness caused by noroviruses?

Illness caused by norovirus infection has several names, including the following:

- Stomach flu—this "stomach flu" is not related to the flu (or influenza), which is a respiratory illness caused by influenza virus
- Viral gastroenteritis—the most common name for illness caused by norovirus, gastroenteritis refers to an inflammation of the stomach and intestines
- Acute gastroenteritis
- Nonbacterial gastroenteritis
- Food poisoning (although there are other causes of food poisoning)
- Calicivirus infection

How serious is norovirus disease?

People may feel very sick and vomit many times a day, but most people get better within one or two days, and they have no long-term health effects related to their illness. However, sometimes people are unable to drink enough liquids to replace the liquids they lost because of vomiting and diarrhea. These persons can become dehydrated and may need special medical attention. This problem with dehydration is usually only seen among the very young, the elderly, and persons with weakened immune systems.

How do people become infected with noroviruses?

Noroviruses are found in the stool or vomit of infected people. People can become infected with the virus in several ways:

- Eating food or drinking liquids that are contaminated with norovirus
- Touching surfaces or objects contaminated with norovirus, and then placing their hand in their mouth
- Having direct contact with another person who is infected and showing symptoms (for example, when caring for someone with illness, or sharing foods or eating utensils with someone who is ill)

Persons working in day care centers or nursing homes should pay special attention to children or residents who have norovirus illness. This virus is very contagious and can spread rapidly throughout such environments.

When do symptoms appear?

Symptoms of norovirus illness usually begin about 24 to 48 hours after ingestion of the virus, but they can appear as early as 12 hours after exposure.

Are noroviruses contagious?

Noroviruses are very contagious and can spread easily from person to person. Both stool and vomit are infectious. Particular care should be taken with young children in diapers who may have diarrhea.

How long are people contagious?

People infected with norovirus are contagious from the moment they begin feeling ill to at least three days after recovery. Some people may be contagious for as long as two weeks after recovery. Therefore, it is particularly important for people to use good hand-washing and other hygienic practices after they have recently recovered from norovirus illness.

Who gets norovirus infection?

Anyone can become infected with these viruses. There are many different strains of norovirus, which makes it difficult for a person's body to develop long-lasting immunity. Therefore, norovirus illness can recur throughout a person's lifetime. In addition, because of differences in genetic factors, some people are more likely to become infected and develop more severe illness than others.

What treatment is available for people with norovirus infection?

Currently, there is no antiviral medication that works against norovirus and there is no vaccine to prevent infection. Norovirus infection cannot be treated with antibiotics. This is because antibiotics work to fight bacteria and not viruses.

Norovirus illness is usually brief in healthy individuals. When people are ill with vomiting and diarrhea, they should drink plenty of fluids to prevent dehydration. Dehydration among young children, the elderly, and the sick can be common, and it is the most serious health effect that can result from norovirus infection. By drinking oral rehydration fluids (ORF), sports drinks, juice, or water, people can reduce their chance of becoming dehydrated. These liquids do not replace the nutrients and minerals lost during this illness.

Can norovirus infections be prevented?

You can decrease your chance of coming in contact with noroviruses by following these preventive steps:

- Frequently wash your hands, especially after toilet visits and changing diapers and before eating or preparing food.
- Carefully wash fruits and vegetables, and steam oysters before eating them.
- Thoroughly clean and disinfect contaminated surfaces immediately after an episode of illness by using a bleach-based household cleaner.
- Immediately remove and wash clothing or linens that may be contaminated with virus after an episode of illness (use hot water and soap).
- Flush or discard any vomit and/or stool in the toilet and make sure that the surrounding area is kept clean.

Persons who are infected with norovirus should not prepare food while they have symptoms and for three days after they recover from their illness. Food that may have been contaminated by an ill person should be disposed of properly.

Chapter 39

Acrylamide from High-Temperature Cooking

What is acrylamide?

Acrylamide is a chemical that can form in some foods during high-temperature cooking processes, such as frying, roasting, and baking. Acrylamide in food forms from sugars and an amino acid that are naturally present in food; it does not come from food packaging or the environment.

Is acrylamide found anywhere else? Does it have industrial uses?

Acrylamide is produced industrially for use in products such as plastics, grouts, water treatment products, and cosmetics. Acrylamide is also found in cigarette smoke.

Is acrylamide something new in food? When was acrylamide first detected in food?

Acrylamide has probably always been present in cooked foods. However, acrylamide was first detected in certain foods in April 2002.

This section includes "Acrylamide Questions and Answers" and "Additional Information on Acrylamide, Diet, and Food Storage and Preparation," U.S. Food and Drug Administration (www.cfsan.fda.gov), May 22, 2008.

Is there a risk from eating foods that contain acrylamide?

Acrylamide caused cancer in animals in studies where animals were exposed to acrylamide at very high doses. Acrylamide causes nerve damage in people exposed to very high levels at work. FDA [Food and Drug Administration] has not yet determined the exact public health impact, if any, of acrylamide from the much lower levels found in foods. FDA is conducting research studies to determine whether acrylamide in food is a potential risk to human health.

What kinds of cooking lead to acrylamide formation? In what foods?

High-temperature cooking, such as frying, roasting, or baking, is most likely to cause acrylamide formation. Boiling and steaming do not typically form acrylamide. Acrylamide is found mainly in foods made from plants, such as potato products, grain products, or coffee. Acrylamide does not form, or forms at lower levels, in dairy, meat, and fish products. Generally, acrylamide is more likely to accumulate when cooking is done for longer periods or at higher temperatures.

Should I stop eating foods that are fried, roasted, or baked?

No, all these foods are part of a regular diet. FDA's best advice for acrylamide and eating is that consumers adopt a healthy eating plan, consistent with the dietary guidelines for Americans, that emphasizes fruits, vegetables, whole grains, and fat-free or low-fat milk and milk products; includes lean meats, poultry, fish, beans, eggs, and nuts; and is low in saturated fats, trans fats, cholesterol, salt (sodium), and added sugars.

Are acrylamide levels in organic foods different from levels in other foods?

Since acrylamide is formed through cooking, acrylamide levels in cooked organic foods should be similar to levels in cooked nonorganic foods.

What can I do if I want to decrease the amount of acrylamide in foods that I cook or eat?

FDA's best advice for acrylamide and eating is that consumers adopt a healthy eating plan, consistent with the dietary guidelines for Americans, that emphasizes fruits, vegetables, whole grains, and fat-free or low-fat milk and milk products; includes lean meats, poultry, fish, beans, eggs, and nuts; and is low in saturated fats, trans fats, cholesterol, salt (sodium), and added sugars. FDA is waiting for new research results before considering whether new advice on acrylamide is needed.

However, consumers who want to reduce acrylamide levels in their diet now may find the following information helpful.

Food Choice and Acrylamide Exposure

- Acrylamide has been found primarily in food made from plants, such as potatoes, grain products, and coffee. Acrylamide is not typically associated with meat, dairy, or seafood products.
- Acrylamide is typically found in plant-based foods cooked with high heat (e.g., frying, roasting, and baking), not raw plant-based foods or foods cooked by steaming or boiling.
- Some foods are larger sources of acrylamide in the diet, including certain potato products (especially french fries and potato chips), coffee, and foods made of grains (such as breakfast cereal, cookies, and toast). These foods are all part of a regular diet. However, if you want to lower acrylamide intake, reducing consumption of these foods is one way to do so, keeping in mind that it's best to limit intake of foods that are high in saturated fats, trans fats, cholesterol, salt (sodium), and added sugars. FDA does not recommend reducing intake of healthful grain products (e.g., whole grain cereals) that are a good source of whole grains and fiber.

Food Storage and Preparation Methods

- Comparing frying, roasting, and baking potatoes, frying causes the highest acrylamide formation. Roasting potato pieces causes less acrylamide formation, followed by baking whole potatoes. Boiling potatoes and microwaving whole potatoes with skin on to make "microwaved baked potatoes" does not produce acrylamide.
- Soaking raw potato slices in water for 15–30 minutes before frying or roasting helps reduce acrylamide formation during cooking. (Soaked potatoes should be drained and blotted dry before cooking to prevent splattering or fires.)

- Storing potatoes in the refrigerator can result in increased acrylamide during cooking. Therefore, store potatoes outside the refrigerator, preferably in a dark, cool place, such as a closet or a pantry, to prevent sprouting.
- Generally, more acrylamide accumulates when cooking is done for longer periods or at higher temperatures. Cooking cut potato products, such as frozen french fries or potato slices, to a golden yellow color rather than a brown color helps reduce acrylamide formation. Brown areas tend to contain more acrylamide.
- Toasting bread to a light brown color, rather than a dark brown color, lowers the amount of acrylamide. Very brown areas should be avoided, since they contain the most acrylamide.
- Acrylamide forms in coffee when coffee beans are roasted, not when coffee is brewed at home or in a restaurant. So far, scientists have not found good ways to reduce acrylamide formation in coffee.

What is FDA doing about acrylamide in food?

FDA has initiated a broad range of activities on acrylamide since the discovery of acrylamide in food in April 2002. FDA accomplishments include the following:

- Developed an action plan outlining FDA's goals and planned activities on acrylamide in food
- Convened two meetings of FDA's Food Advisory Committee/ Subcommittee for input on FDA's acrylamide program
- Developed a sensitive method for measuring acrylamide in food and posted the method on FDA's website
- Analyzed and posted acrylamide testing results for approximately 2,600 food samples
- Launched a comprehensive research program to study acrylamide toxicology
- Published peer-reviewed research on acrylamide toxicology and detection methods
- Conducted research on ways to reduce acrylamide in food
- Prepared assessments of consumer exposure to acrylamide

- Posted Q&As and consumer information on acrylamide on FDA's website

What FDA data are available on acrylamide levels in U.S. foods?

FDA has posted its current data on acrylamide in foods on the CFSAN website at Acrylamide in Food (www.cfsan.fda.gov/%7Elrd/pestadd.html#acrylamide). The most recent data were added to the website in 2006.

Chapter 40

Aflatoxins

Aflatoxin contamination damages human health, animal health, the food supply, and world markets. Researchers are actively looking for methods to control aflatoxin contamination in susceptible crops. Classical plant disease prevention methods and routine technologies for controlling plant pathogens have generally been unsuccessful. Cooperative efforts to establish control strategies began in 1988 with the start of the annual Aflatoxin Elimination Workshop. The latest published conference report, "Aflatoxin/Fumonisin Workshop 2000," can be found on the USDA/ARS website (www.ars.usda.gov/SP2UserFiles/Place/53254100/AFW2Kproc.pdf).

Aflatoxin Research Areas

- Fungal ecology and development of biological control agents
- Crop resistance through conventional breeding or genetic engineering techniques
- Crop management and fungal relationship
- Processing and new methods of sampling and toxin detection in crops
- Natural compounds that inhibit fungal growth and influence aflatoxin synthesis

---

"A Focus on Aflatoxin Contamination," Food Safety Research Information Office, U.S. Department of Agriculture (fsrio.nal.usda.gov), December 2005.

FDA Action Levels for Aflatoxins

Food and Drug Administration (FDA) has established action levels for aflatoxin present in food or feed to protect human and animal health.

Levels must not exceed the following:

- 20 ppb [parts per billion] for corn and other grains intended for immature animals (including immature poultry) and for dairy animals, or when its destination is not known
- 20 ppb for animal feeds, other than corn or cottonseed meal
- 100 ppb for corn and other grains intended for breeding beef cattle, breeding swine, or mature poultry
- 200 ppb for corn and other grains intended for finishing swine of 100 pounds or greater
- 300 ppb for corn and other grains intended for finishing (i.e., feedlot) beef cattle and for cottonseed meal intended for beef cattle, swine, or poultry

General Facts about Aflatoxins

- Aflatoxins are naturally occurring toxins that are metabolic byproducts of fungi, *Aspergillus flavus* and *Aspergillus parasiticus*, which grow on many food crops under favorable conditions.
- Aflatoxin is a mycotoxin, which literally means poison from a fungi; mycotoxins are named on the basis of the fungus that produces them, thus *Aflatoxin* uses the *A* for *Aspergillus* and *fla* for the species *flavus* along with the word *toxin*.
- Adverse impact on animal and human health with acute toxicological effects such as liver damage and cancer can occur.
- The major types of aflatoxins are B1, B2, G1, G2, and M1, with aflatoxin B1 being the most toxic and usually predominant. Aflatoxin B1 is a very potent carcinogen to humans and animals.
- Aflatoxins can invade the food supply at anytime during production, processing, transport, or storage.
- Conditions that contribute to fungal growth and the production of aflatoxins are the following: a hot and humid climate, kernel

moisture, favorable substrate characteristics, and factors that decrease the host plant's immunity (insect damage, poor fertilization, and drought).

- Food and food crops most prone to contamination are corn and corn products, cottonseed, peanuts and peanut products, tree nuts (pistachio nuts, pecans, walnuts, Brazil nuts), and milk.

Aflatoxicosis and Health Effects

Aflatoxicosis is a condition that results from ingestion of aflatoxin-contaminated food or feed. It is primarily a hepatic disease affecting animals and humans. In animals the condition occurs worldwide. The health impact is usually only seen in third-world countries, and there have not been any cases of aflatoxicosis reported in the United States.

Effect on Animal Health

- Aflatoxins are both teratogenic and carcinogenic; the liver is the principal organ affected in most species. Aflatoxin B1 is considered a carcinogen by the International Agency for Research on Cancer.

- Lactating mothers excrete aflatoxins in their milk, thereby directly affecting the nursing animal. All species of animals are susceptible; however, susceptibility to aflatoxicosis depends on the species, age, and nutritional status of the animal. Young members of the species are usually more susceptible to the acute effects of the disease.

- Adverse effects on animals may be expressed as liver damage, gastrointestinal dysfunction, anemia, reduced feed consumption, reduced reproductivity, immune suppression, decreased milk and egg production, and overall retarded growth and development.

Effect on Human Health

- Unlike third-world countries, where large outbreaks have occurred from the lack of regulatory measures and high exposure levels, the United States has no reported human outbreaks of acute aflatoxicosis.

- The clinical syndrome of aflatoxicosis is characterized by abdominal pain, vomiting, pulmonary edema, convulsions, coma, liver damage, and death.

- Aflatoxin B1 is positively associated with liver cell cancer, supported by epidemiological studies done in Asia and Africa.
- Susceptibility to aflatoxicosis may be influenced by age, sex, nutritional status, health, and the level and duration of exposure.
- Long-term exposure to low levels of aflatoxins in the food supply may have adverse effects over time to humans.
- Humans can become sick by consuming unsafe levels of aflatoxin-contaminated food and food products from grains, nuts, and milk.

Impact on Agriculture

- According to the FAO [Food and Agriculture Organization], each year millions of tons of foodstuffs are lost as a direct result of mycotoxin infestation of the world's food grain crops.
- Stricter regulatory limits (lowering threshold action levels) have been imposed on commodities of many countries intended for use as food and feed, greatly impacting world export markets.
- A significant problem for the U.S. feed industry is that corn contaminated with more than 20 ppb of aflatoxins (1 oz in 3,125 tons) is no longer fit for the feed of immature animals or milk-producing animals.
- Within a few days of eating aflatoxin-contaminated feeds, there is a significant reduction in the milk yield of lactating cows.
- Aflatoxins can cause great economic losses of livestock through impaired animal health.

Chapter 41

Perchlorate

Study of Perchlorate Exposure and Thyroid Function in the U.S. Population

- CDC [Centers for Disease Control and Prevention] researchers recently reported the results of a study on the relationship between exposure to low doses of perchlorate in the U.S. population and thyroid hormone levels. This study is the first to examine the relationship between perchlorate and thyroid function in women with lower urine iodine levels (levels less than 100 micrograms per liter). The study is also much larger than either of the two previous studies of perchlorate and thyroid function that targeted or included women.
- The study involved 2,299 men and women aged 12 years and older. Researchers found an association between levels of perchlorate in urine and decreased thyroid function in women 12 years old and older.
- The relationship was strongest in women with lower iodine intake; that is, in women who had levels of iodine in their urine less than 100 micrograms per liter (µg/L).
- The study did not find a similar association for men.

"Perchlorate Fact Sheet," Centers for Disease Control and Prevention (www.cdc.gov), January 7, 2009.

- For women with lower iodine levels, perchlorate exposure was associated with small-to-moderate size changes in levels of thyroxine, the thyroid hormone that helps regulate the body's metabolism and in levels of thyroid stimulating hormone (TSH), which is responsible for stimulating the production of thyroxine.
- About 36% of women in the United States have these lower iodine levels.
- Among women with higher levels of iodine in their urine (above 100 µg/L), CDC found a statistically significant association between perchlorate and TSH levels but not between levels of perchlorate and thyroxine levels.
- The study was published on October 5, 2006, in the peer-reviewed journal *Environmental Health Perspectives*. It is available online at www.ehponline.org.

How Perchlorate Affects People's Health

- When perchlorate enters the body it can block the thyroid gland from taking up iodine. The thyroid gland needs iodine to make the thyroid hormones that regulate how the body uses energy.
- Deficiency of iodine or conditions that prevent its use in making thyroid hormone lead to decreased amounts of thyroid hormone circulating in the blood, which can manifest as symptoms of hypothyroidism.
- Maintaining sufficient intake of dietary iodine is important for good thyroid health. A good source of iodine is iodized salt. Only a small amount of iodized salt, about half a teaspoon per day, will supply an adequate amount of iodine.
- Scientists continue to conduct research into the health effects of low-dose exposure to perchlorate.

Sources of Perchlorate and How People Are Exposed

- Perchlorate is a chemical most commonly used in rocket fuel. The chemical is also used in explosives and fireworks. A combination of human activity and natural sources has led to the widespread presence of perchlorate in the environment.
- People are exposed to perchlorate by drinking water or eating food containing perchlorate or by working in the manufacture of products containing perchlorate.

Chapter 42

Consumer Beverages

Chapter Contents

Section 42.1

Benzene in Commercial Beverages

"Benzene in Beverages," Food and Drug Administration (www.fda.gov), 2006.

The Food and Drug Administration [FDA] is working with the beverage industry to ensure that benzene levels in soft drinks and other beverages are as low as possible. Benzene is a chemical used in dyes and detergents and in some plastics. It's also released into the air from automobile emissions and results from burning coal and oil. Benzene may be produced in soft drinks and other beverages with certain ingredient combinations. High levels of benzene in workplace air have caused cancer in workers.

The FDA has no regulatory limits for benzene in beverages other than bottled water. The U.S. Environmental Protection Agency has established a maximum contaminant level for benzene of five parts per billion (ppb) in drinking water. The FDA has adopted this level for bottled water as a quality standard. Based on results from a recent survey of soft drinks and other beverages conducted by the FDA's Center for Food Safety and Applied Nutrition (CFSAN), most beverage samples analyzed contained either no detectable benzene or levels below the five ppb limit for drinking water, and do not suggest a safety concern, says Judith Kidwell, a consumer safety officer in the CFSAN's Office of Food Additive Safety.

How Benzene May Form in Soft Drinks

In 1990, the FDA learned that benzene was present in some soft drinks. The FDA and industry initiated research and discovered that exposure to heat and light can stimulate the formation of low levels of benzene in some beverages that contain both benzoate salts, such as sodium benzoate or potassium benzoate, and vitamin C (ascorbic acid).

Sodium benzoate or potassium benzoate may be added to beverages to prevent the growth of bacteria, yeasts, and molds. Benzoate salts also are naturally present in some fruits and their juices, such as cranberries. Vitamin C may be naturally present in beverages or added to prevent spoilage or to provide additional nutrients.

"The presence of benzoates and vitamin C as ingredients in a product doesn't mean that elevated levels of benzene have formed or will form," Kidwell says.

A Recent Survey

In November 2005, the FDA received private laboratory results reporting low levels of benzene in a small number of soft drinks that contain benzoate preservatives and vitamin C. In response to these findings, the FDA began collecting and analyzing samples of beverages with a focus on products that contain both benzoate and vitamin C.

From the start of the survey in November through April 2006, the FDA tested more than 100 soft drinks and other beverages. Beverage samples were collected from retail stores in Maryland, Virginia, and Michigan. The survey is not a reflection of the distribution of benzene in beverages in the U.S. food supply. The data cover a limited number of products and brands, and limited geographic areas. Even though the data are limited, Kidwell says, the FDA believes that the results indicate that benzene levels are not a safety concern for consumers. In May 2006, the FDA released results of the survey through April 20, 2006.

Almost all the samples analyzed in the CFSAN's survey contained either no benzene or levels below five ppb. "And benzene levels in hundreds of samples tested by other government agencies and the beverage industry are consistent with CFSAN's findings," Kidwell says.

The CFSAN found benzene levels above five ppb in five of the beverage products tested: Crystal Light Sunrise Classic Orange, Crush Pineapple, Safeway Select Diet Orange Soda, AquaCal Strawberry Flavored Water Beverage, and Giant Light Cranberry Juice Cocktail.

Additional Actions

The FDA has contacted those firms whose products were found to contain more than five ppb benzene in the CFSAN survey. Manufacturers have reformulated the products to reduce or eliminate benzene, and some have sent samples to the CFSAN for analysis. Thus far, the CFSAN has tested a few of the reformulated products provided by the manufacturers and found that benzene levels were less than one ppb; additional testing is ongoing.

The International Council of Beverages Associations and the American Beverage Association have developed guidance for all beverage manufacturers on ways to minimize benzene formation.

The FDA will continue to collect and analyze beverage samples for the presence of benzene and will continue to follow up with manufacturers as survey results warrant. "Once the FDA has completed its beverage survey we will determine whether further action is necessary to protect the public health," Kidwell says.

Section 42.2

Unpasteurized Juice

"Preventing Health Risks Associated with Drinking Unpasteurized or Untreated Juice," Centers for Disease Control and Prevention (www.cdc.gov), November 17, 2005.

Orange, apple, grape, or cranberry juices come in many different flavors. Juice provides essential nutrients that help keep people healthy. Consumers today have numerous choices when it comes to drinking juice. One of the decisions they must make is whether to buy pasteurized or unpasteurized juice. Though illness due to juice is rare, several outbreaks of diarrheal illness due to juice have been reported in the United States in the last decade. Most outbreaks of illness due to juice have been linked to untreated or inadequately treated juice products. Most juice sold in the United States is treated. One of the most common treatments used is pasteurization.

Some outbreaks of foodborne illness linked to juice include the following:

- 1996: outbreak of *E. coli* O157:H7 infections linked to untreated apple juice sold in multiple states
- 2003: outbreak of *Cryptosporidium* infections linked to apple cider inadequately treated with ozone

- 2005: outbreak of *Salmonella* infections linked to inadequately treated orange juice marketed as "fresh squeezed" and sold in multiple states

Pasteurized juice is heated to a high temperature for a short time before it is sold. By pasteurizing juice, pathogens (germs) that may be present in the liquid are killed. Most juice concentrate sold in grocery stores has been heat treated as part of the concentration process and this is equivalent to pasteurization. About 98% of all juices sold in the United States are pasteurized. Pasteurized juice can be found as frozen concentrate, displayed at room temperature, or in the refrigerated section of your supermarket. Pasteurized juice products may say "Pasteurized" on their labels. Besides pasteurization, some juices are treated with other processes.

Treated juice, more commonly found in health-food stores and farm markets, has been treated to kill pathogens that may be present in the juice through a method other than pasteurization, such as UV irradiation, surface treatment of the fruit, or high-pressure treatment. Some types of treated juice may be marketed as "fresh squeezed."

The methods used to treat the juice must have been proven to work and verified by the FDA. These processes must be carried out properly for the treatment to be successful. If these requirements are not met, the treatment may not be effective in killing pathogens and people who consume the juice may become ill. There have been two recent outbreaks of illness related to inadequately treated juices. One was related to inadequate treatment with ozone and the other to inadequate surface treatment of the fruit. Treated juice products do not say "Pasteurized" and do not have a warning label such as on untreated juice. Treated unpasteurized juice is safe if it has been properly processed by a proven effective treatment method such as UV irradiation.

Untreated (raw) juice has not been treated in any way to kill pathogens that may be present. This type of juice may be found in the refrigerated sections of grocery stores, health-food stores, cider mills, and farm markets. Another form of untreated juice is untreated cider. One way to make this cider safer is to heat it to at least 170° F. Prepackaged, untreated juice must bear a warning label that looks similar to this one: "WARNING: This product has not been pasteurized and therefore may contain harmful bacteria that can cause serious illness in children, the elderly, and persons with weakened immune systems."

To minimize health risk, young children, the elderly, and people with weakened immune systems should not consume packaged juice that bears this warning label or any other form of juice that is known to be untreated (e.g., untreated juice served by the glass at a roadside cider stand). Anyone who wishes to reduce their risk may follow this recommendation.

If it is unclear that a juice has been treated to destroy harmful bacteria, avoid drinking it.

Chapter 43

Technologically Altered Foods

Chapter Contents

Section 43.1

FDA Regulations on Genetically Engineered Foods

"FDA Issues Final Guidance on Regulation of Genetically Engineered Animals," Food and Drug Administration (www.fda.gov), January 15, 2009.

The Food and Drug Administration (FDA) has issued final guidance on its approach to regulating genetically engineered (GE) animals.

The guidance is aimed at industry; however, FDA believes it may also help the public gain a better understanding of this important and developing area. The guidance explains the process by which FDA is regulating GE animals.

FDA invited public comments for 60 days after the release of its draft guidance on regulating GE animals in September 2008. The agency received comments from groups and individuals ranging from consumers and animal advocates, to food producers and trade associations, to academics and researchers. FDA considered the approximately 28,000 public comments in producing the final guidance.

Genetic Engineering

Genetic engineering is a process in which scientists use recombinant DNA (rDNA) technology to introduce desirable traits into an organism. DNA is the chemical inside the nucleus of a cell that carries the genetic instructions for making living organisms. Scientists use rDNA techniques to manipulate DNA molecules.

Genetic engineering involves producing and introducing a piece of DNA (the rDNA construct) into an organism so new or changed traits can be given to that organism. The rDNA construct can either come from another existing organism or be synthesized in a laboratory. Although conventional breeding methods have been used for a long time to select for desirable traits in animals, genetic engineering is a much more targeted and powerful method of actually introducing specific desirable traits into animals.

Genetic engineering is not a new technology. It has been widely used in agriculture, for example, to make crops like corn and soy resistant to pests or tolerant to herbicides. In medicine, genetic engineering is used to develop microbes that can produce pharmaceuticals. And in food, genetic engineering is used to produce enzymes that aid in baking, brewing, and cheese making.

Benefits of GE Animals

GE animals hold great promise for human and animal health, the environment, and agriculture.

- **Health protection of animals:** Animals are under development to be more resistant to very painful and harmful diseases, such as infection of the udder (mastitis) in dairy cows and "mad cow" disease (bovine spongiform encephalopathy) in all cattle.
- **New source of medicines:** Animals can be engineered to produce particular substances, such as human antibodies, to make infection-fighting drugs for people. These "biopharm" animals can change the way we treat chronic diseases, such as bleeding disorders, by providing large quantities of safe, health-restoring proteins that previously were available only from human cadavers.
- **Transplantation:** Pigs are being engineered so that their cells, tissues, or organs could be transplanted into humans with a reduced risk of immune rejection.
- **Less environmental impact:** Food animals are being engineered to grow more quickly, require less feed, or leave behind less environmentally damaging waste.
- **Healthier food:** Food animals, such as pigs, are under development to contain increased levels of omega-3 fatty acids, providing a more healthful product. Livestock can also be engineered to provide leaner meat or more milk.

GE Animals Regulated under New Animal Drug Provisions

FDA regulates GE animals under the "new animal drug" provisions of the Federal Food, Drug, and Cosmetic Act (FFDCA), and the agency must approve them before they are allowed on the market. The FFDCA defines a drug as "an article (other than food) intended to affect the structure or any function of the body of man or other animals." Therefore, the rDNA construct is a drug because it is intended to change the structure or function of the body of the GE animal.

FDA will review food and animal feed from GE animals before the food or feed can be marketed. "We want the public to understand that food from GE animals will not enter the food supply unless FDA has determined that it is safe," says Bernadette Dunham, DVM, PhD, the director of FDA's Center for Veterinary Medicine.

FDA may exercise "enforcement discretion" over some GE animals, based on their potential risk and on a case-by-case basis. This means that the agency may not require premarket approval for a low-risk animal. For example, the agency is not requiring premarket approval for GE lab animals used for research, and did not require approval of a GE aquarium fish that glows in the dark. FDA does not expect to exercise enforcement discretion for animal species traditionally consumed as food.

The guidance will help industry comply with FDA's requirements and will help the public understand FDA's oversight of GE animals and food from such animals.

Section 43.2

Cloned Meat and Dairy

"Cloned Food: What it Means to Eat Meat and Dairy from Cloned Animals," © 2008 Friends of the Earth. Reprinted with permission. The complete text of this document, including references, is available at http://www.foe.org/pdf/FOE_Cloned_Food_Factsheet.pdf/.

The FDA has lifted a voluntary ban on allowing cloned animal products from entering the human food supply. Based upon flawed studies, the FDA has claimed that eating meat and dairy from cloned animals or their offspring is harmless to human health.

Cloned animals have a much higher rate of genetic abnormalities than sexually reproduced animals. Most cloned animals die immediately after birth because the intricacies of the cloning process are still not well understood. Dolly, the first cloned sheep, died only six years after her birth of premature arthritis and lung disease. Obviously there are many genetic complications with cloned animals. Why would we want to ingest something that is known to be genetically flawed and diseased?

The FDA has also rejected requests for labeling food from cloned animals and their offspring. You may be able to know if your milk is hormone-free, but you won't be able to tell if it comes from a normal dairy cow or a clone.

The FDA study did not look at the long-term health effects of consuming cloned animal products. Eating genetically abnormal clones may cause human health abnormalities, leading to cancer and other late-onset degenerative diseases. Genetically abnormal clones will also interact freely with the environment, causing unknown downstream effects to other parts of the ecosystem. Creating a livestock population that is genetically identical due to cloning is not sustainable because it reduces genetic diversity, putting the entire livestock population at risk for disease.

Companies that are pursuing animal cloning are the same companies who are pursuing human cloning. By approving and endorsing animal cloning, we are taking a huge ethical jump towards permitting human cloning. Animal cloners want to create a superior animal breed. Perfecting that process will lead to a resurgence of eugenics like never before to create a superior human race.

Senator Barbara Mikulski (D-MD) has taken the lead in Congress on trying to prohibit cloned food from entering our food supply. Her amendment to the Farm Bill (H.R. 2419) to halt the FDA's endorsement of cloned food until two studies were completed by the National Academy of Sciences and the United States Department of Agriculture passed in the Senate. She also included language in the 2008 omnibus package which strongly encouraged the FDA to delay any major decision on cloned food until further study. Senator Mikulski has also introduced into the Senate the Cloned Food Labeling Act (S. 414) which would require labeling of all food products from cloned animals or their offspring. Legislation has been introduced in at least 10 states (CA, KY, MA, MI, MO, NJ, NY, NC, TN, and WA) that would require the labeling of cloned animal products.

Facts on Using Cloned Animals for Food

Destructive Technology

Cloning results in the death at least 95% of all created embryos. The process of cloning drastically increases the chance of fatal disease for both the clone and the mother. Most studies of cloned animals show that there are significant genetic abnormalities in animal clones. This can pose food safety risks.

Flawed Risk-Assessment

The FDA found NO peer-reviewed studies examining the safety of the meat or milk from the offspring of cow clones, cloned pigs or their offspring, cloned goats or their offspring, or meat of cloned cows and only three peer-reviewed studies of milk from cloned cows.

Taking Away Consumer Choice

The FDA lifted a voluntary ban in January 2008 which now permits meat and dairy from cloned cows, pigs, and goats and their offspring to enter the human food supply. There is no labeling or tracking requirement on cloned animals.

The Decision Was Bought

The Biotechnology Industry Organization spent over $1.9 million lobbying in the first quarter of 2008 to get the FDA to lift the voluntary ban on allowing cloned meat and dairy in the human food supply.

Global Resistance

The European Union is waiting for more information before making a decision on using cloned animals for food, and does not yet see convincing arguments to justify the production of food from clones or their offspring. Japan prohibits selling cloned animal products to consumers. South Korea has already banned imported beef from the U.S. due to fear of mad cow disease. South Korea will almost certainly prohibit importing cloned meat from the U.S. as well.

Many other countries are likely to ban using cloned animals for food, which would shut down the U.S. international meat and dairy markets.

Public Does Not Want It

Seventy-seven percent of American consumers are "not comfortable" with eating cloned animal products, and 81% of American consumers believe that cloned foods should be labeled.

Zero percent of participants in an FDA-sponsored study would feed cloned animal foods to their children.

Editor's Note: The information in this section represents the opinion of the copyright holder and is presented as one viewpoint on a complex subject.

Section 43.3

Nanoparticles in Food

This section excerpted from "Out of the Laboratory and onto Our Plates: Nanotechnology in Food and Agriculture," 2nd Edition, April 2008. The complete text of this report, including references, is available at http://www.foe.org/pdf/nano_food.pdf.

In the absence of mandatory product labeling, public debate, or laws to ensure their safety, products created using nanotechnology have entered the food chain. Manufactured nanoparticles, nano-emulsions, and nano-capsules are now found in agricultural chemicals, processed foods, food packaging, and food contact materials including food storage containers, cutlery, and chopping boards. Friends of the Earth has identified 104 of these products, which are now on sale internationally. However given that many food manufacturers may be unwilling to advertise the nanomaterial content of their products, we believe this to be just a small fraction of the total number of products now available worldwide.

Nanotechnology has been provisionally defined as relating to materials, systems, and processes which exist or operate at a scale of 100 nanometers (nm) or less. It involves the manipulation of materials and the creation of structures and systems at the scale of atoms and molecules, the nanoscale. The properties and effects of nanoscale particles and materials differ significantly from larger particles of the same chemical composition.

Nanoparticles can be more chemically reactive and more bioactive than larger particles. Because of their very small size, nanoparticles also have much greater access to our bodies, so they are more likely than larger particles to enter cells, tissues, and organs. These novel properties offer many new opportunities for food industry applications, for example as potent nutritional additives, stronger flavorings and colorings, or antibacterial ingredients for food packaging. However these same properties may also result in greater toxicity risks for human health and the environment.

There is a rapidly expanding body of scientific studies demonstrating that some of the nanomaterials now being used in foods and agricultural products introduce new risks to human health and the environment. For example, nanoparticles of silver, titanium dioxide, zinc, and zinc oxide, materials now used in nutritional supplements, food packaging, and food contact materials, have been found to be highly toxic to cells in test tube studies. Preliminary environmental studies also suggest that these substances may be toxic to ecologically important species such as water fleas. Yet there is still no nanotechnology-specific regulation or safety testing required before manufactured nanomaterials can be used in food, food packaging, or agricultural products.

Early studies of public opinion show that given the ongoing scientific uncertainty about the safety of manufactured nanomaterials in food additives, ingredients, and packaging, people do not want to eat nanofoods. But because there are no laws to require labeling of manufactured nano ingredients and additives in food and packaging, there is no way for anyone to choose to eat nano-free.

Nanotechnology also poses broader challenges to the development of more sustainable food and farming systems. At a time when global sales of organic food and farming are experiencing sustained growth, nanotechnology appears likely to entrench our reliance on chemical and energy-intensive agricultural technologies. Against the backdrop of dangerous climate change, there is growing public interest in reducing the distances that food travels between producers and consumers, yet nanotechnology appears likely to promote transport of fresh and processed foods over even greater distances. The potential for nanotechnology to further concentrate corporate control of global agriculture and food systems and further erode local farmers' control of food production is also a source of concern.

Given the potentially serious health and environmental risks and social implications associated with nanofood and agriculture, Friends of the Earth Australia, Europe, and United States are calling for:

- A moratorium on the further commercial release of food products, food packaging, food contact materials, and agrochemicals that contain manufactured nanomaterials until nanotechnology-specific safety laws are established and the public is involved in decision making.
- Nanomaterials must be regulated as new substances.
    - All deliberately manufactured nanomaterials must be subject to new safety assessments as new substances, even where the properties of their larger scale counterparts are well-known.

    - All deliberately manufactured nanomaterials must be subject to rigorous nano-specific health and environmental impact assessment and demonstrated to be safe prior to approval for commercial use in foods, food packaging, food contact materials, or agricultural applications.

- The size-based definition of nanomaterials must be extended.
    - All particles up to 300 nm in size must be considered to be "nanomaterials" for the purposes of health and environment assessment, given the early evidence that they pose similar health risks as particles less than 100 nm in size which have to date been defined as "nano."
- Transparency in safety assessment and product labeling is essential.
    - All relevant data related to safety assessments, and the methodologies used to obtain them, must be placed in the public domain.
    - All manufactured nano ingredients must be clearly indicated on product labels to allow members of the public to make an informed choice about product use.
- Public involvement in decision making is required.
    - The public, including all stakeholder groups affected, must be involved in all aspects of decision making regarding nanotechnology in food and agriculture. This includes in the development of regulatory regimes, labeling systems, and prioritization of public funding for food and agricultural research. People's right to say no to nanofoods must be recognized explicitly.
- Support for sustainable food and farming is needed.
    - The assessment of food and agricultural nanotechnology, in the context of wider societal needs for sustainable food and farming, must be incorporated into relevant decision-making processes.

Editor's Note: The information in this section represents the opinion of the copyright holder and is presented as one viewpoint on a complex subject.

Part Six

Consumer Products and Medical Hazards

Chapter 44

Teflon (Perfluorochemicals, or PFCs)

Toxic Chemicals in Food Packaging and DuPont's Greenwashing

What Are Perfluorochemicals [PFCs]?

They're found in carpets and on clothes, on fast-food wrappers, and on the inner lining of pet food bags. You might know them as Teflon®, Scotchgard™, Stainmaster® and Gore-Tex®. They pollute water, are persistent in the environment, and remain in the human body for years. Companies that manufacture PFCs have agreed to phase out one variety, called PFOA [perfluorooctanoic acid], by 2015. Unfortunately, there's no evidence that the chemicals being used to replace it are any safer.

What Problems Are Associated with PFCs?

PFCs are associated with smaller birth weight and size in newborn babies, elevated cholesterol, abnormal thyroid hormone levels, liver inflammation, and weaker immune defense against disease—all good reasons to reduce your exposure.

This section includes "Credibility Gap: Toxic Chemicals in Food Packaging and DuPont's Greenwashing: EWG's Guide to PFCs," and "Teflon Chemical Linked to Increased Cholesterol Levels," © 2008 Environmental Working Group (http://www.ewg.org). Reprinted with permission.

How to Avoid PFCs

- Forgo the optional stain treatment on new carpets and furniture. Find products that haven't been pretreated, and if the couch you own is treated, get a cover for it.
- Choose clothing that doesn't carry Teflon® or Scotchgard™ tags. This includes fabric labeled stain- or water-repellent. When possible, opt for untreated cotton and wool.
- Avoid nonstick pans and kitchen utensils. Opt for stainless steel or cast iron instead.
- Cut back on greasy packaged and fast foods. These foods often come in treated wrappers.
- Use real plates instead of paper.
- Pop popcorn the old-fashioned way on the stovetop. Microwaveable popcorn bags are often coated with PFCs on the inside.
- Choose personal care products without "PTFE" or "perfluoro" in the ingredients. Use EWG's Skin Deep at cosmeticsdatabase.com to find safer choices.

Teflon Chemical Linked to Increased Cholesterol Levels

A chemical used to make Teflon, food wrappers, and dozens of other consumer products is linked to higher levels of cholesterol, according to the latest findings of a multiyear study of 69,000 West Virginians and Ohioans whose drinking water was contaminated by a DuPont manufacturing plant in Washington, West Virginia, along the Ohio River.

Perfluorooctanoic acid, commonly known as PFOA or C8, is one of a class of PFCs that the Centers for Disease Control and Prevention has detected in the urine and blood of nearly all Americans tested in bioassays.

"This latest report is just more evidence that this Teflon chemical is far more toxic than originally thought and is dangerous at levels found in the population at large," said Environmental Working Group (EWG) Senior Scientist Olga Naidenko. "The only way to protect future generations of Americans is to change fundamentally the way this country regulates toxic chemicals. We must require industry to prove chemicals are safe before they're used in consumer products."

A team from West Virginia University [WVU] is leading the most extensive study of its kind, funded by DuPont's $107.5 million settlement in a lawsuit over PFOA releases from its West Virginia plant.

A panel of internationally recognized scientists, known as the C8 science panel and charged with overseeing the WVU study, reported last week [October 2008] that levels of total cholesterol, low density lipoprotein (LDL, often called "bad" cholesterol), and triglycerides were all greater in people with high exposures to PFOA.

But, the panel said, those people did not benefit from a corresponding increase in high density lipoprotein (HDL, known as "good" cholesterol). Increased total and low LDL cholesterol levels can lead to heart disease and other chronic ailments later in life.

The panel cautioned that the study did not prove that PFC exposure caused bad cholesterol levels to spike because there were no cholesterol readings for people participating in the study prior to their exposure to PFOA. It added that studies now underway may answer the question of a cause-and-effect relationship between PFOA and cholesterol.

The data produced so far by the unprecedented study is cause for serious concern. The initial results, made public last May [2008], indicated that exposure to PFOA may harm the immune system, liver, and thyroid and cause higher cholesterol in children. WVU findings buttress occupational health studies linking industrial exposure to PFOA to elevated cholesterol levels and higher risk of heart disease, stroke, and cancer.

The chemical industry has agreed to remove PFOA from the market by 2015, but other PFCs will remain available, and the chemical industry is constantly introducing new members of the PFC family.

Editor's Note: The information in this chapter represents the opinion of the copyright holder and is presented as one viewpoint on a complex subject.

Chapter 45

Insect Repellent

DEET (chemical name, N,N-diethyl-meta-toluamide) is the active ingredient in many insect repellent products. It is used to repel biting pests such as mosquitoes and ticks, including ticks that may carry Lyme disease. Every year, approximately one-third of the U.S. population is expected to use DEET. Products containing DEET currently are available to the public in a variety of liquids, lotions, sprays, and impregnated materials (e.g., wrist bands). Formulations registered for direct application to human skin contain from 4 to 100% DEET. Except for a few veterinary uses, DEET is registered for use by consumers, and it is not used on food.

DEET is designed for direct application to human skin to repel insects, rather than kill them. After it was developed by the U.S. Army in 1946, DEET was registered for use by the general public in 1957. Approximately 140 products containing DEET are currently registered with EPA by about 39 different companies.

Safety Review of DEET Completed in 1998

After completing a comprehensive reassessment of DEET, EPA [Environmental Protection Agency] concluded that, as long as consumers follow label directions and take proper precautions, insect repellents containing DEET do not present a health concern. Human

---

"The Insect Repellent DEET," Environmental Protection Agency (www.epa.gov), March 23, 2007.

exposure is expected to be brief, and long-term exposure is not expected. Based on extensive toxicity testing, the agency believes that the normal use of DEET does not present a health concern to the general population. EPA completed this review and issued its reregistration decision (called a RED) in 1998.

How to Use DEET Products Safely

Consumers can reduce their own risks when using DEET by reading and following product labels. All DEET product labels include the following directions:

- Read and follow all directions and precautions on this product label.
- Do not apply over cuts, wounds, or irritated skin.
- Do not apply to hands or near eyes and mouth of young children.
- Do not allow young children to apply this product.
- Use just enough repellent to cover exposed skin and/or clothing.
- Do not use under clothing.
- Avoid overapplication of this product.
- After returning indoors, wash treated skin with soap and water.
- Wash treated clothing before wearing it again.
- Use of this product may cause skin reactions in rare cases.

The following additional statements will appear on the labels of all aerosol and pump spray formulation labels:

- Do not spray in enclosed areas.
- To apply to face, spray on hands first and then rub on face. Do not spray directly onto face.

Using DEET on Children

DEET is approved for use on children with no age restriction. There is no restriction on the percentage of DEET in the product for use on children, since data do not show any difference in effects between young animals and adult animals in tests done for product registration. There also are no data showing incidents that would lead EPA to believe there is a need to restrict the use of DEET. Consumers are always advised to read and follow label directions in using any pesticide product, including insect repellents.

What to Do in the Event of a Potential Reaction to DEET

If you suspect that you or your child is having an adverse reaction to this product, discontinue use of the product, wash treated skin, and call your local poison control center or physician for help. If you go to a doctor, take the repellent container with you.

Benefits of DEET Products

DEET's most significant benefit is its ability to repel potentially disease-carrying insects and ticks. The Centers for Disease Control (CDC) receives more than 20,000 reports of Lyme disease (transmitted by deer ticks) and 100 reports of encephalitis (transmitted by mosquitoes) annually. Both of these diseases can cause serious health problems or even death in the case of encephalitis. Where these diseases are endemic, the CDC recommends use of insect repellents when out of doors. Studies submitted to EPA indicate that DEET repels ticks for about three to eight hours, depending on the percentage of DEET in the product.

Chapter 46

Antibacterial Soap (Triclosan)

Triclosan is an antimicrobial agent found in a broad variety of products, ranging from hospital and household liquid hand soap, detergents, and other sanitizing products, to toothpaste and hair products, pesticides, and plastic and foam products like cutting boards and shoe insoles. The popularity of antibacterial consumer products has led to increased consumer use of triclosan. This antimicrobial agent is marketed under a variety of trademarked names as well, including Microban, Irgasan DP-300, Lexol 300, Ster-Zac, Cloxifenolum, Biofresh, and others.

Triclosan has been detected in human breast milk and blood samples from the general population, and in the urine of 61% of 90 girls ages six to eight tested in a recent study spearheaded by Mount Sinai School of Medicine. EWG [Environmental Working Group]-led biomonitoring studies have detected triclosan in 17 of 21 people tested. Scientists recently found triclosan in 58% of 85 streams across the U.S., the likely result of its presence in discharges of treated wastewater.

The amount of triclosan in the wastewater stream is estimated to be as much as three to five milligrams per person per day from residences alone; in addition, substantial discharges of this antimicrobial agent are

---

The information in this chapter is excerpted from "Down the Drain: Sources of Hormone-Disrupting Chemicals in San Francisco Bay," © 2007 Environmental Working Group. Reprinted with permission. The complete text of this report including references is available at http://www.ewg.org/reports/downthedrain.

expected from laundries, hair salons, medical facilities, and many other commercial and industrial sites. Optimal water treatment can result in degradation and removal of 95% of triclosan; however, small amounts may pass through the treatment plants to receiving waters.

Triclosan kills microbes by disrupting protein production, and also by binding to the active site of a critical carrier protein reductase that is essential for fatty acid synthesis. This target enzyme is present in microbes but not in humans. Though triclosan is known to be acutely toxic to certain types of aquatic organisms, available studies do not indicate it causes cancer or birth defects in humans. Products containing triclosan may occasionally cause skin irritation in people with a specific sensitivity.

Triclosan has the tendency to bioaccumulate, or become more concentrated in the fatty tissues of humans and other animals that are exposed to this chemical. The chemical structure of triclosan is similar to that of DES [diethylstilbestrol], a nonsteroidal estrogen linked to cancer development in those exposed in utero, raising concerns about its potential to act as an endocrine disruptor. A recent study on fish showed that triclosan had weakly androgenic effects, but no estrogenic effects.

In contrast, another study found that low levels of triclosan in combination with thyroid hormones triggered rapid transformation of tadpoles into frogs. Rather than mimicking the thyroid hormone, triclosan, in concentrations of less than one part per billion commonly measured in U.S. streams, appeared to make thyroid hormones more potent. This hormone signaling mechanism is similar in frogs and humans, suggesting that triclosan could potentially disrupt the human thyroid system.

The evolving interaction between microbes and antiseptic agents has led to concern that use of specific antimicrobial ingredients may provoke the development of strains of bacteria that are resistant to disinfection. Studies have described strains of bacteria that have acquired reduced susceptibility to triclosan. The identification of a triclosan-resistant bacterial enzyme suggests that resistance to this antiseptic ingredient may develop more readily than to other agents. In addition, exposing specific bacterial strains to triclosan appears to result in selection favoring bacteria that are resistant to multiple antibiotics.

The American Medical Association has advanced an official recommendation against using antibacterial products in the home due to concern about antimicrobial resistance. A Food and Drug Administration panel reviewed the existing research and found no evidence that households that use antibacterial products are healthier than households that use soap and water and other typical cleansing products.

Studies indicate that in surface waters, triclosan can interact with sunlight and microbes to form methyl triclosan, a chemical that may bioacummulate in wildlife and humans. A recent European study found methyl triclosan in fish, especially concentrated in fatty tissue. Triclosan also can degrade into a form of dioxin, a class of chemicals linked to a broad range of toxicities including cancer. New research shows that triclosan in tap water can react with residual chlorine from standard water disinfecting procedures to form a variety of chlorinated byproducts at low levels, including chloroform, a suspected human carcinogen.

Editor's Note: The information in this chapter represents the opinion of the copyright holder and is presented as one viewpoint on a complex subject.

Chapter 47

Plastics

Chapter Contents

Section 47.1

Bisphenol A

This section begins with questions and answers from "Bisphenol A (BPA)," National Institute of Environmental Health Sciences (www.niehs.nih.gov), September 2008. Additional information from the Environmental Working Group is cited separately within the section.

What is BPA [Bisphenol A]?

BPA is a high production volume chemical used primarily in the production of polycarbonate plastics and epoxy resins.

Where is BPA found?

Polycarbonate plastics have many applications including use in some food and drink packaging, e.g., water and infant bottles, compact discs, impact-resistant safety equipment, and medical devices. Epoxy resins are used as lacquers to coat metal products such as food cans, bottle tops, and water supply pipes. Some dental sealants and composites may also contribute to BPA exposure.

How does BPA get into the body?

The primary source of exposure to BPA for most people is through the diet. While air, dust, and water are other possible sources of exposure, BPA in food and beverages accounts for the majority of daily human exposure.

BPA can leach into food from the protective internal epoxy resin lining of canned foods and from consumer products such as polycarbonate tableware, food storage containers, water bottles, and baby bottles. The degree to which BPA leaches from polycarbonate bottles into liquid may depend more on the temperature of the liquid or bottle than the age of the container.

Why are people concerned about BPA?

One reason people may be concerned about BPA is because human exposure to BPA is widespread. The 2003–2004 National Health and

Nutrition Examination Survey (NHANES) conducted by the Centers for Disease Control and Prevention (CDC) found detectable levels of BPA in 93% of 2,517 urine samples from people six years and older. The CDC NHANES data are considered representative of exposures in the United States. Another reason for concern, especially for parents, may be because some animal studies report effects in fetuses and newborns exposed to BPA.

Why did the National Toxicology Program (NTP) evaluate BPA?

The NTP Center for the Evaluation of Risks to Human Reproduction (CERHR) conducted the BPA evaluation. BPA was selected for evaluation because of the following factors:

- Widespread human exposure from use and occurrence in the environment
- Growing public concern
- Amount of BPA produced
- Extensive database of animal studies on reproductive and developmental effects

What did the NTP conclude about BPA?

The NTP has "some concern" for effects on the brain, behavior, and prostate gland in fetuses, infants, and children at current human exposures to BPA.

The NTP has "minimal concern" for effects on the mammary gland and an earlier age for puberty for females, in fetuses, infants, and children at current human exposures to BPA.

More research is clearly needed to understand exactly how these findings relate to human health and development, but at this point we can't dismiss the possibility that the effects we're seeing in animals may occur in humans.

The NTP has "negligible concern" that exposure of pregnant women to BPA will result in fetal or neonatal mortality, birth defects, or reduced birth weight and growth in their offspring.

The NTP has "negligible concern" that exposure to BPA will cause reproductive effects in nonoccupationally exposed adults and "minimal concern" for workers exposed to higher levels in occupational settings.

Explain the levels of concern used by the NTP. What does "some concern" mean?

"Some concern" represents the midpoint of a five-level scale of concern used by the NTP. The likelihood of an adverse effect resulting from human exposure is expressed as a level of concern. The levels from highest to lowest are the following:

- Serious concern
- Concern
- Some concern
- Minimal concern
- Negligible concern

In the case of BPA, the NTP expressed "some concern" for potential exposures to the fetus, infants, and children. There are insufficient data from studies in humans to reach a conclusion on reproductive or developmental hazards presented by current exposures to BPA, but there is limited evidence of developmental changes occurring in some animal studies at doses that are experienced by humans. It is uncertain if similar changes would occur in humans, but the possibility of adverse health effects cannot be dismissed.

The NTP conclusions are based on the weight of scientific evidence and integrate toxicity and exposure information.

How will the NTP conclusions be used?

The NTP shares the results widely. For example, "The NTP-CERHR Monograph," which includes the "NTP Brief on BPA," the "Expert Panel Report," and the public comments on the "Panel Report," are added to the NTP/CERHR and NIEHS [National Institute of Environmental Health Sciences] websites and distributed to federal and state agencies and interested individuals and organizations. It is also indexed in PubMed.

What can I do to prevent exposure to BPA?

If you are concerned, you can make personal choices to reduce exposure:

- Don't microwave polycarbonate plastic food containers. BPA is strong and durable, but over time it may break down from repeated use at high temperatures.

- Avoid plastic containers with the #7 on the bottom (www.recyclenow.org/r_plastics.html).
- Don't wash polycarbonate plastic containers in the dishwasher with harsh detergents.
- Reduce your use of canned foods. Eat fresh or frozen foods.
- When possible, opt for glass, porcelain, or stainless steel containers, particularly for hot food or liquids.
- Use infant formula bottles that are BPA free and look for toys that are labeled BPA free.

FDA's Flawed Assessment of Bisphenol A Safety Underscores the Need for State and Federal Legislation

"EWG Questions FDA Verdict on Plastic Chemical," © 2008 Environmental Working Group (http://www.ewg.org). Reprinted with permission.

An Environmental Working Group (EWG) analysis of FDA [Food and Drug Administration]'s draft assessment of BPA revealed a number of critical flaws and built-in assumptions that biased the agency's evaluation and ensured that the FDA would find current exposure levels in the population to be safe.

Laboratory studies show BPA harms brain development, raising concerns about its presence in baby bottles and other products that could expose babies and young children.

1. The FDA limited its assessment to studies that conformed to rigid, 50-year-old study designs that feed animals high amounts of BPA and analyze the animals for overt signs of poisoning and toxicity. FDA admits in their assessment that the studies they use to set the safety level do not adequately address the impacts of early life exposure to the developing brain, behavior, and the reproductive system. Notably, the only studies that conformed to these 50-year-old study designs were those funded by industry.
2. By adhering to what it euphemistically calls studies that follow "good laboratory practices," the FDA ignores more than 100 studies, including many funded by the National Toxicology Program, showing toxic effects of BPA at very low doses.

3. FDA's so-called 2,000-fold margin of safety evaporates if current exposures are compared to any of the low-dose studies, particularly the 12 studies the National Toxicology Program highlights in their April 14, 2008 BPA assessment as raising concerns for the safety of infant exposure to BPA.
4. FDA's exposure calculations underestimate infant ingestion. They calculate formula intake for the average infant instead of focusing on babies who eat the most, thus underestimating risks for half of all infants. They also assume that liquid formula has 2.5 parts per billion (ppb) BPA, even though their own testing of just 14 liquid formulas found up to five times more than this (13 ppb). These errors contradict the accepted risk assessment practice of focusing on risks to the most highly exposed population. FDA claims that its analysis was comprehensive, but in reality it underestimates risks to the most vulnerable infants by a wide margin.

When FDA evaluates new drugs for approval they are required to consider all available evidence of toxicity, not just the findings of studies that conform to standard designs of past decades. In this case they disregard studies showing that BPA exposure harms the developing brain and reproductive system, and encourage parents to continue exposing their children to BPA when safer alternatives exist. Given FDA's reckless disregard for children's health, state and federal actions are needed to protect children from avoidable contaminants in baby bottles and infant formula.

Editor's Note: The information in this section represents the opinion of the copyright holder and is presented as one viewpoint on a complex subject.

Section 47.2

Phthalates and Polyvinyl Chloride (PVC)

This section excerpted from "Pass up the Poison Plastic: The PVC-Free Guide for Your Family & Home," © 2008 Center for Health, Environment, and Justice (www.besafenet.com). Reprinted with permission. The full report, including references, is available online.

Introduction

The Center for Health, Environment, and Justice (CHEJ) has written this section to empower you to make smarter, healthier shopping choices for your family, home, and environment.

We're faced with a seemingly infinite number of choices when shopping for products, yet often have little information about the toxic chemicals used to manufacture them. We have the right to know what chemicals are in the products we are purchasing and if chemicals pose health risks for our families, the workers, and communities where they're manufactured and disposed in.

Corporations need to take action to phase out highly toxic chemicals that poison workers and communities from production to disposal. They have a fundamental responsibility to ensure chemicals and products are not harmful to their workers, neighbors, and global environment. As consumers, we also need to take personal responsibility for the health and environmental impacts of the products we purchase—and think more holistically about their lifecycle. The health and well-being of communities where products are manufactured and dumped impact our collective quality of life. Moreover, with finite resources available, many people are asking themselves the hard question of whether or not we really need all of these products that clutter our lives.

Polyvinyl chloride (PVC or vinyl) is the worst plastic for our health and environment, releasing dangerous chemicals that can cause cancer from manufacture to disposal. PVC products often contain dangerous toxic additives such as phthalates and lead, which can leach out and pose dangers to consumers. The vast majority of PVC manufactured is used in the production of building materials, however it's also used in many other consumer products such as children's toys, shower curtains, office supplies, and packaging.

The Center for Health, Environment, and Justice put together "Pass Up the Poison Plastic" to empower you to find safer solutions to polyvinyl chloride, the poison plastic. This section lists the most common consumer products made out of PVC and safer PVC-free alternatives.

A growing number of companies have committed to phase PVC out of their products and have vowed to create safer and healthier alternatives for their customers. Visit CHEJ's PVC Campaign website to learn about these initiatives: www.besafenet.com/pvc.

Safer and cost-effective alternatives are already available for virtually every PVC product on the market. Alternative products can be made from safer plastics, sustainable bio-based materials, and most importantly organic materials instead of hazardous PVC.

You can help build consumer consciousness and demand for safer, healthier products by purchasing PVC-free products. By doing so, we can all help to phase out PVC and promote safer substitutes.

Top 10 Reasons to Buy PVC-Free Products

PVC plastic poses serious environmental and health threats at all stages of its lifecycle: from manufacturing to use to disposal. Here are the top 10 reasons consumers should look for PVC-free products.

1. **The Production of PVC Involves Cancer-Causing Chemicals:** PVC products are made from toxic chemicals. Three chemicals are at the core of PVC production: chlorine gas is converted into ethylene dichloride (EDC), which is then converted into vinyl chloride monomer (VCM), which is then converted into PVC. Both VCM and EDC are extremely hazardous. Vinyl chloride, the key building block of PVC, causes a rare form of liver cancer, and damages the liver and central nervous system. Vinyl chloride is one of the few chemicals the U.S. EPA classifies as a known human carcinogen. EDC is a probable human carcinogen that also affects the central nervous system and damages the liver.

2. **PVC Leads to Dioxin Formation:** The formation of dioxin is a major concern in PVC's lifecycle. When PVC is manufactured or burned as a waste material, or accidentally in landfill fires or building and motor vehicle fires, numerous dioxins are formed and released into the air or water. The term "dioxin"

refers to a family of chemicals that are unintentionally made. They are generated as by-products during production and disposal of chlorinated compounds including PVC. Dioxins are a highly toxic group of chemicals that build up in the food chain, cause cancer, and can harm the immune and reproductive systems. Dioxins have been targeted for global phase out by the Stockholm Convention on Persistent Organic Pollutants. Dioxins have also been targeted for virtual elimination in the Great Lakes through the U.S. and Canadian Great Lakes Binational Toxics Strategy.

3. **PVC is Harmful to Workers:** Studies have documented links between working in PVC facilities and the increased likelihood of developing diseases including angiosarcoma, a rare form of liver cancer, brain cancer, lung and liver cancer, lymphomas, leukemia, and liver cirrhosis. Workplace exposures in PVC facilities have been significantly reduced from the levels of the 1960s, however there is no threshold below which VCM, a major constituent in PVC production, does not increase the risk of cancer. Thus, current exposures in the U.S. continue to pose cancer hazards to workers. Furthermore, occupational exposure to VCM remains extremely high in some facilities in Eastern Europe and Asia. There is also evidence of increased risk of developing cancer for workers exposed to dioxins in PVC plants. In addition to chronic diseases, PVC workers face deadly hazards from accidents and explosions on the job at PVC manufacturing plants.

4. **PVC Pollutes the Air and Groundwater of Surrounding Communities:** PVC chemical plants are often located in or near low-income neighborhoods and communities of color, such as Mossville, Louisiana, making the production of PVC a major environmental justice concern. Reveilletown, Louisiana, was once a small African American town adjacent to a PVC facility owned by Georgia-Gulf. In the 1980s, after a groundwater toxic plume of vinyl chloride began to seep under homes, Georgia-Gulf agreed to permanently evacuate the entire community of 106 residents. In Pottstown, Pennsylvania, chemical waste dumped in lagoons at the OxyChem PVC plant contaminated groundwater and is now targeted for cleanup under the federal Superfund program. In Point Comfort, Texas, vinyl chloride was discovered in wells near a Formosa PVC chemical plant, and the company had to spend one million dollars cleaning up contaminated groundwater.

5. **PVC: Second Largest User of Mercury Globally:** Mercury is used to produce chlorine gas. In China and Russia, mercury is also used to make vinyl chloride monomer, the basic building block of PVC. This use accounts for an astonishing 20% of global mercury consumption (700 tons), the second largest sector globally. Mercury is a potent neurological and reproductive toxin that accumulates primarily as methyl mercury in aquatic food chains. The PVC industry's use of mercury has been increasing in recent years despite the fact that the dangers of mercury are well-known. In 2002, the Chinese PVC industry used 354 tons of mercury. Within two years, that had increased to 610 tons of mercury, growing at an annual rate of 31.4%. It's been estimated that mercury usage will continue to increase to over 1,000 tons by 2010. Assuming PVC accounts for 40% of the global chlorine production, between chlorine and vinyl chloride monomer production, the PVC industry currently accounts for 27.2% of the world's mercury consumption, the second largest user of mercury in the entire world.

6. **PVC Production Sites a Target for Terrorists:** A 2002 Rand report for the U.S. Air Force identified the transport and storage of chlorine gas as among the top chemical targets for a terrorist attack and cited examples of threats and attacks already carried out around the world. As a prime feedstock for PVC, chlorine makes the PVC industry and the trains that deliver the chlorine highly vulnerable to terrorist attacks. The U.S. Naval Research Laboratory estimated that as many as 100,000 Americans could be killed or injured in just 30 minutes as a result of a terrorist attack on railways carrying lethal chlorine. The *Washington Post* reported that a classified study conducted by the U.S. Army Surgeon General dated October 29, 2001, found that a terrorist attack resulting in a chemical release in a densely populated area could injure or kill as many as 2.4 million people. The best security would be to switch to safer materials that don't require chlorine. Since PVC production is the largest single use of chlorine, reducing its use represents the most important step we can take to reduce the risk of accidental or intentional chlorine disasters.

7. **PVC Products Contain and Leach Toxic Additives:** PVC products often contain toxic additives such as phthalates, lead, and cadmium. Many of these additives are not chemically bound to the plastic and can migrate out of the product posing potential

hazards to consumers. In some cases, these additives can be released from the product into the air inside your home. Some phthalates have been linked to reproductive problems including shorter pregnancy duration, premature breast development in girls, sperm damage, and impaired reproductive development in males. Certain phthalates have now been banned in children's toys in the United States effective February 2009. Lead has been used to stabilize and is found in many different PVC products.

8. **Burning PVC Leads to Dioxin Formation:** A major concern about PVC is the formation of dioxins whenever it is burned. This is due to the relationship between PVC, chlorine, and dioxin. PVC is a significant source of the chlorine necessary for dioxin formation during the combustion of municipal and household waste in incinerators, burn barrels, landfills, an estimated one million building and motor vehicle fires, and open dumps. The strongest evidence of dioxin formation during combustion comes from laboratory studies showing that PVC content in the waste stream fed to incinerators is linked to elevated levels of dioxins in stack air emissions and in residual incinerator ash. Dioxins also form when PVC products and materials are burned in accidental building and vehicle fires.

9. **Discarding PVC in Landfills Poses Risks:** The land disposal of PVC product waste, especially flexible materials, also poses environmental and public health risks. As flexible PVC degrades in a landfill, toxic additives leach out of the waste into groundwater, which is especially problematic for unlined landfills. These additives also contribute to the formation of landfill gases, which are formed in municipal waste landfills. In addition, there are over 8,400 landfill fires reported every year in the U.S. These fires burn PVC waste and contribute to dioxin formation. Land disposal is the final fate of between two and four billion pounds of PVC that are discarded every year at some 1,800 municipal waste landfills in the U.S.

10. **PVC Contaminates and Ruins Recyclable Plastics:** PVC packaging has a national recycling rate far lower than other plastics. Just 0.7% of PVC bottles were recycled in 2006, compared to 23.5% for PET [polyethylene terephthalate] plastic bottles and 26.4% for HDPE [high-density polyethylene] bottles. According to the Association of Postconsumer Plastics Recyclers,

"PVC is a major contaminant to the PET bottle recycling stream." One PVC bottle can contaminate and ruin a recycling load of 100,000 recyclable PET bottles, if the PVC cannot be separated from the PET. This is because PET and PVC behave very differently when they are processed for recycling. PVC burns at a lower temperature than PET. It burns at the temperature that simply melts PET. When this occurs, "black spots" get into the PET resin contaminating the batch and ruining or seriously downgrading the quality of recycled PET residue.

Quick Tips for Avoiding PVC, the Poison Plastic

To rid your home of PVC, we've compiled these quick tips for avoiding PVC in common consumer and household products. These tips are by no means exhaustive or complete, but will help you embark down the road towards safer PVC-free products.

In general, we recommend looking for nonplastic products whenever available. When choosing plastic items, be sure to not only avoid PVC but also polycarbonate (PC), polystyrene (PS), and acrylonitrile butadiene styrene (ABS) plastics.

How to Identify PVC, the Poison Plastic: In order to avoid PVC products, consumers need to know how to identify PVC products and how to find safer alternatives.

PVC products are often labeled with the words "vinyl" on the packaging, such as vinyl three-ring binders. PVC packaging can be identified by looking for the number "3" inside, or the letters "V" or "PVC" underneath the universal recycling symbol, indicating the product is made out of PVC. Just remember—bad news comes in threes, don't buy PVC.

For some products, it is not easy to determine whether they contain PVC because it's not properly labeled. If you're uncertain, contact the manufacturer or retailer and ask what type of plastic their product is made of. You have a right to know.

Five Easy Steps to Begin Going PVC-Free in Your Home

1. When remodeling your home, use PVC-free building materials.
2. Buy PVC-free baby products and toys for your children, grandchildren, and relatives.
3. Replace your PVC shower curtain.

4. Shop for PVC-free electronics.
5. Don't buy products that are packaged in PVC. Just remember: bad news comes in threes, don't buy PVC.

Clothing/Accessories

- Look for PVC-free materials in rainwear, prints on clothing, and accessories (such as handbags and belts).
- In purchasing accessories like purses and jewelry, look for fabrics and other materials rather than plastics. Choices include jacquards, velvets, crinkled crepes, satins, wood, metals, pearls, rhinestones, etc.
- Be cautious of products usually made of or coated with PVC, which can include various items such as bibs, hats, bags, raingear, and shoes.
- Avoid jewelry with plastic cords, dull metallic components, or white fake pearls, which can contain lead.

Children's Products and Toys

- Look for toys and infant products labeled PVC-, phthalate-, and lead-free.
- Look for toys made with materials like organic cotton and sustainably harvested wood.
- Choose PVC-free pacifiers and teethers. Silicone pacifiers are available; many companies have stopped using PVC for teethers.
- Avoid modeling clays made of PVC (polymer clays such as Fimo and Sculpey). Look for clays made without PVC, or make your own (recipes are available online such as at www.theholidayzone.com/recipes/dough.html).
- Consult online resources such as www.healthytoys.org, www.thesoftlanding.com, and www.zrecommends.com.

Christmas Trees

- Almost all fake Christmas trees are made with PVC. Purchase vintage aluminum trees, or real, locally grown, and sustainably harvested organic trees. You can also purchase a live tree in a pot, which can later be planted outside.

Credit Cards

- Credit cards are often made of PVC but PVC-free cards are available. Just ask your bank.

Electronics

- Avoid electronics manufacturers who have not committed to phasing out PVC and other toxic chemicals in their production (consult the latest edition of Greenpeace's "Greener Electronics Guide").
- Buy electronics from companies who have pledged to responsibly "take it back" at the end of its useful life.

Food Wrap

- When buying food wrap, choose butcher paper, waxed paper, parchment paper, low density polyethylene (LDPE), or cellulose bags.
- Ask the manager of your grocery store to stock PVC-free food wrap for meats and cheeses in the deli.

Halloween Costumes

- Shop for PVC-free costumes and costumes that are made from materials like cotton. Try to avoid costumes with shiny prints that often contain PVC.
- Make your own Halloween costumes instead of buying them. Go to local thrift stores to find clothes to make into costumes.

Home Repair and Construction Materials

Flooring and Carpeting

- Avoid vinyl flooring; choose Forest Stewardship Council (FSC)-certified wood, ceramic tiles, bamboo, cork, or linoleum instead.
- Watch out for PVC in carpet padding and backing.

Piping

- Avoid PVC piping, especially for pipes carrying drinking water; choose safer alternatives like HDPE (high density polyethylene), iron, steel, concrete vitrified clay, and copper.

Roofing Membranes

- Look for PVC-free roofing made out of thermoplastic polyolefin (TPO), ethylene propylene diene monomer (EPDM), nitrile butadiene polymer (NBP), and low-slope metal roofing.

Siding

- Purchase fiber-cement board; stucco; recycled, reclaimed, or FSC-certified wood; oriented strand board (OSB); brick; or polypropylene (PP) siding.

Shutters

- Choose shutters made of wood, aluminum, or PVC-free plastic.

Wall Coverings

- Instead of vinyl wallpaper, choose paint, paper-based wallpaper, or wood paneling.

Windows and Doors

- Purchase wood, metal, or fiberglass windows instead of vinyl.
- Instead of vinyl roller shades, choose metal or wood blinds.
- Window treatments/drapes can be made of fabric, wood, bamboo, or many other materials.

Lunch Boxes

- Use cloth lunch bags or metal lunch boxes rather than plastic lunch boxes, many of which are made of PVC.

Mattresses, Couches, and Padded Chairs

- Avoid products such as inflatable furniture, PVC-coated fabrics, and vinyl furniture covers.
- Choose furniture made from solid wood (FSC certified), metal, and glass.

Office and School Supplies

- Avoid backpacks with shiny plastic designs that often contain PVC and may contain lead.

- Look for backpacks like the original fabric models.
- Stick to the plain metal paperclips, as colored paper clips are coated with PVC.
- Most three-ring binders are vinyl; look for cardboard, fabric-covered, or polypropylene binders.

Outdoor Products

- When shopping for nonvinyl garden hoses, look for those labeled "drinking-water safe." Hoses with this label are PVC-free.
- Avoid plastic outdoor furniture, but if desired, look for recycled PE types. Otherwise, opt for metals and FSC-certified woods.

Packaging

- Avoid the three-arrow "recycling" symbol with the number 3 and/or the initials PVC, indicating it's made with PVC. If neither symbol is present, call the manufacturer's question/comment line (usually a toll-free 800 number) listed on the package to find out what it's made of.
- Avoid products packaged in unlabeled plastics, such as clamshells and blister packs, which are often PVC.
- Choose products with packaging made from more easily recycled materials like paper (look for those with higher post-consumer recycled content), glass, and metal.
- Avoid single-use disposable packaging whenever possible.

Shower Curtains

- Choose curtains and liners made of cotton (organic is preferable), polyester, polyethylene vinyl acetate (PEVA), ethylene vinyl acetate (EVA), or nylon.

Utensils and Dishware

- Use stainless steel utensils; if you require disposable dinnerware, look for biobased (i.e., made with polylactic acid (PLA) or polyhydroxyalkanoates (PHA) plastics) cutlery and plates.
- Never microwave with cling wrap or plastic containers; use glass, stoneware, or ceramic dishware and containers instead.

Heating plastic increases the chances of chemical additives leaching into food and beverages.

- Choose drinking containers made of glass or stainless steel; or if plastic is necessary, be sure to avoid PVC, polystyrene (PS), and polycarbonate (PC) plastics.

Editor's Note: The information in this section represents the opinion of the copyright holder and is presented as one viewpoint on a complex subject.

Chapter 48

Contaminants in Consumer Products

Chapter Contents

Section 48.1

An Action Plan for Import Safety

"Action Plan for Import Safety," Food and Drug Administration (www.fda.gov), 2008.

On November 6, 2007, the Interagency Working Group on Import Safety (Working Group), established by Executive Order 13439, issued an "Action Plan for Import Safety: A Roadmap for Continual Improvement" (Action Plan). The Action Plan is based on the principles of prevention, intervention, and response and contains 14 broad recommendations and 50 specific short- and long-term action steps to better protect consumers and enhance the safety of the increasing volume of imports entering the United States.

1. **Prevention:** Prevent harm in the first place. The U.S. government must work with the private sector and foreign governments to adopt an approach to import safety that builds safety into the manufacturing and distribution processes. This effort will reduce the risks to consumers from otherwise dangerous imported products.

2. **Intervention:** Intervene when risks are identified. Federal, state, local, and foreign governments, along with foreign producers and the importing community, must adopt more effective techniques for identifying potential product hazards. When problems are discovered, government officials must act swiftly, and in a coordinated manner, to seize, destroy, or otherwise prevent dangerous goods from advancing beyond the point-of-entry. For foreign countries, taking steps to ensure the safety of products exported to the United States will benefit them by facilitating trade.

3. **Response:** Respond rapidly after harm has occurred. In the event that an unsafe import makes its way into domestic commerce, swift actions must be taken to limit potential exposure and harm to the American public.

Since the release of the Action Plan, the FDA [Food and Drug Administration] has collaborated with many partners to improve the safety of imported products. The following is a list of FDA accomplishments since issuance of the Action Plan.

Prevention

- **Signed memoranda of agreement (MOA) with China.** FDA signed two MOAs with China and held bilateral talks with the Chinese regulatory agencies to work toward creation of a certification program to help ensure items exported to the United States meet Department of Health and Human Services (HHS) and FDA safety standards. Additionally, these MOAs provide a streamlined process for facilitating FDA inspections conducted in China. This aspect of the agreement has already proven effective in giving FDA prompt access to conduct inspections.
- **Issued "Report on the Use of Standards."** FDA issued its "Annual Report on the Use of Standards" by the agency. This report describes the agency's involvement in standards-setting activities during 2007.
- **Expanded FDA's international outreach.** FDA provided a briefing to Washington, DC–based foreign embassy personnel on FDA actions under the Action Plan and the FDA "Food Protection Plan." Additionally, FDA discussed import safety with counterparts from Australia, New Zealand, the European Union, India, Vietnam, and several other countries. These discussions support new capacity building, new bilateral agreements, and continued efforts to expand FDA's foreign presence.
- **Released self-assessment tools for industry.** FDA worked domestically with industry to strengthen existing safety standards by releasing self-assessment tools for industry to minimize the risk of intentional contamination of food and cosmetics.
- **Participated in Food and Agriculture Organization (FAO)/World Health Organization (WHO) activities.** FDA participated in FAO/WHO activities to establish the Scientific Basis for International Standards and Guidance for Residues, Chemical Contaminants, and Pathogens in Fresh Produce, Seafood, and Other Commodities. This included the completion of a risk assessment on *Vibrio parahaemolyticus*, which can cause gastrointestinal illness in humans.

- **Participated in the Codex Alimentarius Commission (Codex) activities to promote international food safety standards and guidance through Codex Alimentarius.** FDA provided the U.S. delegate or alternate delegate to 14 Codex committees including those that developed standards in the areas of food hygiene, food additives, contaminants, nutrition, food labeling, biotechnology, and food import and export inspection and certification systems.

- **Participated in the WHO International Medical Products Anti-Counterfeiting Task Force (IMPACT).** FDA provided the U.S. delegate or alternate delegate to the WHO IMPACT, which aims to build coordinated action across and between countries in order to halt the production, trading, and selling of counterfeit medical products around the globe. IMPACT is a coalition comprised of all the major anticounterfeiting players, including international organizations, nongovernmental organizations, medicines regulatory authorities, enforcement authorities, associations representing pharmaceutical manufacturers, wholesalers, health professionals, and patients.

- **Published draft compliance policy guide (CPG) on *Listeria monocytogenes*.** FDA published a draft CPG on *Listeria monocytogenes* and held a public meeting to solicit public comment and encourage discussion on the CPG.

- **Issued draft guidance for industry on control of *Listeria monocytogenes*.** The draft guidance is intended to assist processors in controlling *Listeria monocytogenes* in the food processing environment during the manufacture of refrigerated or frozen, ready-to-eat foods. The draft guidance for industry, when finalized, will complement FDA's current good manufacturing practices regulations.

- **Issued fresh-cut produce guidance.** FDA issued guidance on fresh-cut produce to advise industry on how to limit contamination of fresh-cut fruits and vegetables.

- **Issued amended Interim Final Rule on Use of Materials Derived from Cattle in Human Food and Cosmetics.** FDA issued an amended interim final rule that permits the agency to designate a country as not subject to certain bovine spongiform encephalopathy (BSE)-related restrictions upon written request and if the country demonstrates and provides supporting documentation that its current controls make such restrictions unnecessary.

- **Issued a federal register notice for food and feed third-party certification programs.** FDA issued a federal register notice that sought public comment on the existence and use of third-party certification programs to better understand how they can be used to help to ensure that food products are safe, secure, and meet FDA requirements.

- **Provided technical assistance to China.** FDA provided training on regulatory requirements and technical assistance training to Chinese regulatory agencies.

- **Hired leadership for an FDA office in China.** FDA received approval and has hired leadership for a new FDA office in China.

- **Provided technical assistance to South Africa.** FDA's Office of Cosmetics and Colors (OCAC) in the Center for Food Safety and Applied Nutrition participated in a U.S. Department of Agriculture/Foreign Agriculture Service workshop for South African regulators and industry representatives. OCAC gave a seminar on regulatory requirements for marketing cosmetics in the United States, which included specific information on imports and labeling.

- **Sought to establish an FDA presence in India.** An FDA delegation visited Indian counterparts to discuss requirements for an FDA presence in India. Results are promising for future collaboration.

- **Continued International Cooperation on Cosmetics Regulation (ICCR).** FDA continued to participate in ICCR activities, including strengthening the mechanisms for participating cosmetics regulatory authorities to keep each other apprised of emerging product-related safety issues.

- **Issued a federal register notice on animal feed safety.** FDA issued a federal register notice for a public meeting to present changes to the Animal Feed Safety System project and the ranking of feed hazards according to the risk they pose to animal and public health.

- **Issued Final Rule on Substances Prohibited from Use in Animal Food or Feed.** FDA issued a final rule to expand protections against bovine spongiform encephalopathy (BSE) by prohibiting certain material in all animal feed that can carry the agent that causes BSE.

- **Participated in HHS delegation to Vietnam.** FDA accompanied an HHS delegation to Vietnam to discuss a cooperative arrangement with the Ministry of Health covering food, feed, and medical products.

- **Sought to establish an FDA presence in the Middle East.** The FDA commissioner traveled to Jordan to explore expanding FDA's presence in the Middle East.

- **Coordinated food safety exchange of information.** FDA led the Security and Prosperity Partnership of North America Health Working Group with Canada and Mexico to coordinate and exchange information on food safety investigations and follow-up activities.

- **Negotiated a plan to leverage inspectional resources.** The FDA negotiated a plan for leveraging inspectional resources of the European Union. The initial effort is to establish a pilot program to coordinate inspection planning.

- **Protected American consumers from potentially harmful products.** Between November 7, 2007, and May 20, 2008, HHS/FDA refused admission of 8,543 entry lines, each line representing a distinct product type, that appeared to be adulterated, misbranded, processed under unsanitary conditions, or unapproved new drugs. The refusal of these potentially harmful products prevented them from being distributed to the American public.

Intervention

- **Collaborated on an interagency agreement to determine the survivability of *Bacillus anthracis* (causative agent of anthrax).** FDA entered into an agreement with the U.S. Department of Agriculture and the Department of Homeland Security to determine the survivability of *Bacillus anthracis* in processed liquid egg products, which includes whole eggs, egg yolks, and egg whites.

- **Established a memorandum of understanding (MOU) to develop forensic tools.** FDA entered into an MOU with the Department of Homeland Security to develop forensic tools to allow the identification and differentiation of individual strains of foodborne bacteria.

- **Modernized FDA's Mission Accomplishments and Regulatory Compliance Services (MARCS).** The MARCS program manages the integration, re-engineering, and enhancement of the legacy systems that support FDA field activities. MARCS was recently upgraded to include international mail courier information collection and photographic capture of parcels and contents.

- **Enabled single sign-on for import systems.** The FDA enabled a single sign-on capability for the Field Accomplishments and Compliance Tracking System and the Operational and Administrative System for Import Support. By not having to log on to multiple systems, it will be easier for agency staff to use these systems in accomplishing their work.

- **Improved interagency interaction.** Representatives from Customs and Border Protection, Department of Justice, U.S. Department of Agriculture, Department of Commerce, Consumer Protection Safety Commission, FDA, Environmental Protection Agency, and Department of Transportation held a series of meetings to identify ways to improve upon agency interaction during the cargo clearance process and to maximize the sharing of critical data among agencies.

- **Developed a platform for rapid detection of pathogens in food.** FDA developed a rapid detection method using flow cytometry to identify *E. coli* and *Salmonella* in food. This system is being used in poultry-processing facilities to detect and prevent bacterial contamination during food processing.

- **Approved the use of cetylpyridinium chloride (CPC) as an antimicrobial agent.** FDA approved CPC as an antimicrobial agent applied in solution to raw poultry carcasses to prevent contamination with *Salmonella* or *E. coli*.

- **Developed a cell-based cytotoxicity assay.** FDA developed a cell-based cytotoxicity assay to assess the biological activity of the bioterrorism agents ricin and abrin in infant formulas, fruit juices, and yogurt. This assay can be used to assess other chemicals that may be used by terrorists to contaminate the food supply.

- **Developed a flow cytometry–based system.** In collaboration with outside parties, FDA developed a flow cytometry–based system which uses probes to identify bacteria according to genus, species, or serotype (e.g., differentiating normal *E. coli* from *E. coli* O157), depending on the level of specificity desired. This system has been successfully commercialized and is being used in poultry-processing facilities to detect and prevent bacterial contamination.
- **Employed a new detection method for *Salmonella*.** FDA is using genetic analysis to identify hundreds of *Salmonella enterica* strains from seafood imports. The analysis provides information that can be used to trace more quickly outbreaks of *Salmonella enterica* and implement surveillance programs to ensure the safety of imported seafood.
- **Developed a new detection method for mycotoxins.** FDA developed a method to detect mycotoxins in distiller's grains.
- **Developed portable x-ray fluorescence (XRF) devices.** FDA has developed the analytical capabilities using handheld XRF devices to detect lead and other heavy metals in a variety of products and media. More than 80 elements can be rapidly screened that could be extended to the field and used in remote sites outside the laboratory. To date a cadre of investigators and analysts has been trained to screen a variety of products.
- **Upgraded eLEXNET portal collaboration and user interface tools.** FDA has upgraded the Electronic Laboratory Exchange Network (eLEXNET) user interface to more effectively provide information and stimulate interactive information exchange amongst users. eLEXNET is a seamless, integrated, web-based information network that allows health officials at multiple government agencies engaged in food safety activities to compare, share, and coordinate laboratory analysis findings. This network provides the necessary infrastructure for an early warning system that identifies potentially hazardous foods and enables health officials to assess risks and analyze trends.

- **Developed a real-time polymerase chain reaction assay for the detection of *Salmonella* and *E. coli* in multiple food matrices.** FDA developed a method which was AOAC International validated to rapidly screen large numbers of samples for *Salmonella* and *E. coli* in 24 hours. FDA has also developed a method to rapidly screen large numbers of samples within 30 hours.

- **Issued a compliance program for select imported biologic regulated products (CP 7342.007).** FDA issued a comprehensive compliance program for select biologic imports (www.fda.gov/cber/cpg/7342007.htm). The new compliance program gives the field comprehensive instructions for reviewing import entries of select biologic products. It outlines what regulatory requirements apply and what steps to take if a product does not comply.

- **Expedited entry of stem cells for transplantation.** The FDA, Customs and Border Protection, and the National Marrow Donor Program entered into an agreement for expedited entry of hematopoietic stem cells for transplantation. Hematopoietic stem cells are used for transplantation into immune-compromised individuals, particularly those individuals who have cancer and require donated stem cell transplant material as part of their treatment protocol.

- **Responded to adverse events associated with heparin.** After discovering an increase in adverse reactions to certain heparin sodium products, FDA designed, validated, and publicized test methods for analyzing heparin for contamination. FDA began inspections of domestic and foreign facilities and suppliers to determine the presence and cause of the contamination, map the supply route of contaminated products, and gauge the inspected firms' compliance with current good manufacturing practices. Working relationships developed through the memoranda of agreement with China helped speed and facilitate HHS/FDA visas and inspections in responding to the heparin crisis. HHS/FDA was joined in the facilities by representatives from the Chinese State Food and Drug Administration and continues to have conversations with them as they conduct their testing so that any findings are shared.

- **Completed PREDICT pilot.** The PREDICT prototype for improved, risk-based electronic screening of imports was pilot tested using seafood entries at five ports in metropolitan Los Angeles. The test was successful. Using PREDICT, the "hit rate" of violative findings for field exams increased to 7.0% from 3.7%. For samples, the violation rate increased to 19.3% from 14.4%. FDA is now expanding the prototype to include automated database lookups with regards to marketing status, and to add more types of products for PREDICT screening.

Response

- **Collaborated with states.** FDA held a conference call with the state commissioners of agriculture and health to discuss collaboration between the states and the agency regarding food safety. The FDA commissioner announced that a 50-state meeting will be held to develop implementation strategies for the implementation of the "Food Protection Plan," the Action Plan, and the FDA Amendments Act (FDAAA) between federal, state, and local partners.
- **Issued federal register notices for pharmaceutical serialization, track and trace, and authentication.** FDA published two federal register (FR) notices pursuant to section 913 of the FDA Amendments Act of 2007 to seek public comment on standards for pharmaceutical serialization, track and trace, and authentication, as well as to seek public comment on technologies used for track and trace and authentication of pharmaceuticals. Track-and-trace technologies can be used as anticounterfeiting and antidiversion tools by tracking a product throughout the supply chain.
- **Developed a recall template.** FDA developed a template for public notification of recalls and presented it to the FDA Risk Communications Advisory Committee.
- **Issued a request for applications for states interested in establishing food hazard rapid response teams (RRT).** The goal of developing and sustaining an RRT is in concert with long-term goals to enhance the food inspection and foodborne illness response programs; to increase the ability to inspect and obtain compliance for firms in their jurisdiction involved in the processing, manufacturing, distribution, transportation and warehousing of food; and to verify compliance with the state laws and regulations, good manufacturing practices, food defense, and other food protection requirements.

Section 48.2

Health Concerns over U.S. Imports of Chinese Products

"Health and Safety Concerns over U.S. Imports of Chinese Products: An Overview," Congressional Research Service, October 17, 2008.

China is a major source of U.S. imports of consumer products (such as toys) and an increasingly important supplier of various food products. Reports of unsafe seafood, pet food, toys, tires, and other products imported from China over the past year or so have raised concern in the United States over the health, safety, and quality of imported Chinese products. This section provides an overview of this issue and implications for U.S.–China trade relations.

In 2007, China overtook Canada to became the largest source of U.S. imports (at $322 billion); about 17% of all U.S. imports now come from China. Over the past year or so, numerous recalls and warnings have been issued by U.S. firms over various products imported from China, due to health and safety concerns. This has led many U.S. policymakers to question the adequacy of China's regulatory environment in ensuring that its exports to the United States meet U.S. standards for health, safety, and quality; as well as the ability of U.S. government regulators, importers, and retailers to identify and take action against unsafe imports (from all countries) before they enter the U.S. market.

Warnings, Recalls, and Detentions

The FDA in March 2007 issued warnings and announced voluntary recalls on certain pet foods (and products used to manufacture pet food and animal feed) from China believed to have caused the sickness and deaths of numerous pets in the United States. In May 2007, the FDA issued warnings on certain toothpaste products (some of which were found to be counterfeit) found to originate in China that contained poisonous chemicals. In June 2007, the FDA announced import controls on all farm-raised catfish, basa, shrimp, dace (related to carp), and eel from China after antimicrobial agents, which are not approved in the United States for use in farm-raised aquatic animals, were found. Such shipments will be detained until they are proven to be free of contaminants. On January 25, 2008, the FDA posted on its website a notice by Baxter Healthcare Corporation that it had temporarily halted the manufacture of its multiple-dose vials of heparin (a blood thinner) for injection because of recent reports of serious adverse events (including an estimated 81 deaths and hundreds of complications) associated with the use of this drug. On February 18, 2008, the *New York Times* reported that a Chinese firm that produces an active ingredient used to produce heparin was not certified by the Chinese government to make the drug and had not undergone FDA inspection; many have speculated that the Chinese plant is likely the source of the problem. On September 12, 2008, the FDA issued a health information advisory on infant formula in response to reports of contaminated milk-based infant formula manufactured and sold in China, and later issued a warning on other products containing milk imported from China.

The National Highway Traffic Safety Administration (NHTSA) in June 2007 was informed by Foreign Tire Sales Inc., an importer of foreign tires, that it suspected that up to 450,000 tires (later reduced to 255,000 tires) made in China may have a major safety defect (i.e., missing or insufficient gum strip inside the tire). The company was ordered by the NHTSA to issue a recall. The Chinese government and the manufacturer have maintained that the tires in question meet or exceed U.S. standards.

The Consumer Product Safety Commission (CPSC) issued alerts and announced voluntary recalls by U.S. companies on numerous products made in China in 2007. From January–December 2007, over four-fifths of CPSC recall notices involved Chinese products. Over this period, roughly 17.6 million toy units were recalled because of excessive lead levels. Recalls were also issued on 9.5 million Chinese-made toys (because of the danger of loose magnets), 4.2 million "Aqua Dots" toys (because beads contain a chemical that can turn toxic if ingested), and 1 million toy ovens (due to potential finger entrapment and burn hazards).

U.S. Imports of Products of Concern from China

Table 48.1 lists products imported from China in 2007 that have been the subject of recent U.S. health and safety concerns, such as toys, seafood, tires, animal foods, organic chemicals and pharmaceuticals, and toothpaste. It indicates that China was a major source of imports for many of these products. For example, China was the largest supplier of imported toys (89% of total), seafood products (15%), and tires (26%); the second largest foreign supplier of animal food products (24%); the sixth largest supplier of toothpaste (1%); and the ninth largest source of imported pharmaceuticals and organic chemicals (3%). The table also indicates that, despite health and safety concerns, U.S. imports of most of the products listed (with the exception of toothpaste) increased in 2007 over 2006 levels. For example, toy imports from China grew by 33.4%.

Table 48.1. U.S. Imports of Selected Products from China in 2007

Product Description	Imports from China ($ millions)	China's Rank as a Source of Imported Product	Imports from China as a % of Total U.S. Imports (%)	Percentage Change in Imports in 2007 over 2006 (%)
Dolls, toys, and games	19,460.5	1	89.4	33.4
Fish and other seafood products	2,054.3	1	14.9	4.8
Tires	2,436.4	1	26.0	28.5
Animal foods	163.0	2	24.0	19.3
Toothpaste	1.3	6	1.0	-59.6
Organic chemicals and pharmaceutical products	3,235.3	9	3.4	25.0
Total imports from China	321,507.8	1	16.5	11.7

Source: USITC DataWeb using various classifications systems and digit levels.

China's Poor Regulatory System

Many analysts contend that China's health and safety regime for manufactured goods and agricultural products is fragmented and ineffective. Problems are seen as including weak consumer protection laws and poorly enforced regulations, lack of inspections and ineffective penalties for code violators, underfunded and understaffed regulatory agencies and poor interagency cooperation, the proliferation of fake goods and ingredients, the existence of numerous unlicensed producers, falsified export documents, extensive pollution, intense competition that often induces firms to cut corners, the relative absence of consumer protection advocacy groups, failure by Chinese firms to closely monitor the quality of their suppliers' products, restrictions on the media, and extensive government corruption and lack of accountability, especially at the local level.

Chinese officials contend that most Chinese-made products are safe and note that U.S. recalls for health and safety reasons have involved a number of countries (as well as U.S. products). They also argue that some of the blame for recalled products belongs to U.S. importers or designers. They further contend that some U.S. products imported into China have failed to meet Chinese standards. However, they have acknowledged numerous product health and safety problems in China, as reflected in reports that have appeared in China's state-controlled media. For example, in June 2004, the Chinese *People's Daily* reported that fake baby formula had killed 50 to 60 infants in China. In June 2006, the *China Daily* reported that 11 people had died from a tainted injection used to treat gall bladders. In August 2006, *Xinhua News Agency* reported that a defective antibiotic drug killed seven people and sickened many others.

China has announced a number of initiatives to improve and strengthen food and drug safety supervision and standards, increase inspections, require safety certificates before some products can be sold, and to crack down on government corruption:

- In May 2007, the *Xinhua News Agency* reported that former director of China's State Food and Drug Administration had been sentenced to death for taking bribes (equivalent to $850,000) in return for approving untested and/or fake medicines (he was executed on July 10, 2007). On the same day, the *Xinhua News Agency* reported that the Chinese government had announced that it would, by the end of 2007, complete regulations for setting up a national food recall system that would ban the sale of toys that failed to pass a national compulsory safety certification.

- On June 27, 2007, the *China Daily* reported that a nationwide inspection of the food production industry had found that a variety of dangerous industrial raw materials had been used in the production of flour, candy, pickles, biscuits, black fungus, melon seeds, bean curd, and seafood. As a result, the government reportedly closed 180 food factories found to be producing unsafe products and/or making fake commodities. It also reported that in 2006, the government had conducted 10.4 million inspections, uncovering problems in 360,000 food businesses, and had closed 152,000 unlicensed food businesses.

- On July 4, 2007, the *China Daily* reported that the government had finished making amendments to all food safety standards and had established an emergency response mechanism among several ministries to deal with major problems regarding food safety.

- On August 9, 2007, *China Daily* reported that the government had pledged to spend $1 billion by 2010 to improve drug and food safety.
- On August 15, 2007, a spokesperson from the Chinese embassy in Washington, DC, said that China would require that every food shipment be inspected for quality by the government by September 1, 2007.
- On August 20, 2007, the Chinese government announced that it had created a 19-member cabinet-level panel to oversee product quality and food safety (headed by Vice-Premier Wu Yi) and would start a four-month nationwide campaign to improve the quality of goods and food.
- On December 5, 2007, the government stated that during the first 10 months of the year, it had shut down 47,800 food factories without operating licenses.
- On January 15, 2008, China announced it had inspected over 3,000 export-oriented toy manufacturers and had revoked licenses for 600 firms that failed to meet quality standards.

Despite these efforts, reports of tainted products persist. For example, in January 2008, dozens of people in Japan reportedly became ill from eating dumplings imported from China that contained pesticide. In September 2008, the Chinese government reported that infant formula that was tainted with melamine had killed 4 children and sickened 53,000 others (13,000 of whom had to be hospitalized). The government announced on September 22, 2008, that China's chief quality supervisor had stepped down from his post over the incident. Other local and provincial officials have reportedly been sacked for trying to cover up incident. At least 22 Chinese baby formula companies have been found to have tainted products. Press reports indicate that other milk products made in China may have been contaminated as well. On October 15, 2008, the government ordered a blanket recall of all dairy products made before September 14, 2008. Several countries have banned the sale of Chinese-made milk products.

The United States and China reached a number of agreements in 2007 to address health and safety concerns:

- On September 11, 2007, the CPSC and its Chinese counterpart, the General Administration of Quality Supervision, Inspection, and Quarantine (AQSIQ), signed a joint statement on enhancing consumer product safety. China pledged to implement a comprehensive plan to intensify efforts (such as increased inspections, efforts to educate Chinese manufacturers, bilateral technical personal exchanges and training, regular meetings to exchange information with U.S. officials, and the development of a product tracking system) to prevent exports of unsafe products to the United States, especially in regard to lead paint and toys.

- On September 12, 2007, the NHTSA signed a memorandum of cooperation with its Chinese counterpart on enhanced cooperation and communication on vehicles and automotive equipment safety.
- On December 11, 2007, the U.S. HHS announced that it had signed two MOAs with its Chinese counterparts; the first covering specific food and feed items that have been of concern to the United States, and the second covering drugs and medical devices. Both MOAs would require Chinese firms that export such products to the United States to register with the Chinese government and to obtain certification before they can export. Such firms would also be subject to annual inspections to ensure they meet U.S. standards. The MOAs also establish mechanisms for greater information sharing, increase access of production facilities by U.S. officials, and create a working group in order to boost cooperation. On March 13, 2008, the FDA announced that it planned to place eight FDA staffers in China. Some members of Congress have proposed placing a CPSC official at the U.S. embassy in Beijing.

Economic Implications

Many members of Congress have called for tighter rules (such as increased inspections, certification requirements, and mandatory standards for toys) and increased funding for U.S. product safety agencies. On December 19, 2007, the House passed H.R. 4040 (Rush): *The Consumer Product Safety Modernization Act*. On March 6, 2008, the Senate passed its version of H.R. 4040 as a substitute amendment (S. 2263: *The CPSC Reform Act*). House and Senate Conferees reached a compromise agreement on H.R. 4040 on July 28, 2008, and the bill was signed into law (P.L. 110-314) on August 14.

Concerns over the health, safety, and quality of Chinese products could have a number of important economic implications. Both the United States and China have accused each other of using health and safety concerns as an excuse to impose protectionist measures and some observers contend that this issue could lead to growing trade friction between the two sides. International concerns over the safety of Chinese exports may diminish the attractiveness of China as a destination for foreign investment in export-oriented manufacturing, as well as for foreign firms that contract with Chinese firms to make and export products under their labels (such as toys). Efforts by China to restore international confidence in the health and safety of its exports through increased inspections, certification requirements, mandatory testing, etc., could have a significant impact on the cost of doing business in China, which could slow the pace of Chinese exports and hurt employment in the export sector. Moreover, international concerns over the safety of Chinese products could prove to be a setback to the government's efforts to develop and promote internationally recognized Chinese brands (such as cars), which it views as important to the country's future economic development. Thus, it is very likely the Chinese government will take this issue very seriously. However, it is unclear how long it will take for the central government to effectively address the numerous challenges it faces (especially government corruption and counterfeiting) to ensure that its exports comply with the health and safety standards of the United States and other trading partners. Additionally, a sharp decrease in purchases by U.S. consumers of Chinese products could negatively impact U.S. firms that import and/or sell such products and may raise prices of some commodities as firms attempt to rectify various safety problems.

The current crisis in China over melamine-tainted milk (which can cause kidney stones) and the growing number of children who have reportedly have become ill have seriously challenged the government's assertions that most products made in China are safe and that an effective regulatory regime has been established.

Section 48.3

Melamine

"Frequently Asked Questions and Answers on Melamine and Melamine Contamination," Food and Drug Administration (www.fda.gov), 2009.

What is melamine?

Melamine is a small, nitrogen-containing molecule that has a number of industrial uses, including as a binding agent, flame retardant, and as part of a polymer in the manufacture of cooking utensils and plates, plastic resins, and components of paper, paperboard, and industrial coatings. Melamine is not approved for direct addition to human or animal foods marketed in the United States.

Melamine also has been used as a fertilizer in some parts of the world. It is not registered for use as a fertilizer in the United States.

Melamine-related compounds are in the same family of chemicals as melamine, and include cyanuric acid, ammeline, and ammelide. (Melamine-related compounds are also known as melamine analogues.) Melamine and its related compounds have no approved use as direct ingredients in human or animal food in the United States.

What is the risk of giving your child infant formula from China?

The Chinese government has found some infant formula, milk, and products made with milk-derived ingredients from China to be contaminated with melamine and melamine-related compounds. Melamine is a chemical that if ingested in sufficient amounts can result in kidney failure and death. Tragically, reports indicate that over 52,000 children in China have become ill, more than 12,000 have been hospitalized, and several have died as a result of consuming Chinese infant formula made with contaminated milk. Many of the infants who became ill are suffering from kidney stones, a condition that is rare in infants.

Have any illnesses linked to melamine in Chinese food products been reported in the United States?

No. FDA is not aware of any such illnesses in the United States.

Is there any Chinese-made infant formula offered for sale in the United States?

No Chinese manufacturers of infant formula have fulfilled the requirements to sell infant formula in the United States. To help verify that no Chinese-made infant formula is for sale in the U.S., FDA—in conjunction with state and local officials—began a nationwide effort to check Asian markets for Chinese-manufactured infant formula. In particular, this effort has focused on areas of the country with large Chinese communities, such as Los Angeles, San Francisco, Seattle, and New York. To date, federal, state, and local investigators have visited more than 1,800 retail markets and have not found Chinese-manufactured infant formula present on shelves in these markets.

What should I do if I have fed my child infant formula made in China?

Individuals who have fed their infants formula made in China should contact their health care professional if they have questions regarding their infant's health or note any changes in their infant's health status. FDA recommends that you replace any such product with an appropriate infant formula manufactured in the United States.

Do companies that manufacture infant formula for the United States market use any milk-derived ingredients from China in their formula?

FDA has contacted the companies that manufacture infant formula for distribution in the United States. The companies informed FDA that they do not import formula or milk-derived ingredients from China.

Are any bulk shipments of potentially contaminated milk-derived ingredients from China entering the United States?

Milk-derived ingredients include whole milk powder, nonfat milk powder, whey powder, lactose powder, and casein. The FDA is sampling and testing these products when offered for import from Chinese sources to determine if they contain melamine.

What are the adverse effects from consuming a food that contains melamine?

FDA's "Safety and Risk Assessment of Melamine and Melamine-Related Compounds" provides information about the levels of these contaminants that do not raise public health concerns. When products with melamine contamination above these levels are consumed, individuals are at risk of conditions such as kidney stones, kidney failure, and death.

What is FDA's "Safety and Risk Assessment of Melamine and Melamine-Related Compounds" in human foods and what did it conclude?

A safety/risk assessment is the product of a scientifically based methodology used to estimate the risk to human health from exposure to specified compounds. It is based on available data and certain scientific assumptions in the absence of data. The purpose of the FDA's "Interim Safety and Risk Assessment of Melamine and its Analogues in Food for Humans" was to identify the level of melamine and melamine-related compounds in food which would not raise public health concerns. The interim safety/risk assessment evaluated the melamine exposure in infant formula and in other foods.

The safety/risk assessment, prompted by reports of melamine contamination of milk-derived ingredients and finished food products containing milk manufactured in China, was conducted by scientists from FDA's Center for Food Safety and Applied Nutrition and the Center for Veterinary Medicine. The FDA reviewed scientific literature on melamine toxicity.

Infant Formula: FDA is currently unable to establish any level of melamine and melamine-related compounds in infant formula that does not raise public health concerns. In large part, this is because of gaps in our scientific knowledge about the toxicity of melamine and its analogues in infants, including the following:

- The consequences of the continuous use of infant formulas as the sole source of nutrition for infants
- The uncertainties associated with the possible presence and co-ingestion of more than one melamine analogue
- For premature infants with immature kidney function, the possibility that parents might feed them these formulas as the sole

source of nutrition and, thus, these infants could, on a body weight basis, experience greater levels of intake for a longer time than full-term infants

There is too much uncertainty to set a level in infant formula and rule out any health concern. However, it is important to understand this does not mean that any exposure to any detectable level of melamine and melamine-related compounds in formula will result in harm to infants.

Other Food Products: In food products other than infant formula, the FDA concludes levels of melamine and melamine-related compounds below 2.5 parts per million (ppm) do not raise health concerns. This conclusion assumes a worst-case exposure scenario in which 50% of a person's diet is contaminated at this level, and applies a tenfold safety factor to the tolerable daily intake (TDI) to account for any uncertainties. The TDI is an estimate of the maximum amount of an agent to which an individual could be exposed on a daily basis over the course of a lifetime without an appreciable health risk.

Will FDA's "Safety and Risk Assessment of Melamine and Melamine-Related Compounds" in human foods be subject to peer review?

Through an independent contractor, FDA is identifying a group of experts who will be charged with peer reviewing the risk assessment. This group will also be asked to contribute to future scientific analysis related to the risk of melamine and melamine-related compounds to humans and animals.

What if high levels of melamine are detected in products?

FDA is testing bulk shipments of milk and milk-derived ingredients from China, finished food products from China made with milk or milk-derived ingredients, and finished food products from other countries that may contain milk or milk-derived ingredients from China. If products contain melamine and/or a melamine-related compound, the agency will take appropriate action.

What are the symptoms and signs of melamine poisoning?

Irritability, blood in urine, little or no urine, signs of kidney infection, and high blood pressure can all be signs of melamine poisoning.

Is it just products made with milk or milk-derived ingredients from China that are being reported contaminated?

Reports from China and other countries, as well as U.S. testing, suggest that the melamine contamination is limited to products containing milk or milk-derived ingredients from China.

Are products being recalled in the United States because of melamine contamination?

Yes. Companies have recalled products and the FDA is advising consumers not to consume certain products because of melamine contamination. For a complete list of those products, please visit FDA's website at www.fda.gov/oc/opacom/hottopics/melamine.html. The FDA has also issued a product-specific import alert, which prevents certain products from entering U.S. commerce because of melamine contamination, at www.fda.gov/ora/fiars/ora_import_ia9931.html.

Chapter 49

Fragrance Additives

Indoor air quality in health care settings is under scrutiny by numerous environmental health and nursing organizations because patients, nurses, and others have experienced health problems in those settings. Health Care Without Harm, Environmental Working Group, American Nurses Association, Maryland State Nurses Association, University of Maryland School of Nursing, and Massachusetts Nurses Association are leaders in the movement to improve healthcare environments. Research has documented a direct connection between impaired health status and some chemical exposures. Harmful chemicals in the healthcare workplace include PVCs [polyvinyl chloride], disinfectants such as ethylene oxide and glutaraldehyde, DEHP [Di(2-ethylhexyl)phthalate]-containing products, natural rubber latex, mercury, and pesticides, to name just a few.

Some individuals and groups of individuals are especially affected by fragrance exposure. Infants and children with immature immune systems and elders with weakened immune systems are particularly susceptible to harmful chemicals. In addition, people with asthma, allergies, migraines, compromised immune systems, and those who have been chemically injured are particularly vulnerable. Some patients are expressing frustration because their right to access health

---

This chapter excerpted from "Campaign for Fragrance-Free Health Care in the U.S.," by Peggy Wolff, MS, APRN, HNC, *The Maryland Nurse*, February-March-April 2006. © 2006 Maryland Nurses Association. Reprinted by permission via Copyright Clearance Center.

care is affected by toxic chemicals in health care environments. *Sometimes they even have to choose between not getting health care and being exposed to harmful chemicals.* Individuals of reproductive age are at heightened risk of chemical body burden that can be transmitted to the unborn, while new mothers are torn between the positive and negative effects of breastfeeding their infants because hazardous chemicals are consistently being detected in the breast milk of a majority of women.

Nurses may be at even greater risk than patients because they experience cumulative exposure. For an increasing number of nurses, fragrance use in their workplace is a barrier to employment. The Job Accommodation Network [JAN], a group concerned with employment rights for people with disabilities, has reported a sharp increase in the number of complaints related to fragrance and work. Between 1992–1995 JAN handled 37 cases related to fragrance while between 1995–2000, 567 cases were handled. Lessenger reported a case of a medical assistant developing acute anaphylactic reaction after being sprayed by perfume and cautions health care providers that this type of assault is becoming more common.

This section focuses on the harmful chemicals in synthetic fragrance, another important and prevalent cause of poor indoor air quality in health care settings. The following questions will be answered: What are the health effects of fragrance exposure? What are some of the harmful chemicals commonly found in fragrance?

Health Effects of Synthetic Fragrance

At present one in five people in the U.S. experience adverse health effects from fragrance exposure. These effects range from mild to serious with fatalities reported in a very small number of cases. Each and every system of the body may be adversely affected. An example related to the respiratory system occurs when a person has a flare up in their asthma or even has an asthma attack when exposed to fragrance. In one study 72% of asthmatics had negative reactions to perfumes. Few nurses are aware that fragrance can cause respiratory problems. Respiratory problems can occur because fragrance is a known respiratory irritant. High levels of respiratory irritants can cause asthma or asthma-like conditions according to Betty Bridges, R.N., owner of an informative website on fragrance and health. In one tragic situation, a nurse practitioner died due to complications from an allergic reaction to perfume in 2002 at Inova Fairfax Hospital. Many symptoms such as irritability, impaired concentration, headaches, ataxia, and dizziness may develop when the central nervous system is involved. The most common site for allergic reactions to fragrance is the skin, with between 5 and 20% of the population experiencing such effects. Dermatitis, itchy or burning skin, may occur. Cosmetics and fragranced products can also pose high risks for breast cancer and other illnesses. See Table 49.1 for the Environmental Protection Agency's list of adverse health effects associated with fragrance chemicals.

Table 49.1. Common Health Effects from Exposure to Synthetic Fragrance

According to the Environmental Protection Agency, the following health problems have been associated with fragrance exposure:

asthma,
reactive airway disease (RADS),
difficulty breathing,
coughing,
fatigue,
eye irritation,
sinusitis,
rhinitis,
inflammation of mucous membranes,
skin problems including dermatitis,
immune system damage,
nausea,
vomiting,
abdominal pain,
changes in blood pressure,
cancer,

and even death in severe cases due to respiratory failure.

Effects on the brain and nervous system include:

convulsions,
headaches/migraines,
depression,
dizziness,
irritability,
confusion,
panic attacks,
anxiety,
memory loss,
impaired concentration,
drowsiness,
insomnia,
impaired vision,
ataxia,
stupor,
spaciness,
giddiness,
slurred speech,
twitching muscles,
tingling in the limbs,

and loss of muscular coordination.

1991 EPA [Environmental Protection Agency] study by Larry Wallace. "Identification of Polar Volatile Organic Compounds in Consumer Products and Common Microenvironments."

Harmful Chemicals in Synthetic Fragrance and Their Health Effects

What is in fragrance that could lead to this myriad of symptoms/ health problems? For the past 50 years, 80–90% of fragrances have been synthesized from petroleum, not from natural sources, as advertisers might like us to believe. A few of the commonly found harmful chemicals in fragranced products are acetone, benzene, phenol, toluene, benzyl acetate, and limonene. See Table 49.2 for some of the health effects associated with each of these chemicals. Only a small sampling of chemicals and some of their health effects are provided because of space constraints.

Harmful health effects of fragrance are caused not only by the chemicals mentioned previously and a few thousand other individual chemicals, but each fragrance may well contain hundreds of different chemicals in combination. Only a small minority of individual chemicals have been tested for respiratory and neurotoxic effects and rarely have chemical combinations been tested for their health effects. Since fragrance ingredients are protected under trade secret laws, the consumer is kept in the dark about many of the harmful chemicals that make up fragrance.

Table 49.2. Fragrance Chemicals and Their Related Health Problems

Acetone—dryness of the mouth and throat; dizziness, nausea, lack of coordination, slurred speech, drowsiness, and in severe cases coma; it acts primarily as a CNS [central nervous system] depressant

Benzene—irritation of the eyes and respiratory system; decrease in white blood cells; headaches, impaired judgment, and menstrual disorders

Phenol—eye, nose, and throat irritation, abdominal pain; cardiac arrhythmias and failure, cardiovascular collapse, chromosomal aberrations and damage; cold sweats, collapse, confusion, headaches, hemolytic anemia, profuse sweating, and ringing in the ear

Toluene—skin, eye, and respiratory irritant; CNS depressant; liver and kidney disorders; and toxic brain dysfunction

Benzyl acetate—skin, eye, respiratory, and gastrointestinal irritant; vomiting, diarrhea, tissue damage, and abnormal EEGs [electroencephalographies]

Limonene—skin and eye irritant and sensitizer; stomach irritant, albumin and blood in urine; and many CNS effects

Irritants in fragrance can initiate a *sensitizing process* as the immune system "learns" to recognize materials that will later prompt a reaction when re-exposure occurs. Breakdown products of limonene, a-pinene, and benzaldehyde are known sensitizers commonly found in fragrance. Phthalates and synthetic musk compounds are two groups of chemicals frequently found in fragrance products that are known to cause serious and long-term health effects. Phthalates have been shown to cause endocrine disruption and are frequently found in fragrance products. Synthetic musk compounds used in fragrance can accumulate in fat tissue and be found in breast milk. These same compounds have also been shown to contribute to water contamination, harming aquatic and other wildlife.

Where Is Fragrance Found?

Fragrance is ubiquitous in our society. In addition to being in obvious products like perfume and cologne, fragrance is in most personal care, laundry, and cleaning products unless labeled "fragrance free." Fragrance may also be in bath tissue, candles, markers, and numerous other widely used products. Air "fresheners" usually contain synthetic fragrance; rather than freshening the air, they significantly compromise air quality.

Chapter 50

Beauty Products

Section 50.1

Cosmetics

This section excerpted from "Unmasked: 10 Ugly Truths behind the Myth of Cosmetic Safety," http://safecosmetics.org/downloads/Unmaskedbrochure_2007.pdf.

1. Toxic chemicals are in our beauty products—and in our bodies.

Every day we use multiple personal care products—from shampoo to deodorant, lotion to makeup—that contain chemical ingredients that are absorbed through the skin, inhaled, or ingested. So it's not surprising that potentially harmful chemicals have gotten into our bodies, our breast milk, and our children. Some of these chemicals are linked to cancer, birth defects, learning disabilities, and other health problems that are epidemic in our society. Astonishingly, in the United States, one in two men and one in three women are expected to develop cancer during their lifetimes, according to the National Cancer Institute.

2. Small exposures can add up to harm.

The cosmetics industry says it's safe to put toxic chemicals linked to cancer, infertility, or other health problems into personal care products because the amount in each product is too small to matter. But none of us use just one product. Think about how many products you use in a single day—from toothpaste to soap, shampoo, hair conditioner, deodorant, body lotion, shaving products, and makeup—and how many products you use in a year, and over a lifetime. Small amounts of toxic chemicals add up and can accumulate in our bodies. Chemicals linked to cancer and birth defects do not belong in personal care products, period.

Ingredients Banned from Cosmetics

- United States: 10
- European Union: 1,100+

3. The government should be protecting us, but it's not.

Major loopholes in federal law prevent the U.S. Food and Drug Administration (FDA) or any other government agency from approving the safety of cosmetics and body care products before they can be sold. The European Union now bans more than 1,100 chemicals from personal care products because they may cause cancer, birth defects, or reproductive problems. In stark contrast, just 10 ingredients are banned from cosmetics in the United States.

One-third of personal care products contain at least one chemical linked to cancer, according to the Skin Deep report by the Environmental Working Group, a partner in the Campaign for Safe Cosmetics.

4. You can't believe industry safety claims.

Manufacturers say their products are safe. But what do those claims really mean? It may mean that the company has tested the ingredients it uses—but only to determine if the chemicals cause rashes, swelling, or other acute reactions. Companies are not required to test the ingredients in their products to determine if they cause long-term, negative health effects, such as cancer or the inability to have a healthy child. Since there is no government standard for safety, companies can say whatever they want about the safety of their products.

- Ingredients in personal care products in the U.S.: 10,500
- Portion of chemical ingredients in cosmetics that have been assessed for health and safety by the industry's self-policing safety panel: 11%

5. The $50 billion U.S. cosmetics industry routinely opposes laws that would protect consumers and the environment.

The Cosmetics, Toiletry, and Fragrance Association (CTFA) has lobbied against laws that would control pollution at cosmetics manufacturing plants, require recycled content in packaging, or add more consumer safety information on labels. The industry says it doesn't need laws because it can voluntarily regulate itself. An industry-funded panel called the Cosmetics Ingredient Review panel—not the FDA or any other government agency—is currently in charge of reviewing the safety of cosmetics.

6. We have to protect ourselves until we convince the government to protect us.

According to Skin Deep, the highest-concern product categories are:

- hair color and bleach;
- hair relaxer;
- nail polish;
- skin lightener;
- nail treatment.

But even in these highest-concern categories, some brands are safer than others. Consumers can research these products to find the safest alternatives by clicking on the Skin Deep link at www.safecosmetics.org.

7. Two of the highest-concern cosmetics are marketed to African American women.

Products promising lighter skin and straighter hair are problematic because of their message about what is considered beautiful. But the Skin Deep report shows that some hair relaxers and skin lighteners share a second problem: they contain ingredients such as hydroquinone, placenta, and petroleum by-products that are linked to cancer, reproductive and hormonal problems, and some of them sensitize the skin, which means that dangerous ingredients are more likely to penetrate into the body.

8. Even ingredients that are known to cause harm can be put into personal care products.

Few ingredients have been assessed for long-term health impacts, but those that have—and are known or suspected to be toxic—are still allowed in cosmetics. Seven of the most problematic are:

Mercury: Often listed as thimerosal on ingredient labels, mercury is a possible human carcinogen, and a human reproductive or developmental toxin. Found in some eye drops, ointments, and mascaras.

Placenta: Placenta produces progesterone, estrogen, and other hormones that can interfere with the body's normal hormone functions and can lead to serious health problems—like breast cancer—when used in cosmetics. Sometimes used in hair relaxers, moisturizers, and toners.

Lead Acetate: This compound of lead is a known human reproductive and developmental toxin. Prohibited from use in cosmetics in the European Union. Found in some hair dyes and cleansers.

Petrochemicals: These by-products of crude oil (appearing on labels as petrolatum, mineral oil, and paraffin) may contain known or suspected human carcinogens as well as harmful breakdown products or impurities from manufacturing processes (such as 1,4-dioxane), which are not listed on ingredient labels. Found in some hair relaxers, shampoos, anti-aging creams, mascaras, perfumes, foundations, lipsticks, and lip balms.

Phthalates: These plasticizing chemicals are probable human reproductive or developmental toxins and endocrine disruptors. Two phthalates often used in cosmetics (dibutyl and diethylhexyl) have been banned in the European Union. Found in some nail polishes, fragrances, and hair sprays.

Hydroquinone: A possible carcinogen and probable neurotoxin and skin sensitizer, hydroquinone can also cause a skin disease called ochronosis, which leaves irreversible black-blue lesions on skin. Found in some skin lightening products and moisturizers.

Nanoparticles: Extremely tiny particles which are largely untested and unlabeled in personal care products, capable of being absorbed directly into the bloodstream. Found in some eye shadows, bronzers, sunscreens, and lotions.

9. Men are not immune to these problems.

Two products marketed to men to color gray hair (EBL GreyBan and Grecian Formula 16) contain lead acetate, which can harm fertility and impact the development of a child before birth. Clairol Herbal Essences True Intense Hair Color for Men is among the highest concern hair color products in Skin Deep. Some aftershave lotions, antidandruff shampoos, tooth whiteners, sunless tanning products, men's hair-removal products, and colognes are also in the highest-concern category. Skin Deep lists many safer alternatives in each category.

10. The word "natural" on a product label doesn't mean it's safe—or natural.

Neutrogena After Sun Treatment with Natural Soy has one of the highest hazard ratings of the lotions in Skin Deep. What's so "natural" about a product with more than 10 different ingredients that raise health concerns? Neutrogena is owned by Johnson & Johnson, which markets its products as superior because of their "natural" properties and recommendations from health care providers. Another example: Barielle 10 Piece Natural Nail Care System contains several ingredients of high concern including dibutyl phthalate, fragrance, and urea, despite the word "natural" in the product name.

Here's What You Can Do

1. Sign up for the latest news about cosmetics and your health.

The Campaign for Safe Cosmetics sends e-mail news and action alerts once or twice a month. We'll tell you what's happening right now with cosmetic safety and how you can make a difference. Sign up at www.safecosmetics.org/join.

2. Choose safer products.

Visit Skin Deep, the world's largest searchable database of ingredients in cosmetics, by clicking on the link at www.safecosmetics.org. Find out if your favorite products contain hazardous chemicals and find safer alternatives. Then use this section on your next shopping trip to help you make sense of ingredient labels and avoid the most toxic products.

3. Tell your cosmetics companies you want safe products.

Call, write, or e-mail the companies that make your favorite products to let them know you want safe products now! Look on product packaging for a customer service hotline or website. Meanwhile, patronize the companies that have signed the Compact for Safe Cosmetics. The complete list of Compact signers is available at www.safecosmetics.org.

4. Spread the word.

Tell your friends, co-workers, and family about toxic chemicals in cosmetics and tell them how they can learn more and take action. You can even host your own Healthy Cosmetics House Party. Download useful materials, including our Campaign in a Box, from www.safecosmetics.org or contact us for assistance.

Editor's Note: The information in this section represents the opinion of the copyright holder and is presented as one viewpoint on a complex subject.

Section 50.2

Sunscreen

"CDC: Americans Carry Body Burden of Toxic Sunscreen Chemical,"

A new study by the U.S. Centers for Disease Control (CDC) reveals that 97% of Americans are contaminated with a widely used sunscreen ingredient called oxybenzone that has been linked to allergies, hormone disruption, and cell damage. A companion study published just one day earlier revealed that this chemical is linked to low birth weight in baby girls whose mothers are exposed during pregnancy. Oxybenzone is also a penetration enhancer, a chemical that helps other chemicals penetrate the skin.

Although oxybenzone is most common in sunscreen, companies also use the chemical in at least 567 other personal care products.

Environmental Working Group [EWG] identified nearly 600 sunscreens sold in the U.S. that contain oxybenzone, including products by Hawaiian Tropic, Coppertone, and Banana Boat (see the full list of 588 sunscreens at skindeep.ewg.org/browse.php?category=sunscreen&ingred06=704372) as well as 172 facial moisturizers, 111 lip balms, and 81 different types of lipstick.

The Food and Drug Administration [FDA] has failed miserably in its duty to protect the public from toxic chemicals like oxybenzone in personal care products. At the request of industry lobbyists, including Supreme Court Chief Justice John Roberts, who represented the Cosmetic Toiletry and Fragrance Association, the agency has delayed final sunscreen safety standards for nearly 30 years. FDA issued a new draft of the standards last October under pressure from EWG, but continues to delay finalizing them at the behest of the regulated industry.

EWG research shows that 84% of 910 name-brand sunscreen products offer inadequate protection from the sun, or contain ingredients, like oxybenzone, with significant safety concerns.

The last safety review for oxybenzone was done in the 1970s, and does not reflect a wealth of information developed since that time indicating increased toxicity concerns and widespread human exposure. A recent review in the European Union found that sufficient data were not available to assess if oxybenzone in sunscreen was safe for consumers.

Environmental Working Group again calls on FDA to review the safety of oxybenzone, given this new data on widespread contamination of the U.S. population, and to finalize its sunscreen safety standards so that consumers can be certain that sunscreen products they purchase are safe and effective.

CDC Study of Oxybenzone Signals Concern

Top scientists from CDC published results March 21, 2008, from a national survey of 2,500 Americans, age six and up, showing that oxybenzone readily absorbs into the body and is present in 97% of Americans tested. Oxybenzone, also known as benzophenone-3, was detected in the urine of nearly every study participant. Typically, women and girls had higher levels of oxybenzone in their bodies than men and boys, likely a result of differences in use of body care products including sunscreens.

A companion study released a day earlier revealed that mothers with high levels of oxybenzone in their bodies were more likely to give birth to underweight baby girls. Low birth weight is a critical risk factor linked to coronary heart disease, hypertension, type 2 diabetes, and other diseases in adulthood.

Oxybenzone Damages and Penetrates the Skin

Among common sunscreen chemicals, oxybenzone is most likely to be associated with allergic reactions triggered by sun exposure. In a study of 82 patients with photoallergic contact dermatitis, over one quarter showed photoallergic reactions to oxybenzone; another study reported one in five allergic reactions to photopatch tests resulted from exposure to oxybenzone.

Sunlight also causes oxybenzone to form free radical chemicals that may be linked to cell damage, according to two of three studies.

A less visible but more alarming concern, this chemical absorbs through the skin in significant amounts, as indicated by the CDC study. A previous biomonitoring study reported that 96% of six-to-eight-year-old girls had detectable amounts of oxybenzone in their urine. An earlier study detected oxybenzone in the urine of all 30 adult participants.

Studies on human volunteers indicate a wide variation in the level of oxybenzone absorbed into the body, with some individuals absorbing at least 9% of the applied dose, as measured in excretions in urine. Volunteers continued to excrete oxybenzone many days after the last application of the chemical, an indication of its tendency to accumulate in fatty tissues in the body.

In addition to its ability to absorb into the body, oxybenzone is also a penetration enhancer, a chemical that helps other chemicals penetrate the skin.

Oxybenzone May Disrupt the Human Hormone System

Studies on cells and laboratory animals indicate that oxybenzone and its metabolites, the chemicals the body makes from oxybenzone in an attempt to detoxify and excrete it, may disrupt the hormone system. Under study conditions, oxybenzone and its metabolites cause weak estrogenic and anti-androgenic effects. Oxybenzone displays additive hormonal effects when tested with other sunscreen chemicals. Laboratory study also suggests that oxybenzone may affect the adrenal hormone system.

One human study coapplying three sunscreen active ingredients (oxybenzone, 4-MBC, and octinoxate) suggested a minor, intermittent, but statistically significant drop in testosterone levels in men during a one-week application period. Researchers also detected statistically significant declines in estradiol levels in men; other hormonal differences detected could not be linked to sunscreen use due to differences in baseline hormone levels before and during treatment.

Outdated Health Protections Do Not Take into Account These and Other Adverse Effects

A 2006 European Union review concluded that a rigorous exposure assessment of oxybenzone was impossible, due to lack of information about the levels of absorption into the body. The levels of contamination reported in this latest CDC study indicate that absorption may be significant, consistent with previous, small-scale biomonitoring reports. A decades-old evaluation by FDA, as well as more recent review by the cosmetics industry's own safety panel, do not consider concerns regarding hormone disruption, nor the implications of the ability of oxybenzone to penetrate the skin. At present, no health-based standards exist for safe levels of oxybenzone in the body.

Additional cautions must be employed when considering the effects of oxybenzone on children. The surface area of a child's skin relative to body weight is greater than adults. As a result, the potential dose of a chemical following dermal exposure is likely to be about 1.4 times greater in children than in adults. In addition, children are less able than adults to detoxify and excrete chemicals, and children's developing organ systems are more vulnerable to damage from chemical exposures, and more sensitive to low levels of hormonally active compounds. Children also have more years of future life in which to develop disease triggered by early exposure to chemicals. Despite these well-documented concerns regarding children's sensitivity to harmful substances, no special protections exist regarding ingredients in personal care products marketed for babies and children.

The fraction of oxybenzone that is not absorbed into the human body often contaminates water, washed from the skin during swimming and water play or while bathing. Wastewater treatment removes only a fraction of this sunscreen chemical, resulting in detection of oxybenzone in treated wastewater, in lake and sea waters due to recreational use or to discharges from water treatment facilities, and even in fish. Studies show oxybenzone can trigger outbreaks of viral infection in coral reefs and can cause feminization of male fish. Despite significant ecological concerns, there are no measures in place to protect sensitive ecosystems from damage caused by this contaminant.

EWG to FDA: Oxybenzone Investigation Is Long Overdue

FDA last reviewed the safety of oxybenzone in the 1970s, republishing its evaluation in 1978, at the same time it announced plans to develop comprehensive standards for sunscreen safety and effectiveness. Thirty years later, the agency has yet to issue final regulations. Instead, it encourages manufacturers to follow draft guidelines that the agency has delayed finalizing at the behest of the sunscreen industry. As a result, sunscreen manufacturers in the U.S. are free to market products containing ingredients like oxybenzone that have not been proven safe for people.

Found in over half of the 910 name-brand sunscreen products we reviewed, oxybenzone is tied to significant health concerns that must be scrutinized. Instead, FDA's refusal to re-examine this ingredient keeps sunscreens containing oxybenzone on the market. Petitions for review of newly developed sunscreen ingredients approved for use in other countries, and with far fewer health concerns, have been met with similar inattention, blocking Americans' access to better products.

FDA foot-dragging has left the U.S. without enforceable standards for sunscreen safety and effectiveness for decades. EWG demands that FDA finalize the latest version of its monograph on sunscreen products immediately, and launch an investigation into the safety of the sunscreen ingredient oxybenzone.

Editor's Note: The information in this section represents the opinion of the copyright holder and is presented as one viewpoint on a complex subject.

Chapter 51

X-Rays

X-rays refer to radiation, waves or particles that travel through the air like light or radio signals. X-ray energy is high enough that some radiation passes through objects (such as internal organs, body tissues, and clothing) and onto x-ray detectors (such as film or a detector linked to a computer monitor). In general, objects that are more dense (such as bones and calcium deposits) absorb more of the radiation from the x-rays and don't allow as much to pass through them. These objects leave a different image on the detector than less dense objects. Specially trained or experienced physicians can read these images to diagnose medical conditions or injuries.

Procedures

Medical x-rays are used in many types of examinations and procedures. Some examples include the following:

- X-ray radiography (to find orthopedic damage, tumors, pneumonias, foreign objects, etc.)
- Mammography (to image the internal structures of breasts)
- CT (computed tomography, to produce cross-sectional images of the body)

"Medical X-Rays," Food and Drug Administration (www.fda.gov), January 6, 2009.

- Fluoroscopy (to dynamically visualize the body for example to see where to remove plaque from coronary arteries or where to place stents to keep those arteries open)
- Radiation therapy in cancer treatment

Risks/Benefits

Medical x-rays have increased the ability to detect disease or injury early enough for a medical problem to be managed, treated, or cured. When applied and performed appropriately, these procedures can improve health and may even save a person's life.

X-ray energy also has a small potential to harm living tissue. The most significant risks are the following:

- A small increase in the possibility that a person exposed to x-rays will develop cancer later in life
- Cataracts and skin burns only at very high levels of radiation exposure and in only very few procedures

The risk of developing cancer from radiation exposure is generally small, and it depends on at least three factors—the amount of radiation dose, the age at exposure, and the sex of the person exposed:

- The lifetime risk of cancer increases the larger the dose and the more x-ray exams a patient undergoes.
- The lifetime risk of cancer is larger for a patient who received x-rays at a younger age than for one who receives them at an older age.
- Women are at a somewhat higher lifetime risk than men for developing radiation-associated cancer after receiving the same exposures at the same ages.

Information for Patients

You can reduce your radiation risks and contribute to your successful examination or procedure by following these practices:

- Keeping a "medical x-ray history" with the names of your radiological exams or procedures, the dates and places where you had them, and the physicians who referred you for those exams

- Making your current health care providers aware of your medical x-ray history
- Asking your health care provider about whether or not alternatives to x-ray exams would allow the provider to make a good assessment or provide appropriate treatment for your medical situation
- Providing interpreting physicians and referring physicians with recent x-ray images and radiology reports
- Informing radiologists or x-ray technologists in advance if you are pregnant or think you may be pregnant

Part Seven

Additional Help and Information

Chapter 52

Glossary of Terms Related to Environmental Health

absorption: The uptake of water, other fluids, or dissolved chemicals by a cell or an organism (as tree roots absorb dissolved nutrients in soil).

acid deposition: A complex chemical and atmospheric phenomenon that occurs when emissions of sulfur and nitrogen compounds and other substances are transformed by chemical processes in the atmosphere, often far from the original sources, and then deposited on earth in either wet or dry form. The wet forms, popularly called "acid rain," can fall to earth as rain, snow, or fog. The dry forms are acidic gases or particulates.

activated carbon: A highly adsorbent form of carbon used to remove odors and toxic substances from liquid or gaseous emissions. In waste treatment, it is used to remove dissolved organic matter from waste drinking water. It is also used in motor vehicle evaporative control systems.

acute exposure: A single exposure to a toxic substance that may result in severe biological harm or death. Acute exposures are usually characterized as lasting no longer than a day, as compared to longer, continuing exposure over a period of time.

This glossary contains terms from the U.S. Environmental Protection Agency (www.epa.gov/OCEPAterms/).

agricultural waste: Poultry and livestock manure, and residual materials in liquid or solid form generated from the production and marketing of poultry, livestock or fur-bearing animals; also includes grain, vegetable, and fruit harvest residue.

air pollutant: Any substance in air that could, in high enough concentration, harm man, other animals, vegetation, or material. Pollutants may include almost any natural or artificial composition of airborne matter capable of being airborne. They may be in the form of solid particles, liquid droplets, gases, or in combination thereof. Generally, they fall into two main groups: 1) those emitted directly from identifiable sources and 2) those produced in the air by interaction between two or more primary pollutants, or by reaction with normal atmospheric constituents, with or without photoactivation. Exclusive of pollen, fog, and dust, which are of natural origin, about 100 contaminants have been identified. Air pollutants are often grouped in categories for ease in classification; some of the categories are the following: solids, sulfur compounds, volatile organic chemicals, particulate matter, nitrogen compounds, oxygen compounds, halogen compounds, radioactive compound, and odors.

airborne particulates: Total suspended particulate matter found in the atmosphere as solid particles or liquid droplets. Chemical composition of particulates varies widely, depending on location and time of year. Sources of airborne particulates include the following: dust, emissions from industrial processes, combustion products from the burning of wood and coal, combustion products associated with motor vehicle or nonroad engine exhausts, and reactions to gases in the atmosphere.

algal blooms: Sudden spurts of algal growth, which can affect water quality adversely and indicate potentially hazardous changes in local water chemistry.

background level: 1) The concentration of a substance in an environmental media (air, water, or soil) that occurs naturally or is not the result of human activities. 2) In exposure assessment, the concentration of a substance in a defined control area during a fixed period of time before, during, or after a data-gathering operation.

bacteria: (singular: bacterium) Microscopic living organisms that can aid in pollution control by metabolizing organic matter in sewage, oil spills, or other pollutants. However, bacteria in soil, water, or air can also cause human, animal, and plant health problems.

bioconcentration: The accumulation of a chemical in tissues of a fish or other organism to levels greater than in the surrounding medium.

biological pesticides: Certain microorganism, including bacteria, fungi, viruses, and protozoa, that are effective in controlling pests. These agents usually do not have toxic effects on animals and people and do not leave toxic or persistent chemical residues in the environment.

body burden: The amount of a chemical stored in the body at a given time, especially a potential toxin in the body as the result of exposure.

chronic exposure: Multiple exposures occurring over an extended period of time or over a significant fraction of an animal's or human's lifetime (usually seven years to a lifetime).

concentration: The relative amount of a substance mixed with another substance. An example is five ppm [parts per million] of carbon monoxide in air or one mg [milligram] per liter of iron in water.

contamination: Introduction into water, air, and soil of microorganisms, chemicals, toxic substances, wastes, or wastewater in a concentration that makes the medium unfit for its next intended use. Also applies to surfaces of objects, buildings, and various household and agricultural use products.

disinfectant: A chemical or physical process that kills pathogenic organisms in water, air, or on surfaces. Chlorine is often used to disinfect sewage treatment effluent, water supplies, wells, and swimming pools.

disinfectant by-product: A compound formed by the reaction of a disinfectant such as chlorine with organic material in the water supply; a chemical by-product of the disinfection process.

disposal: Final placement or destruction of toxic, radioactive, or other wastes; surplus or banned pesticides or other chemicals; polluted soils; and drums containing hazardous materials from removal actions or accidental releases. Disposal may be accomplished through use of approved secure landfills, surface impoundments, land farming, deep-well injection, ocean dumping, or incineration.

dosage/dose: 1) The actual quantity of a chemical administered to an organism or to which it is exposed. 2) The amount of a substance that reaches a specific tissue (e.g., the liver). 3) The amount of a substance available for interaction with metabolic processes after crossing the outer boundary of an organism.

environmental equity/justice: Equal protection from environmental hazards for individuals, groups, or communities regardless of race, ethnicity, or economic status. This applies to the development, implementation, and enforcement of environmental laws, regulations, and policies, and implies that no population of people should be forced to shoulder a disproportionate share of negative environmental impacts of pollution or environmental hazard due to a lack of political or economic strength levels.

exposure assessment: Identifying the pathways by which toxicants may reach individuals, estimating how much of a chemical an individual is likely to be exposed to, and estimating the number likely to be exposed.

genetic engineering: A process of inserting new genetic information into existing cells in order to modify a specific organism for the purpose of changing one of its characteristics.

hazardous chemical: An EPA [Environmental Protection Agency] designation for any hazardous material requiring an MSDS [Material Safety Data Sheet] under OSHA's [Office of Safety and Health Administration] Hazard Communication Standard. Such substances are capable of producing fires and explosions or adverse health effects like cancer and dermatitis. Hazardous chemicals are distinct from hazardous waste.

heavy metals: Metallic elements with high atomic weights (e.g., mercury, chromium, cadmium, arsenic, and lead) can damage living things at low concentrations and tend to accumulate in the food chain.

industrial source reduction: Practices that reduce the amount of any hazardous substance, pollutant, or contaminant entering any waste stream or otherwise released into the environment. Also reduces the threat to public health and the environment associated with such releases. Term includes equipment or technology modifications, substitution of raw materials, and improvements in housekeeping, maintenance, training, or inventory control.

landfills: 1) Sanitary landfills are disposal sites for nonhazardous solid wastes spread in layers, compacted to the smallest practical volume, and covered by material applied at the end of each operating day. 2) Secure chemical landfills are disposal sites for hazardous waste, selected and designed to minimize the chance of release of hazardous substances into the environment.

lifetime exposure: Total amount of exposure to a substance that a human would receive in a lifetime (usually assumed to be 70 years).

lowest observed adverse effect level (LOAEL): The lowest level of a stressor that causes statistically and biologically significant differences in test samples as compared to other samples subjected to no stressor.

monitoring: Periodic or continuous surveillance or testing to determine the level of compliance with statutory requirements and/or pollutant levels in various media or in humans, plants, and animals.

mutagen/mutagenicity: An agent that causes a permanent genetic change in a cell other than that which occurs during normal growth. Mutagenicity is the capacity of a chemical or physical agent to cause such permanent changes.

nitrate: A compound containing nitrogen that can exist in the atmosphere or as a dissolved gas in water and that can have harmful effects on humans and animals. Nitrates in water can cause severe illness in infants and domestic animals. A plant nutrient and inorganic fertilizer, nitrate is found in septic systems, animal feed lots, agricultural fertilizers, manure, industrial waste waters, sanitary landfills, and garbage dumps.

organic chemicals/compounds: Naturally occurring (animal- or plant-produced or synthetic) substances containing mainly carbon, hydrogen, nitrogen, and oxygen.

ozone (O_3): Found in two layers of the atmosphere, the stratosphere and the troposphere. In the stratosphere (the atmospheric layer 7 to 10 miles or more above the earth's surface) ozone is a natural form of oxygen that provides a protective layer shielding the earth from ultraviolet radiation. In the troposphere (the layer extending up 7 to 10 miles from the earth's surface), ozone is a chemical oxidant and major component of photochemical smog. It can seriously impair the respiratory system and is one of the most widespread of all the criteria pollutants for which the Clean Air Act required EPA to set standards. Ozone in the troposphere is produced through complex chemical reactions of nitrogen oxides, which are among the primary pollutants emitted by combustion sources; hydrocarbons, released into the atmosphere through the combustion, handling, and processing of petroleum products; and sunlight.

particulates: 1) Fine liquid or solid particles such as dust, smoke, mist, fumes, or smog found in air or emissions. 2) Very small solids suspended in water; they can vary in size, shape, density, and electrical charge and can be gathered together by coagulation and flocculation.

pathogens: Microorganisms (e.g., bacteria, viruses, or parasites) that can cause disease in humans, animals, and plants.

persistence: Refers to the length of time a compound stays in the environment, once introduced. A compound may persist for less than a second or indefinitely.

pesticide: Substances or mixtures thereof intended for preventing, destroying, repelling, or mitigating any pest. Also, any substance or mixture intended for use as a plant regulator, defoliant, or desiccant.

pollution: Generally, the presence of a substance in the environment that because of its chemical composition or quantity prevents the functioning of natural processes and produces undesirable environmental and health effects. Under the Clean Water Act, for example, the term has been defined as the man-made or man-induced alteration of the physical, biological, chemical, and radiological integrity of water and other media.

residential waste: Waste generated in single and multifamily homes, including newspapers, clothing, disposable tableware, food packaging, cans, bottles, food scraps, and yard trimmings other than those that are diverted to backyard composting.

residual: Amount of a pollutant remaining in the environment after a natural or technological process has taken place; e.g., the sludge remaining after initial wastewater treatment, or particulates remaining in air after it passes through a scrubbing or other process.

sediments: Soil, sand, and minerals washed from land into water, usually after rain. They pile up in reservoirs, rivers, and harbors, destroying fish and wildlife habitat and clouding the water so that sunlight cannot reach aquatic plants. Careless farming, mining, and building activities will expose sediment materials, allowing them to wash off the land after rainfall.

sick building syndrome: Building whose occupants experience acute health and/or comfort effects that appear to be linked to time spent therein, but where no specific illness or cause can be identified. Complaints may be localized in a particular room or zone, or may spread throughout the building.

teratogen: A substance capable of causing birth defects.

tolerances: Permissible residue levels for pesticides in raw agricultural produce and processed foods. Whenever a pesticide is registered for use on a food or a feed crop, a tolerance (or exemption from the tolerance requirement) must be established. EPA establishes the tolerance levels, which are enforced by the Food and Drug Administration and the Department of Agriculture.

toxicity: The degree to which a substance or mixture of substances can harm humans or animals. *Acute toxicity* involves harmful effects in an organism through a single or short-term exposure. *Chronic toxicity* is the ability of a substance or mixture of substances to cause harmful effects over an extended period, usually upon repeated or continuous exposure sometimes lasting for the entire life of the exposed organism. *Subchronic toxicity* is the ability of the substance to cause effects for more than one year but less than the lifetime of the exposed organism.

treatment: 1) Any method, technique, or process designed to remove solids and/or pollutants from solid waste, waste-streams, effluents, and air emissions. 2) Methods used to change the biological character or composition of any regulated medical waste so as to substantially reduce or eliminate its potential for causing disease.

vapor: The gas given off by substances that are solids or liquids at ordinary atmospheric pressure and temperatures.

volatile organic compound (VOC): Any organic compound that participates in atmospheric photochemical reactions except those designated by EPA as having negligible photochemical reactivity.

wastewater: The spent or used water from a home, community, farm, or industry that contains dissolved or suspended matter.

Chapter 53

Directory of Environmental Health Organizations and Resources

Environmental Agencies and Organizations

Agency for Toxic Substances and Disease Registry (ATSDR)
Centers for Disease Control and Prevention
4770 Buford Highway NE
Atlanta, GA 30341
Toll-Free: 800-232-4636 (800-CDC-INFO)
TTY: 888-232-6348
E-mail: cdcinfo@cdc.gov
Website: http://www.atsdr.cdc.gov

This chapter contains resources compiled from many sources deemed reliable. Inclusion does not constitute endorsement and there is no implication associated with omission. All contact information was verified in July 2009.

AIRNow
Environmental Protection Agency Office of Air Quality Planning and Standards
Information Transfer Group
Mail Code E143-03
Research Triangle Park, NC 27711
Fax: 919-541-0242
E-mail: AIRNOWComments@epamail.epa.gov
Website: http://airnow.gov

American Council on Science and Health
1995 Broadway, 2nd Floor
New York, NY 10023-5860
Toll-Free: 866-905-2694
Phone: 212-362-7044
Fax: 212-362-4919
E-mail: acsh@acsh.org
Website: http://www.acsh.org

American Lung Association
National Headquarters
1301 Pennsylvania Avenue, NW
Suite 800
Washington, DC 20004
Toll-Free: 800-586-4872
(800-LUNGUSA)
Website: http://www.lungusa.org

Americans with Disabilities Act Hotline
United States Access Board
1331 F Street NW, Suite 1000
Washington, DC 20004-1111
Toll-Free: 800-872-2253
(800-USA-ABLE)
Phone: 202-272-5435
Toll-Free TTY: 800-993-2822
TTY: 202-272-0082
Fax: 202-272-0081
E-mail: info@access-board.gov
Website: http://
www.access-board.gov

Asthma and Allergy Foundation of America
1233 20th Street, NW, Suite 402
Washington, DC 20036
Phone: 800-727-8462
(800-7-ASTHMA)
E-mail: info@aafa.org
Website: http://aafa.org

Autism Society of America
7910 Woodmont Ave., Suite 300
Bethesda, MD 20814-3067
Toll-Free: 800-328-8476
(800-3-AUTISM)
Phone: 301-657-0881
Website: http://
www.autism-society.org

Beyond Pesticides
701 E Street, SE
Suite 200
Washington, DC 20003
Phone: 202-543-5450
Fax: 202-543-4791
E-mail:
info@beyondpesticides.org
Website: http://
www.beyondpesticides.org

Birth Defect Research for Children, Inc.
800 Celebration Avenue
Suite 225
Celebration, FL 34747
Phone: 407-566-8304
Fax: 407-566-8341
Website: http://
www.birthdefects.org

Center for Environmental Health
2201 Broadway
Suite 302
Oakland, CA 94612
Phone: 510-655-3900
Fax: 510-655-9100
Website: http://www.ceh.org

Center for Health, Environment, and Justice
P.O. Box 6806
Falls Church, VA 22040-6806
Phone: 703-237-2249
E-mail: chej@chej.org
Websites: http://www.chej.org,
http://besafenet.com

Center for Science in the Public Interest
1875 Connecticut Ave. NW
Suite 300
Washington, DC 20009
Phone: 202-332-9110
Fax: 202-265-4954
E-mail: cspi@cspinet.org
Website: http://cspinet.org

Chemical Injury Information Network
P.O. Box 301
White Sulphur Springs, MT 59645
Phone: 406-547-2255
Fax: 406-547-2455
Website: http://ciin.org

Children's Environmental Health Network
110 Maryland Avenue NE
Suite 505
Washington, DC 20002
Phone: 202-543-4033
Fax: 202-543-8797
E-mail: cehn@cehn.org
Website: http://cehn.org

The Collaborative on Health and the Environment
c/o Commonweal
P.O. Box 316
Bolinas, CA 94924
E-mail: info@healthandenvironment.org
Website: http://www.healthandenvironment.org

Environment & Human Health, Inc.
1191 Ridge Road
North Haven, CT 06473
Phone: 203-248-6582
Fax: 203-288-7571
E-mail: info@ehhi.org
Website: http://www.ehhi.org

Environmental Defense Fund
257 Park Ave. South
New York, NY 10010
Phone: 212-505-2100
Fax: 212-505-2375
E-mail: members@environmentaldefense.org
Website: http://www.environmentaldefense.org

Environmental Health Network (of California)
P.O. Box 1155
Larkspur, CA 94977-1155
Phone: 415-541-5075
Website: http://ehnca.org

Environmental Justice & Health Union
528 61st Street, Suite A
Oakland, CA 94609
E-mail: ejhu@ejhu.org
Website: http://www.ejhu.org

Environmental Protection Agency (EPA)
Ariel Rios Building
1200 Pennsylvania Avenue, NW
Washington, DC 20460
Phone: 202-272-0167
TTY: 202-272-0165
Website: http://www.epa.gov

EPA National Service Center for Environmental Publications
P.O. Box 42419
Cincinnati, OH 45242-0419
Toll-Free: 800-490-9198 (publications)
Fax: 301-604-3408
E-mail: nscep@bps-lmit.com (e-mail for publication requests)
Website: http://www.epa.gov/ncepihom

Environmental Working Group
1436 U Street NW, Suite 100
Washington, DC 20009
Phone: 202-667-6982
Website: http://www.ewg.org

Federal Emergency Management Agency (FEMA)
500 C Street SW
Washington, DC 20472
Phone: 202-646-2500
Website: http://www.fema.gov

Food and Drug Administration (FDA)
10903 New Hampshire Avenue
Silver Spring, MD 20993-0002
Phone: 888-463-6332 (888-INFO-FDA)
Website: http://www.fda.gov

Food and Water Watch
1616 P Street, NW, Suite 300
Washington, DC 20036
Phone: 202-683-2500
Fax: 202-683-2501
Website: http://foodandwaterwatch.org

Food Safety and Inspection Service
U.S. Department of Agriculture
1400 Independence Avenue SW
Washington, DC 20250-3700
Website: http://www.fsis.usda.gov

Food Safety Research Information Office (FSRIO)
U.S. Department of Agriculture
National Agricultural Library
Room 304B
10301 Baltimore Avenue
Beltsville, MD 20705
Phone: 301-504-5515
Fax: 301-504-7680
Website: http://fsrio.nal.usda.gov

Friends of the Earth
1717 Massachusetts Ave.
Suite 600
Washington, DC 20036
Phone: 202-783-7400
Fax: 202-783-0444
Website: http://foe.org

Greenpeace, USA
702 H Street NW, Suite 300
Washington, DC 20001
Toll-Free: 800-326-0959
Phone: 202-462-1177
E-mail: info@wdc.greenpeace.org
Website: http://www.greenpeaceusa.org

Healthy Child Healthy World
12300 Wilshire Blvd., Suite 320
Los Angeles, CA 90025
Phone: 310-820-2030
Fax: 310-820-2070
Website: http://healthychild.org

Inform, Inc.
318 West 39th Street, 5th Floor
New York, NY 10018
Phone: 212-361-2400
Website: http://informinc.org

Institute for Children's Environmental Health
P.O. Box 991
Freeland, WA 98249
Phone: 360-331-7904
Fax: 360-331-7908
Websites: http://www.iceh.org, www.partnersforchildren.org

Kidshealth.org
Nemours Foundation
Website: http://www.kidshealth.org

March of Dimes
1275 Mamaroneck Avenue
White Plains, NY 10605
Phone: 914-997-4488 (National Office)
Website: http://www.marchofdimes.com

National Cancer Institute (NCI)
NCI Public Inquiries Office
6116 Executive Boulevard, Room 3036A
Bethesda, MD 20892-8322
Toll-Free: 800-422-6237 (800-4-CANCER), Mon. through Fri. 9:00 a.m. to 4:30 p.m., EST
Live chat: http://cissecure.nci.nih.gov/livehelp/welcome.asp
Website: http://www.cancer.gov

National Center for Environmental Health (NCEH)
Centers for Disease Control and Prevention
1600 Clifton Rd.
Atlanta, GA 30333
Toll-Free: 800-232-4636 (800-CDC-INFO)
Toll-Free TTY: 888-232-6348
E-mail: cdcinfo@cdc.gov
Website: http://www.cdc.gov/nceh

National Environmental Health Association (NEHA)
720 S. Colorado Blvd.
Suite 1000-N
Denver, CO 80246-1926
Phone: 303-756-9090
Fax: 303-691-9490
E-mail: staff@neha.org
Website: http://www.neha.org

National Institute for Occupational Safety and Health (NIOSH)
Centers for Disease Control and Prevention
1600 Clifton Rd.
Atlanta, GA 30333
Toll-Free: 800-232-4636 (800-CDC-INFO)
Phone: 404-639-3311
Website: http://www.cdc.gov/niosh

National Institute of Allergy and Infectious Diseases (NIAID)
Office of Communications and Public Liaison
6610 Rockledge Drive, MSC 6612
Bethesda, MD 20892-6612
Toll-Free: 866-284-4107
Phone: 301-496-5717
Toll-Free TDD: 800-877-8339
Fax: 301-402-3573
Website: http://www.niaid.nih.gov

National Institute of Environmental Health Sciences (NIEHS)
Office of Communications and Public Liaison
P.O. Box 12233, MD K3-16
Research Triangle Park, NC 27709
Phone: 919-541-3345
Fax: 919-541-4395
Website: http://www.niehs.nih.gov

National Institute on Aging (NIA)
Building 31, Room 5C27
31 Center Drive, MSC 2292
Bethesda, MD 20892
Phone: 301-496-1752
Toll-Free TTY: 800-222-4225
Fax: 301-496-1072
Website: http://www.nia.nih.gov

National Institutes of Health (NIH)
9000 Rockville Pike
Bethesda, MD 20892
Phone: 301-496-4000
TTY: 301-402-9612
E-mail: NIHinfo@od.nih.gov
Website: http://www.nih.gov

National Library of Medicine
Reference and Web Services
8600 Rockville Pike
Bethesda, MD 20894
Toll-Free: 888-346-3656 (888-FIND-NLM)
Phone: 301-594-5983
Toll-Free TDD: 800-735-2258 (via Maryland Relay Service)
Fax: 301-402-1384
Interlibrary loan fax: 301-496-2809
E-mail: custserv@nlm.nih.gov
Website: http://www.nlm.nih.gov

National Resources Defense Council (NRDC)
40 West 20th Street
New York, NY 10011
Phone: 212-727-2700
Fax: 212-727-1773
E-mail: nrdcinfo@nrdc.org
Website: http://www.nrdc.org

National Safety Council
1121 Spring Lake Dr.
Itasca, IL 60143-3201
Toll-Free: 800-621-7615
Phone: 630-285-1121
Fax: 630-285-1315
E-mail: info@nsc.org
Website: http://www.nsc.org

National Women's Health Information Center
U.S. Department of Health and Human Services
8270 Willow Oaks Corporate Dr.
Fairfax, VA 22031
Toll-Free: 800-994-9662
Toll-Free TTD: 888-220-5446
Website: http://www.womenshealth.gov

Occupational Safety and Health Administration (OSHA)
200 Constitution Ave. NW
Washington, DC 20210
Toll-Free: 800-321-6742 (800-321-OSHA)
Toll-Free TTY: 877-889-5627
Website: http://www.osha.gov

Office of Environmental Health Hazard Assessment (OEHHA)
California Environmental Protection Agency
Phone: 916-323-2514
E-mail: cepacomm@calepa.ca.gov
Website: http://oehha.org

Organic Consumers Association
6771 South Silver Hill Drive
Finland, MN 55603
Phone: 218-226-4164
Fax: 218-353-7652
Website: http://www.organicconsumers.org

Pesticide Action Network North America (PANNA)
49 Powell St., Suite 500
San Francisco, CA 94102
Phone: 415-981-1771
Fax: 415-951-1991
E-mail: panna@panna.org
Website: http://www.panna.org

U.S. Consumer Product Safety Commission
4330 East West Highway
Bethesda, MD 20814
Phone: 301-504-7923 (Mon.–Fri. 8:00 a.m.–4:30 p.m. EST)
Fax: 301-504-0124 and 301-504-0025
Consumer hotline: 800-638-2772 (TTY 800-638-8270). Call to obtain product safety and other agency information and to report unsafe products. Hotline staff may be reached from 8:30 a.m.–5:00 p.m. EST. Messages may be left anytime after these hours. Available 24 hours a day, 7 days a week.
Website: http://www.cpsc.gov

U.S. Department of Agriculture Meat & Poultry Hotline
Toll-Free: 888-674-6854 (888-MPHotline) (10 a.m.– 4 p.m. EST, recorded messages 24/7)
Toll-Free TTY: 800-256-7072
E-mail: MPHotline.fsis@usda.gov
Automated response system: http://AskKaren.gov

U.S. Department of Housing and Urban Development (HUD)
451 7th St. SW
Washington, DC 20410
Phone: 202-708-1112
TTY: 202-708-1455
Website: http://www.hud.gov

Washington State Department of Health
Division of Environmental Health
P.O. Box 47820
Olympia, WA 98504-7820
Website: http://www.doh.wa.gov/ehp

Washington Toxics Coalition
4649 Sunnyside Avenue N
Suite 540
Seattle, WA 98103
Phone: 206-632-1545
E-mail: info@watoxics.org
Website: http://www.watoxics.org

World Health Organization
Avenue Appia 20
1211 Geneva 27
Switzerland
Phone: +41 22 791 21 11
Fax: +41 22 791 31 11
E-mail: info@who.int
Website: http://www.who.int

Environmental Coalitions and Campaigns on the Internet

Alliance for Healthy Homes
50 F Street NW
Suite 300
Washington, DC 20001
Phone: 202-347-7610
Fax: 202-347-0058
E-mail: afhh@afhh.org
Website: http://afhh.org

American Public Information on the Environment
Public Information on the Environment
P.O. Box 676
Northfield, MN 55057-0676
Toll-Free 800-320-2743 (320-APIE)
Fax: 507-645-5724
E-mail: info@americanpie.org
Website: http://www.americanpie.org

Appetite for a Change
Organic Consumers Association
6771 South Silver Hill Drive
Finland MN 55603
Phone: 218-226-4164
Fax: 218-353-7652
Website: http://www.organicconsumers.org/afc.cfm

Be Safe Campaign for Precautionary Action
Center for Health, Environment, and Justice
Main Office
P.O. Box 6806
Falls Church, VA 22040-6806
Phone: 703-237-2249
Fax: 703-237-8389
E-mail: chej@chej.org
Website: http://besafenet.com

Campaign for Safe Cosmetics
E-mail: info@safecosmetics.org
Website: http://
www.safecosmetics.org

Campaign for Tobacco-Free Kids
1400 Eye Street, Suite 1200
Washington DC 20005
Phone: 202-296-5469
Website: http://
www.tobaccofreekids.org

Clean Air Task Force
18 Tremont Street, Suite 530
Boston, MA 02108
Phone: 617-624-0234
Fax: 617-624-0230
E-mail: info@catf.us
Website: http://www.catf.us

Clean Water Fund
1010 Vermont Avenue, NW, Suite 1100
Washington, DC 20005
Phone: 202-895-0432
E-mail: cwf@cleanwater.org
Website: http://
www.cleanwaterfund.org

Environmental Defense Fund
257 Park Avenue South
New York, NY 10010
Phone: 212-505-2100
Fax: 212-505-2375
Website: http://www.edf.org

Environmental Health Strategy Center
E-mail:
info@preventharm.org
Website:
http://www.preventharm.org

Environmental Health Watch
Cleveland Environmental Center
3500 Lorain Avenue
#302
Cleveland, OH 44113
Phone: 216-961-4646
Fax: 216-961-7179
E-mail: e-h-w@ehw.org
Website: http://www.ehw.org

Health and Environment Alliance
28 Boulevard Charlemagne
B1000 Brussels, Belgium
Phone: +32 2 234 3640
Fax: +32 2 234 3649
E-mail:
info@env-health.org
Website:
http://www.env-health.org

Healthy Building Network
927 15th Street, NW, 4th Floor
Washington, DC 20005
Phone: 202-898-1610
Fax: 202-898-1612
E-mail:
info@healthybuilding.net
Website:
http://www.healthybuilding.net

Healthy Toys
E-mail:
HealthyToys@ecocenter.org
Website: http://
www.healthytoys.org

National Council for Science and the Environment
1101 17th Street NW, Suite 250
Washington, DC 20036
Phone: 202-530-5810
Fax: 202-628-4311
E-mail: info@NCSEonline.org
Website: http://ncseonline.org

Physicians for Social Responsibility
1875 Connecticut Avenue, NW
Suite 1012
Washington, DC, 20009
Phone: 202-667-4260
Fax: 202-667-4201
Website: http://
www.envirohealthaction.org

Right-to-Know Network
1742 Connecticut Avenue, NW
Washington, DC 20009
Phone: 202-234-8494
Fax: 202-234-8584
Website: http://www.rtknet.org

Science and Environmental Health Network
Website: http://www.sehn.org

Scorecard
E-mail: scorecard@getactive.com
Website: http://
www.scorecard.org

Skin Deep Cosmetic Safety Database
Environmental Working Group
Website: http://
www.cosmeticsdatabase.com

Stop Toxic Imports
Website: http://
www.stoptoxicimports.org

Union of Concerned Scientists
National Headquarters
Two Brattle Square
Cambridge, MA 02238-9105
Phone: 617-547-5552
Fax: 617-864-9405
Website: http://www.ucsusa.org

Women's Health and the Environment
Website: http://
www.womenshealth
andenvironment.org/

World Resources Institute
10 G Street NE, Suite 800
Washington, DC 20002
Phone: 202-729-7600
Fax: 202-729-7610
Website: http://www.wri.org

Index

Index

Page numbers followed by 'n' indicate a footnote. Page numbers in *italics* indicate a table or illustration.

A

B

C

D

F

I

K

L

M

O

P

Q

R

S

U

V

W

X

Y

Z

Health Reference Series

Complete Catalog

List price $93 per volume. School and library price $84 per volume.

Adolescent Health Sourcebook, 3rd Edition

Basic Consumer Health Information about Adolescent Growth and Development, Puberty, Sexuality, Reproductive Health, and Physical, Emotional, Social, and Mental Health Concerns of Teens and Their Parents, Including Facts about Nutrition, Physical Activity, Weight Management, Acne, Allergies, Cancer, Diabetes, Growth Disorders, Juvenile Arthritis, Infections, Substance Abuse, and More

Along with Information about Adolescent Safety Concerns, Youth Violence, a Glossary of Related Terms, and a Directory of Resources

Edited by Amy L. Sutton. 600 pages. 2010. 978-0-7808-1140-9.

■

Adult Health Concerns Sourcebook

Basic Consumer Health Information about Medical and Mental Concerns of Adults, Including Facts about Choosing Healthcare Providers, Navigating Insurance Options, Maintaining Wellness, Preventing Cancer, Heart Disease, Stroke, Diabetes, and Osteoporosis, and Understanding Aging-Related Health Concerns, Including Menopause, Cognitive Changes, and Changes in the Coronary and Vascular Systems

Along with Tips on Caring for Aging Parents and Dealing with Health-Related Work and Travel Issues, a Glossary, and a Directory of Resources for Additional Help and Information

Edited by Sandra J. Judd. 648 pages. 2008. 978-0-7808-0999-4.

"Provides a thorough list of topics that are important to adult health and for caregivers."

—*CHOICE, Nov '08*

"Written in easy-to-understand language... the content is well-organized and is intended to aid adults in making health care-related decisions."

—*AORN Journal, Dec '08*

■

AIDS Sourcebook, 4th Edition

Basic Consumer Health Information about Human Immunodeficiency Virus (HIV) and Acquired Immunodeficiency Syndrome (AIDS), Featuring Updated Statistics and Facts about Risks, Prevention, Screening, Diagnosis, Treatments, Side Effects, and Complications, and Including a Section about the Impact of HIV/AIDS on the Health of Women, Children, and Adolescents

Along with Tips on Managing Life with AIDS, Reports on Current Research Initiatives and Clinical Trials, a Glossary of Related Terms, and Resource Directories for Further Help and Information

Edited by Ivy L. Alexander. 680 pages. 2008. 978-0-7808-0997-0.

SEE ALSO *Contagious Diseases Sourcebook, 2nd Edition*

■

Alcoholism Sourcebook, 3rd Edition

Basic Consumer Health Information about Alcohol Use, Abuse, and Dependence, Featuring Facts about the Physical, Mental, and Social Health Effects of Alcohol Addiction, Including Alcoholic Liver Disease, Pancreatic Disease, Cardiovascular Disease, Neurological Disorders, and the Effects of Drinking during Pregnancy

Along with Information about Alcohol Treatment, Medications, and Recovery Programs, in Addition to Tips for Reducing the Prevalence of Underage Drinking, Statistics about Alcohol Use, a Glossary of Related Terms, and Directories of Resources for More Help and Information

Edited by Joyce Brennfleck Shannon. 600 pages. 2010. 978-0-7808-1141-6.

SEE ALSO *Drug Abuse Sourcebook, 3rd Edition*

■

Allergies Sourcebook, 3rd Edition

Basic Consumer Health Information about Allergic Disorders, Such as Anaphylaxis,

Hives, Eczema, Rhinitis, Sinusitis, and Conjunctivitis, and Their Triggers, Including Pollen, Mold, Dust Mites, Animal Dander, Insects, Chemicals, Food, Food Additives, and Medications

Along with Advice about the Diagnosis and Treatment of Allergy Symptoms, a Glossary of Related Terms, a Directory of Resources for Help and Information, and Suggestions for Additional Reading

Edited by Amy L. Sutton. 588 pages. 2007. 978-0-7808-0950-5.

SEE ALSO *Asthma Sourcebook, 2nd Edition*

Alzheimer Disease Sourcebook, 4th Edition

Basic Consumer Health Information about Alzheimer Disease, Other Dementias, and Related Disorders, Including Multi-Infarct Dementia, Dementia with Lewy Bodies, Frontotemporal Dementia (Pick Disease), Wernicke-Korsakoff Syndrome (Alcohol-Related Dementia), AIDS Dementia Complex, Huntington Disease, Creutzfeldt-Jacob Disease, and Delirium

Along with Information about Coping with Memory Loss and Forgetfulness, Maintaining Skills, and Long-Term Planning for People with Dementia, and Suggestions Addressing Common Caregiver Concerns, Updated Information about Current Research Efforts, a Glossary of Related Terms, and Directories of Sources for Additional Help and Information

Edited by Karen Bellenir. 603 pages. 2008. 978-0-7808-1001-3.

"An invaluable resource for persons who have received a diagnosis, for caregivers, and for family members dealing with this insidious disease. It is recommended for public, community college, and ready-reference sections in academic libraries."

—*American Reference Books Annual, 2009*

SEE ALSO *Brain Disorders Sourcebook, 3rd Edition*

Arthritis Sourcebook, 3rd Edition

Basic Consumer Health Information about the Risk Factors, Symptoms, Diagnosis, and Treatment of Osteoarthritis, Rheumatoid Arthritis, Juvenile Arthritis, Gout, Infectious Arthritis, and Autoimmune Disorders Associated with Arthritis

Along with Facts about Medications, Surgeries, and Self-Care Techniques to Manage Pain and Disability, Tips on Living with Arthritis, a Glossary of Related Terms, and Resources for Additional Help and Information

Edited by Amy L. Sutton. 600 pages. 2010. 978-0-7808-1077-8.

Asthma Sourcebook, 2nd Edition

Basic Consumer Health Information about the Causes, Symptoms, Diagnosis, and Treatment of Asthma in Infants, Children, Teenagers, and Adults, Including Facts about Different Types of Asthma, Common Co-Occurring Conditions, Asthma Management Plans, Triggers, Medications, and Medication Delivery Devices

Along with Asthma Statistics, Research Updates, a Glossary, a Directory of Asthma-Related Resources, and More

Edited by Karen Bellenir. 581 pages. 2006. 978-0-7808-0866-9.

SEE ALSO *Lung Disorders Sourcebook; Respiratory Disorders Sourcebook, 2nd Edition*

Attention Deficit Disorder Sourcebook

Basic Consumer Health Information about Attention Deficit/Hyperactivity Disorder in Children and Adults, Including Facts about Causes, Symptoms, Diagnostic Criteria, and Treatment Options Such as Medications, Behavior Therapy, Coaching, and Homeopathy

Along with Reports on Current Research Initiatives, Legal Issues, and Government Regulations, and Featuring a Glossary of Related Terms, Internet Resources, and a List of Additional Reading Material

Edited by Dawn D. Matthews. 447 pages. 2002. 978-0-7808-0624-5.

"Recommended reference source."

—*Booklist, Jan '03*

SEE ALSO *Learning Disabilities Sourcebook, 3rd Edition*

Autism and Pervasive Developmental Disorders Sourcebook

Basic Consumer Health Information about Autism Spectrum and Pervasive Developmental Disorders, Such as Classical Autism, Asperger Syndrome, Rett Syndrome, and Childhood Disintegrative Disorder, Including Information about Related Genetic Disorders and Medical Problems and Facts about Causes, Screening Methods, Diagnostic Criteria, Treatments and Interventions, and Family and Education Issues

Along with a Glossary of Related Terms, Tips for Evaluating the Validity of Health Claims, and a Directory of Resources for Additional Help and Information

Edited by Sandra J. Judd. 603 pages. 2007. 978-0-7808-0953-6.

"This book provides a current overview of disorders on the autism spectrum and information about various therapies, educational resources, and help for families with practical issues such as workplace adjustments, living arrangements, and estate planning. It is a useful resource for public and consumer health libraries."

—*American Reference Books Annual, 2009*

SEE ALSO *Learning Disabilities Sourcebook, 3rd Edition*

■

Back and Neck Disorders Sourcebook, 2nd Edition

Basic Consumer Health Information about Spinal Pain, Spinal Cord Injuries, and Related Disorders, Such as Degenerative Disk Disease, Osteoarthritis, Scoliosis, Sciatica, Spina Bifida, and Spinal Stenosis, and Featuring Facts about Maintaining Spinal Health, Self-Care, Pain Management, Rehabilitative Care, Chiropractic Care, Spinal Surgeries, and Complementary Therapies

Along with Suggestions for Preventing Back and Neck Pain, a Glossary of Related Terms, and a Directory of Resources

Edited by Amy L. Sutton. 607 pages. 2004. 978-0-7808-0738-9.

"Recommended... An easy to use, comprehensive medical reference book."

—*E-Streams, Sep '05*

"For anyone who has back or neck problems, this book is ideal. Its easy-to-understand language and variety of topics makes this sourcebook a worthwhile read. The price... is reasonable for the amount of information contained in the book"

—*Occupational Therapy in Health Care, 2007*

■

Blood & Circulatory Disorders Sourcebook, 3rd Edition

Basic Consumer Health Information about Blood and Circulatory System Disorders, Such as Anemia, Leukemia, Lymphoma, Rh Disease, Hemophilia, Thrombophilia, Other Bleeding and Clotting Deficiencies, and Artery, Vascular, and Venous Diseases, Including Facts about Blood Types, Blood Donation, Bone Marrow and Stem Cell Transplants, Tests and Medications, and Tips for Maintaining Circulatory Health

Along with a Glossary of Related Terms and a List of Resources for Additional Help and Information

Edited by Sandra J. Judd. 600 pages. 2010. 978-0-7808-1081-5.

SEE ALSO *Leukemia Sourcebook*

■

Brain Disorders Sourcebook, 3rd Edition

Basic Consumer Health Information about Acquired and Traumatic Brain Injuries, Brain Tumors, Cerebral Palsy and Other Genetic and Congenital Brain Disorders, Infections of the Brain, Epilepsy, and Degenerative Neurological Disorders Such as Dementia, Huntington Disease, and Amyotrophic Lateral Sclerosis (ALS)

Along with Information on Brain Structure and Function, Treatment and Rehabilitation Options, a Glossary of Terms Related to Brain Disorders, and a Directory of Resources for More Information

Edited by Joyce Brennfleck Shannon. 600 pages. 2010. 978-0-7808-1083-9.

SEE ALSO *Alzheimer Disease Sourcebook, 4th Edition*

■

Breast Cancer Sourcebook, 3rd Edition

Basic Consumer Health Information about Breast Health and Breast Cancer, Including Facts about Environmental, Genetic, and Other Risk Factors, Prevention Efforts, Screening and Diagnostic Methods, Surgical Treatment Options and Other Care Choices, Complementary and Alternative Therapies, and Post-Treatment Concerns

Along with Statistical Data, News about Research Advances, a Glossary of Related Terms, and Directories of Resources for Additional Information and Support

Edited by Karen Bellenir. 606 pages. 2009. 978-0-7808-1030-3.

"A very useful reference for people wanting to learn more about breast cancer and how to negotiate their care or the care of a loved one. The third edition is necessary as information/ treatment options continue to evolve."

—*Doody's Review Service, 2009*

SEE ALSO *Cancer Sourcebook for Women, 3rd Edition, Women's Health Concerns Sourcebook, 3rd Edition*

Breastfeeding Sourcebook

Basic Consumer Health Information about the Benefits of Breastmilk, Preparing to Breastfeed, Breastfeeding as a Baby Grows, Nutrition, and More, Including Information on Special Situations and Concerns Such as Mastitis, Illness, Medications, Allergies, Multiple Births, Prematurity, Special Needs, and Adoption

Along with a Glossary and Resources for Additional Help and Information

Edited by Jenni Lynn Colson. 367 pages. 2002. 978-0-7808-0332-9.

SEE ALSO *Pregnancy and Birth Sourcebook, 3rd Edition*

Burns Sourcebook

Basic Consumer Health Information about Various Types of Burns and Scalds, Including Flame, Heat, Cold, Electrical, Chemical, and Sun Burns

Along with Information on Short-Term and Long-Term Treatments, Tissue Reconstruction, Plastic Surgery, Prevention Suggestions, and First Aid

Edited by Allan R. Cook. 604 pages. 1999. 978-0-7808-0204-9.

"This is an exceptional addition to the series and is highly recommended for all consumer health collections, hospital libraries, and academic medical centers."

—*E-Streams, Mar '00*

"This key reference guide is an invaluable addition to all health care and public libraries in confronting this ongoing health issue."

—*American Reference Books Annual, 2000*

SEE ALSO *Dermatological Disorders Sourcebook, 2nd Edition*

Cancer Sourcebook, 5th Edition

Basic Consumer Health Information about Major Forms and Stages of Cancer, Featuring Facts about Head and Neck Cancers, Lung Cancers, Gastrointestinal Cancers, Genitourinary Cancers, Lymphomas, Blood Cell Cancers, Endocrine Cancers, Skin Cancers, Bone Cancers, Metastatic Cancers, and More

Along with Facts about Cancer Treatments, Cancer Risks and Prevention, a Glossary of Related Terms, Statistical Data, and a Directory of Resources for Additional Information

Edited by Karen Bellenir. 1105 pages. 2007. 978-0-7808-0947-5.

"The 5th, updated edition of Cancer Sourcebook should be in every public and health lending library collection... An unparalleled discussion essential for any health collections considering an all-in-one basic general reference."

—*California Bookwatch, Aug '07*

SEE ALSO *Breast Cancer Sourcebook, 3rd Edition, Cancer Survivorship Sourcebook, Leukemia Sourcebook*

Cancer Sourcebook for Women, 4th Edition

Basic Consumer Health Information about Gynecologic Cancers and Other Cancers of Special Concern to Women, Including Cancers of the Breast, Cervix, Colon, Lung, Ovaries, Thyroid, and Uterus

Along with Facts about Benign Conditions of the Female Reproductive System, Cancer Risk

Factors, Diagnostic and Treatment Procedures, Side Effects of Cancer and Cancer Treatments, Women's Issues in Cancer Survivorship, a Glossary of Related Terms, and a Directory of Resources for Additional Help and Information

Edited by Karen Bellenir. 600 pages. 2010. 978-0-7808-1139-3.

SEE ALSO Breast Cancer Sourcebook, 3rd Edition, Women's Health Concerns Sourcebook, 3rd Edition

Cancer Survivorship Sourcebook

Basic Consumer Health Information about the Physical, Educational, Emotional, Social, and Financial Needs of Cancer Patients from Diagnosis, through Cancer Treatment, and Beyond, Including Facts about Researching Specific Types of Cancer and Learning about Clinical Trials and Treatment Options, and Featuring Tips for Coping with the Side Effects of Cancer Treatments and Adjusting to Life after Cancer Treatment Concludes

Along with Suggestions for Caregivers, Friends, and Family Members of Cancer Patients, a Glossary of Cancer Care Terms, and Directories of Related Resources

Edited by Karen Bellenir. 633 pages. 2007. 978-0-7808-0985-7.

"Well organized and comprehensive in coverage, the book speaks to issues encountered both during and after cancer treatment. Recommended for consumer health and public libraries."

—*Library Journal, Aug 1 '07*

"Cancer Survivorship Sourcebook will be useful to anyone who has a friend or loved one with a cancer diagnosis."

—*American Reference Books Annual, 2008*

SEE ALSO *Cancer Sourcebook, 5th Edition, Disease Management Sourcebook*

Cardiovascular Disorders Sourcebook, 4th Edition

Basic Consumer Health Information about Heart and Blood Vessel Diseases and Disorders, Such as Angina, Heart Attack, Heart Failure, Cardiomyopathy, Arrhythmias, Valve Disease, Atherosclerosis, Aneurysms, and Congenital Heart Defects, Including Information about Cardiovascular Disease in Women, Men, Children, Adolescents, and Minorities

Along with Facts about Diagnosing, Managing, and Preventing Cardiovascular Disease, a Glossary of Related Medical Terms, and a Directory of Resources for Additional Information

Edited by Amy L. Sutton. 600 pages. 2010. 978-0-7808-1080-8.

Caregiving Sourcebook

Basic Consumer Health Information for Caregivers, Including a Profile of Caregivers, Caregiving Responsibilities and Concerns, Tips for Specific Conditions, Care Environments, and the Effects of Caregiving

Along with Facts about Legal Issues, Financial Information, and Future Planning, a Glossary, and a Listing of Additional Resources

Edited by Joyce Brennfleck Shannon. 583 pages. 2001. 978-0-7808-0331-2.

"Essential for most collections."

—*Library Journal, Apr 1 '02*

"An ideal addition to the reference collection of any public library. Health sciences information professionals may also want to acquire the Caregiving Sourcebook for their hospital or academic library for use as a ready reference tool by health care workers interested in aging and caregiving."

—*E-Streams, Jan '02*

Child Abuse Sourcebook, 2nd Edition

Basic Consumer Health Information about the Physical, Sexual, and Emotional Abuse of Children, Neglect, Münchhausen Syndrome by Proxy (MSBP), and Shaken Baby Syndrome, and Featuring Facts about Withholding Medical Care, Corporal Punishment, Child Maltreatment in Youth Sports, and Parental Substance Abuse

Along with Information about Child Protective Services, Foster Care, Adoption, Parenting Challenges, Abuse Prevention Programs, and Intervention, Treatment, and Recovery Guidelines, a Glossary of Related Terms, and Resources for Additional Help and Information

Edited by Joyce Brennfleck Shannon. 600 pages. 2009. 978-0-7808-1037-2.

SEE ALSO *Domestic Violence Sourcebook, 3rd Edition*

Childhood Diseases and Disorders Sourcebook, 2nd Edition

Basic Consumer Health Information about the Physical, Mental, and Developmental Health of Pre-Adolescent Children, Including Facts about Infectious Diseases, Asthma, Allergies, Diabetes, and Other Acute and Chronic Conditions Affecting the Gastrointestinal Tract, Ears, Nose, Throat, Liver, Kidneys, Heart, Blood, Brain, Muscles, Bones, and Skin

Along with Reports on Recommended Childhood Vaccinations, Wellness Guidelines, a Glossary of Related Medical Terms, and a List of Resources for Parents

Edited by Sandra J. Judd. 694 pages. 2009. 978-0-7808-1031-0.

"The strength of this source is the wide range of information given about childhood health issues... It is most appropriate for public libraries and academic libraries that field medical questions."

—*American Reference Books Annual, 2009*

SEE ALSO *Healthy Children Sourcebook*

Colds, Flu and Other Common Ailments Sourcebook

Basic Consumer Health Information about Common Ailments and Injuries, Including Colds, Coughs, the Flu, Sinus Problems, Headaches, Fever, Nausea and Vomiting, Menstrual Cramps, Diarrhea, Constipation, Hemorrhoids, Back Pain, Dandruff, Dry and Itchy Skin, Cuts, Scrapes, Sprains, Bruises, and More

Along with Information about Prevention, Self-Care, Choosing a Doctor, Over-the-Counter Medications, Folk Remedies, and Alternative Therapies, and Including a Glossary of Important Terms and a Directory of Resources for Further Help and Information

Edited by Chad T. Kimball. 622 pages. 2001. 978-0-7808-0435-7.

"A good starting point for research on common illnesses. It will be a useful addition to public and consumer health library collections."

—*American Reference Books Annual, 2002*

"Will prove valuable to any library seeking to maintain a current, comprehensive reference collection of health resources... Excellent reference."

—*The Bookwatch, Aug '01*

SEE ALSO Contagious Diseases Sourcebook, 2nd Edition

Communication Disorders Sourcebook

Basic Information about Deafness and Hearing Loss, Speech and Language Disorders, Voice Disorders, Balance and Vestibular Disorders, and Disorders of Smell, Taste, and Touch

Edited by Linda M. Ross. 533 pages. 1996. 978-0-7808-0077-9.

"This is skillfully edited and is a welcome resource for the layperson. It should be found in every public and medical library."

—*Booklist Health Sciences Supplement, Oct '97*

Complementary & Alternative Medicine Sourcebook, 4th Edition

Basic Consumer Health Information about Ayurveda, Acupuncture, Aromatherapy, Chiropractic Care, Diet-Based Therapies, Guided Imagery, Herbal and Vitamin Supplements, Homeopathy, Hypnosis, Massage, Meditation, Naturopathy, Pilates, Reflexology, Reiki, Shiatsu, Tai Chi, Traditional Chinese Medicine, Yoga, and Other Complementary and Alternative Medical Therapies

Along with Statistics, Tips for Selecting a Practitioner, Treatments for Specific Health Conditions, a Glossary of Related Terms, and a Directory of Resources for Additional Help and Information

Edited by Amy L. Sutton. 600 pages. 2010. 978-0-7808-1082-2.

Congenital Disorders Sourcebook, 2nd Edition

Basic Consumer Health Information about Nonhereditary Birth Defects and Disorders

Related to Prematurity, Gestational Injuries, Congenital Infections, and Birth Complications, Including Heart Defects, Hydrocephalus, Spina Bifida, Cleft Lip and Palate, Cerebral Palsy, and More

Along with Facts about the Prevention of Birth Defects, Fetal Surgery and Other Treatment Options, Research Initiatives, a Glossary of Related Terms, and Resources for Additional Information and Support

Edited by Sandra J. Judd. 619 pages. 2007. 978-0-7808-0945-1.

"Congenital Disorders Sourcebook provides an excellent, non-technical overview of many aspects of pregnancy with the focus on congenital disorders."

—*American Reference Books Annual, 2008*

"An excellent readable reference aimed at the lay public for difficult to understand medical problems. An excellent starting point for the interested parent or family member who may then be motivated to seek more information."

—*Doody's Review Service, 2007*

SEE ALSO *Pregnancy and Birth Sourcebook, 3rd Edition*

Contagious Diseases Sourcebook, 2nd Edition

Basic Consumer Health Information about Diseases Spread from Person to Person through Direct Physical Contact, Airborne Transmissions, Sexual Contact, or Contact with Blood or Other Body Fluids, Including Pneumococcal, Staphylococcal, and Streptococcal Diseases, Colds, Influenza, Lice, Measles, Mumps, Tuberculosis, and Others

Along with Facts about Self-Care and Over-the-Counter Medications, Antibiotics and Drug Resistance, Disease Prevention, Vaccines, and Bioterrorism, a Glossary, and a Directory of Resources for More Information

Edited by Joyce Brennfleck Shannon. 600 pages. 2010. 978-0-7808-1075-4.

SEE ALSO *AIDS Sourcebook, 4th Edition, Hepatitis Sourcebook*

Cosmetic and Reconstructive Surgery Sourcebook, 2nd Edition

Basic Consumer Information about Plastic Surgery and Non-Surgical Appearance-Enhancing Procedures, Including Facts about Botulinum Toxin, Collagen Replacement, Dermabrasion, Chemical Peels, Eyelid Surgery, Nose Reshaping, Lip Augmentation, Liposuction, Breast Enlargement and Reduction, Tummy Tucking, and Other Skin, Hair, Facial, and Body Shaping Procedures

Along with Information about Reconstructive Procedures for Congenital Disorders, Disfiguring Diseases, Burns, and Traumatic Injuries, a Glossary of Related Terms, and a Directory of Additional Resources

Edited by Karen Bellenir. 483 pages. 2007. 978-0-7808-0951-2.

"A comprehensive source for people considering cosmetic surgery... also recommended for medical students who will perform these procedures later in their careers; and public librarians and academic medical librarians who may assist patrons interested in this information."

—*Medical Reference Services Quarterly, Fall '08*

"A practical guide for health care consumers and health care workers... This easy-to-read reference guide would be useful for novice and veteran health care consumers, surgical technology students, nursing students, and perioperative nurses new to plastic and reconstructive surgery. It also may be helpful for medical-surgical nurses as a guide for patient teaching in their practices."

—*AORN Journal, Aug '08*

SEE ALSO *Surgery Sourcebook, 2nd Edition*

Death and Dying Sourcebook, 2nd Edition

Basic Consumer Health Information about End-of-Life Care and Related Perspectives and Ethical Issues, Including End-of-Life Symptoms and Treatments, Pain Management, Quality-of-Life Concerns, the Use of Life Support, Patients' Rights and Privacy Issues, Advance Directives, Physician-Assisted Suicide, Caregiving, Organ and Tissue Donation, Autopsies, Funeral Arrangements, and Grief

Along with Statistical Data, Information about the Leading Causes of Death, a Glossary, and Directories of Support Groups and Other Resources

Edited by Joyce Brennfleck Shannon. 626 pages. 2006. 978-0-7808-0871-3.

■

Dental Care and Oral Health Sourcebook, 3rd Edition

Basic Consumer Health Information about Dental Care and Oral Health Throughout the Lifespan, Including Facts about Cavities, Bad Breath, Cold and Canker Sores, Dry Mouth, Toothaches, Gum Disease, Malocclusion, Temporomandibular Joint and Muscle Disorders, Oral Cancers, and Dental Emergencies

Along with Information about Mouth Hygiene, Crowns, Bridges, Implants, and Fillings, Surgical, Orthodontic, and Cosmetic Dental Procedures, Pain Management, Health Conditions that Impact Oral Care, a Glossary of Related Terms, and a Directory of Additional Resources

Edited by Amy L. Sutton. 619 pages. 2008. 978-0-7808-1032-7.

"Could serve as turning point in the battle to educate consumers in issues concerning oral health. Tightly written in terms the average person can understand, yet comprehensive in scope and authoritative in tone, it is another excellent sourcebook in the Health Reference Series... Should be in the reference department of all public libraries, and in academic libraries that have a public constituency."

—*American Reference Books Annual, 2009*

■

Depression Sourcebook, 2nd Edition

Basic Consumer Health Information about Unipolar Depression, Bipolar Disorder, Dysthymia, Seasonal Affective Disorder, Postpartum Depression, and Other Depressive Disorders, Including Facts about Populations at Special Risk, Coexisting Medical Conditions, Symptoms, Treatment Options, and Suicide Prevention

Along with Statistical Data, a Glossary of Related Terms, and a Directory of Resources for Additional Help and Information

Edited by Sandra J. Judd. 646 pages. 2008. 978-0-7808-1003-7.

"Recommended for public libraries."

—*American Reference Books Annual, 2009*

SEE ALSO *Mental Health Disorders Sourcebook, 4th Edition*

■

Dermatological Disorders Sourcebook, 2nd Edition

Basic Consumer Health Information about Conditions and Disorders Affecting the Skin, Hair, and Nails, Such as Acne, Rosacea, Rashes, Dermatitis, Pigmentation Disorders, Birthmarks, Skin Cancer, Skin Injuries, Psoriasis, Scleroderma, and Hair Loss, Including Facts about Medications and Treatments for Dermatological Disorders and Tips for Maintaining Healthy Skin, Hair, and Nails

Along with Information about How Aging Affects the Skin, a Glossary of Related Terms, and a Directory of Resources for Additional Help and Information

Edited by Amy L. Sutton. 617 pages. 2006. 978-0-7808-0795-2.

"Well organized... presents a plethora of information in a manner that is appropriate in style and readability for the intended audience."

—*Physical Therapy, Nov '06*

"Helpfully brings together... sources in one convenient place, saving the user hours of research time."

—*American Reference Books Annual, 2006*

SEE ALSO *Burns Sourcebook*

■

Diabetes Sourcebook, 4th Edition

Basic Consumer Health Information about Type 1 and Type 2 Diabetes Mellitus, Gestational Diabetes, Monogenic Forms of Diabetes, and Insulin Resistance, with Guidelines for Lifestyle Modifications and the Medical Management of Diabetes, Including Facts about Insulin, Insulin Delivery Devices, Oral Diabetes Medications, Self-Monitoring of Blood Glucose, Meal Planning, Physical Activity Recommendations, Foot Care, and Treatment Options for People with Kidney Failure

Along with a Section about Diabetes Complications and Co-Occurring Conditions, a Glossary of Related Terms, and Directories of Resources for Additional Help and Information

Edited by Karen Bellenir. 627 pages. 2008. 978-0-7808-1005-1.

"Completely and comprehensively covering almost everything a student or physician would need to know... well worth the investment."

—*Internet Bookwatch, Dec '08*

SEE ALSO *Endocrine and Metabolic Disorders Sourcebook, 2nd Edition*

Diet and Nutrition Sourcebook, 3rd Edition

Basic Consumer Health Information about Dietary Guidelines and the Food Guidance System, Recommended Daily Nutrient Intakes, Serving Proportions, Weight Control, Vitamins and Supplements, Nutrition Issues for Different Life Stages and Lifestyles, and the Needs of People with Specific Medical Concerns, Including Cancer, Celiac Disease, Diabetes, Eating Disorders, Food Allergies, and Cardiovascular Disease

Along with Facts about Federal Nutrition Support Programs, a Glossary of Nutrition and Dietary Terms, and Directories of Additional Resources for More Information about Nutrition

Edited by Joyce Brennfleck Shannon. 605 pages. 2006. 978-0-7808-0800-3.

"A valuable resource tool for any individual."

—*Journal of Dental Hygiene, Apr '07*

"From different recommended eating habits to reduce disease and common ailments to nutrition advice for those with specific conditions, Diet and Nutrition Sourcebook is especially important because so much is changing in this area, and so rapidly."

—*California Bookwatch, Jun '06*

SEE ALSO *Eating Disorders Sourcebook, 2nd Edition, Vegetarian Sourcebook*

Digestive Diseases and Disorders Sourcebook

Basic Consumer Health Information about Diseases and Disorders that Impact the Upper and Lower Digestive System, Including Celiac Disease, Constipation, Crohn's Disease, Cyclic Vomiting Syndrome, Diarrhea, Diverticulosis and Diverticulitis, Gallstones, Heartburn, Hemorrhoids, Hernias, Indigestion (Dyspepsia), Irritable Bowel Syndrome, Lactose Intolerance, Ulcers, and More

Along with Information about Medications and Other Treatments, Tips for Maintaining a Healthy Digestive Tract, a Glossary, and Directory of Digestive Diseases Organizations

Edited by Karen Bellenir. 323 pages. 2000. 978-0-7808-0327-5.

"An excellent addition to all public or patient-research libraries."

—*American Reference Books Annual, 2001*

"Recommended reference source."

—*Booklist, May '00*

SEE ALSO *Gastrointestinal Diseases and Disorders Sourcebook, 2nd Edition*

Disabilities Sourcebook

Basic Consumer Health Information about Physical and Psychiatric Disabilities, Including Descriptions of Major Causes of Disability, Assistive and Adaptive Aids, Workplace Issues, and Accessibility Concerns

Along with Information about the Americans with Disabilities Act, a Glossary, and Resources for Additional Help and Information

Edited by Dawn D. Matthews. 602 pages. 2000. 978-0-7808-0389-3.

"A must for libraries with a consumer health section."

—*American Reference Books Annual, 2002*

"A much needed addition to the Omnigraphics Health Reference Series. A current reference work to provide people with disabilities, their families, caregivers or those who work with them, a broad range of information in one volume, has not been available until now... It is recommended for all public and academic library reference collections."

—*E-Streams, May '01*

"An excellent source book in easy-to-read format covering many current topics; highly recommended for all libraries."

—*CHOICE, Jan '01*

Disease Management Sourcebook

Basic Consumer Health Information about Coping with Chronic and Serious Illnesses, Navigating the Health Care System, Communicating with Health Care Providers, Assessing Health Care Quality, and Making Informed Health Care Decisions, Including Facts about Second Opinions, Hospitalization, Surgery, and Medications

Along with a Section about Children with Chronic Conditions, Information about Legal, Financial, and Insurance Issues, a Glossary of Related Terms, and Directories of Additional Resources

Edited by Joyce Brennfleck Shannon. 621 pages. 2008. 978-0-7808-1002-0.

"Consumers need to know how to manage their health care the same way they manage anything else in their lives. The text is very readable and is written for the layperson and consumer. The cost is not prohibitive. This book should be in all collections of health care libraries and public libraries."

— American Reference Books Annual, 2009

"The information is very current, and the selection of font and layout make the book easy to read. A hardback that will stand up to much usage, this is an excellent resource for consumers... Recommended. General readers."

—CHOICE, Nov '08

"Intended for lay readers, this resource clarifies the many confusing and overwhelming details associated with chronic disease care. Meticulous and clearly explained, the book even includes diagrams intended to ease comprehension of over-the-counter medication labels. An essential guide to navigating the health-care rapids."

—Library Journal, Aug '08

Domestic Violence Sourcebook, 3rd Edition

Basic Consumer Health Information about Warning Signs, Risk Factors, and Health Consequences of Intimate Partner Violence, Sexual Violence and Rape, Stalking, Human Trafficking, Child Maltreatment, Teen Dating Violence, and Elder Abuse

Along with Facts about Victims and Perpetrators, Strategies for Violence Prevention, and Emergency Interventions, Safety Plans, and Financial and Legal Tips for Victims, a Glossary of Related Terms, and Directories of Resources for Additional Information and Support

Edited by Joyce Brennfleck Shannon. 634 pages. 2009. 978-0-7808-1038-9.

"A recommended pick for any library interested in consumer health and social issues... A 'must' for any serious health collection."

—California Bookwatch, Jul '09

SEE ALSO *Child Abuse Sourcebook, 2nd Edition*

Drug Abuse Sourcebook, 3rd Edition

Basic Consumer Health Information about the Abuse of Cocaine, Club Drugs, Hallucinogens, Heroin, Inhalants, Marijuana, and Other Illicit Substances, Prescription Medications, and Over-the-Counter Medicines

Along with Facts about Addiction and Related Health Effects, Drug Abuse Treatment and Recovery, Drug Testing, Prevention Programs, Glossaries of Drug-Related Terms, and Directories of Resources for More Information

Edited by Joyce Brennfleck Shannon. 600 pages. 2010. 978-0-7808-1079-2.

SEE ALSO *Alcoholism Sourcebook, 3rd Edition*

Ear, Nose, and Throat Disorders Sourcebook, 2nd Edition

Basic Consumer Health Information about Disorders of the Ears, Hearing Loss, Vestibular Disorders, Nasal and Sinus Problems, Throat and Vocal Cord Disorders, and Otolaryngologic Cancers, Including Facts about Ear Infections and Injuries, Genetic and Congenital Deafness, Sensorineural Hearing Disorders, Tinnitus, Vertigo, Ménière Disease, Rhinitis, Sinusitis, Snoring, Sore Throats, Hoarseness, and More

Along with Reports on Current Research Initiatives, a Glossary of Related Medical Terms, and a Directory of Sources for Further Help and Information

Edited by Sandra J. Judd. 631 pages. 2007. 978-0-7808-0872-0.

"A resource book for the general public that provides comprehensive coverage of basic up-to-date medical information about the causes, symptoms, diagnosis, and treatment of diseases and disorders that affect the ears, nose, sinuses, throat, and voice... The majority of information is presented in question and answer format, much like questions a patient might ask of a health care provider. An extensive index facilitates the reader's ability to easily access information on any specific topic."

—*Journal of Dental Hygiene, Oct '07*

"A handy compilation of information on common and some not so common ailments of the ears, nose, and throat."

—*Doody's Review Service, 2007*

Eating Disorders Sourcebook, 2nd Edition

Basic Consumer Health Information about Anorexia Nervosa, Bulimia, Binge Eating, Compulsive Exercise, Female Athlete Triad, and Other Eating Disorders, Including Facts about Body Image and Other Cultural and Age-Related Risk Factors, Prevention Efforts, Adverse Health Effects, Treatment Options, and the Recovery Process

Along with Guidelines for Healthy Weight Control, a Glossary, and Directories of Additional Resources

Edited by Joyce Brennfleck Shannon. 557 pages. 2007. 978-0-7808-0948-2.

"Recommended for the reference collection of large public libraries."

—*American Reference Books Annual, 2008*

"A basic health reference any health or general library needs."

—*Internet Bookwatch, Jun '07*

SEE ALSO *Diet and Nutrition Sourcebook, 3rd Edition, Mental Health Disorders Sourcebook, 4th Edition*

Emergency Medical Services Sourcebook

Basic Consumer Health Information about Preventing, Preparing for, and Managing Emergency Situations, When and Who to Call for Help, What to Expect in the Emergency Room, the Emergency Medical Team, Patient Issues, and Current Topics in Emergency Medicine

Along with Statistical Data, a Glossary, and Sources of Additional Help and Information

Edited by Jenni Lynn Colson. 472 pages. 2002. 978-0-7808-0420-3.

"Handy and convenient for home, public, school, and college libraries. Recommended."

—*CHOICE, Apr '03*

"This reference can provide the consumer with answers to most questions about emergency care in the United States, or it will direct them to a resource where the answer can be found."

—*American Reference Books Annual, 2003*

SEE ALSO *Injury and Trauma Sourcebook*

Endocrine and Metabolic Disorders Sourcebook, 2nd Edition

Basic Consumer Health Information about Hormonal and Metabolic Disorders that Affect the Body's Growth, Development, and Functioning, Including Disorders of the Pancreas, Ovaries and Testes, and Pituitary, Thyroid, Parathyroid, and Adrenal Glands, with Facts about Growth Disorders, Addison Disease, Cushing Syndrome, Conn Syndrome, Diabetic Disorders, Multiple Endocrine Neoplasia, Inborn Errors of Metabolism, and More

Along with Information about Endocrine Functioning, Diagnostic and Screening Tests, a Glossary of Related Terms, and Directories of Additional Resources

Edited by Joyce Brennfleck Shannon. 597 pages. 2007. 978-0-7808-0952-9.

SEE ALSO *Diabetes Sourcebook, 4th Edition*

Environmental Health Sourcebook, 3rd Edition

Basic Consumer Health Information about the Environment and Its Effects on Human Health, Including Facts about Air, Water, and Soil Contamination, Hazardous Chemicals, Foodborne Hazards and Illnesses, Household Hazards Such as Radon, Mold, and Carbon Monoxide, Consumer Hazards from Toxic Products and Imported Goods, and Disorders

Linked to Environmental Causes, Including Chemical Sensitivity, Cancer, Allergies, and Asthma

Along with Information about the Impact of Environmental Hazards on Specific Populations, a Glossary of Related Terms, and Resources for Additional Help and Information.

Edited by Laura Larsen. 600 pages. 2010. 978-0-7808-1078-5

Ethnic Diseases Sourcebook

Basic Consumer Health Information for Ethnic and Racial Minority Groups in the United States, Including General Health Indicators and Behaviors, Ethnic Diseases, Genetic Testing, the Impact of Chronic Diseases, Women's Health, Mental Health Issues, and Preventive Health Care Services

Along with a Glossary and a Listing of Additional Resources

Edited by Joyce Brennfleck Shannon. 648 pages. 2001. 978-0-7808-0336-7.

"Not many books have been written on this topic to date, and the Ethnic Diseases Sourcebook is a strong addition to the list. It will be an important introductory resource for health consumers, students, health care personnel, and social scientists. It is recommended for public, academic, and large hospital libraries."

— *American Reference Books Annual, 2002*

"Will prove valuable to any library seeking to maintain a current, comprehensive reference collection of health resources... An excellent source of health information about genetic disorders which affect particular ethnic and racial minorities in the U.S."

—*The Bookwatch, Aug '01*

Eye Care Sourcebook, 3rd Edition

Basic Consumer Health Information about Eye Care and Eye Disorders, Including Facts about the Diagnosis, Prevention, and Treatment of Refractive Disorders, Cataracts, Glaucoma, Macular Degeneration, and Problems Affecting the Cornea, Retina, and Lacrimal Glands

Along with Advice about Preventing Eye Injuries and Tips for Living with Low Vision or Blindness, a Glossary of Related Terms, and Directories of Resources for More Help and Information

Edited by Amy L. Sutton. 646 pages. 2008. 978-0-7808-1000-6.

"A solid reference tool for eye care and a valuable addition to a collection."

—*American Reference Books Annual, 2009*

Family Planning Sourcebook

Basic Consumer Health Information about Planning for Pregnancy and Contraception, Including Traditional Methods, Barrier Methods, Hormonal Methods, Permanent Methods, Future Methods, Emergency Contraception, and Birth Control Choices for Women at Each Stage of Life

Along with Statistics, a Glossary, and Sources of Additional Information

Edited by Amy Marcaccio Keyzer. 503 pages. 2001. 978-0-7808-0379-4.

"Recommended for public, health, and undergraduate libraries as part of the circulating collection."

—*E-Streams, Mar '02*

"Will prove valuable to any library seeking to maintain a current, comprehensive reference collection of health resources... Excellent reference."

—*The Bookwatch, Aug '01*

SEE ALSO *Pregnancy and Birth Sourcebook, 3rd Edition*

Fitness and Exercise Sourcebook, 3rd Edition

Basic Consumer Health Information about the Physical and Mental Benefits of Fitness, Including Cardiorespiratory Endurance, Muscular Strength, Muscular Endurance, and Flexibility, with Facts about Sports Nutrition and Exercise-Related Injuries and Tips about Physical Activity and Exercises for People of All Ages and for People with Health Concerns

Along with Advice on Selecting and Using Exercise Equipment, Maintaining Exercise Motivation, a Glossary of Related Terms, and a Directory of Resources for More Help and Information

Edited by Amy L. Sutton. 635 pages. 2007. 978-0-7808-0946-8.

"Updates the consumer information on the physical and mental benefits of physical activity throughout the lifespan offered in earlier editions... Recommended. All readers; all levels."

—CHOICE, Oct '07

"An exceptionally well-rounded coverage perfect for any concerned about developing and understanding a fitness program."

—California Bookwatch, Jun '07

SEE ALSO *Sports Injuries Sourcebook, 3rd Edition*

Food Safety Sourcebook

Basic Consumer Health Information about the Safe Handling of Meat, Poultry, Seafood, Eggs, Fruit Juices, and Other Food Items, and Facts about Pesticides, Drinking Water, Food Safety Overseas, and the Onset, Duration, and Symptoms of Foodborne Illnesses, Including Types of Pathogenic Bacteria, Parasitic Protozoa, Worms, Viruses, and Natural Toxins

Along with the Role of the Consumer, the Food Handler, and the Government in Food Safety, a Glossary, and Resources for Additional Help and Information

Edited by Dawn D. Matthews. 327 pages. 1999. 978-0-7808-0326-8.

"Recommended reference source."

—Booklist, May '00

"This book takes the complex issues of food safety and foodborne pathogens and presents them in an easily understood manner. [It does] an excellent job of covering a large and often confusing topic."

— American Reference Books Annual, 2000

Forensic Medicine Sourcebook

Basic Consumer Information for the Layperson about Forensic Medicine, Including Crime Scene Investigation, Evidence Collection and Analysis, Expert Testimony, Computer-Aided Criminal Identification, Digital Imaging in the Courtroom, DNA Profiling, Accident Reconstruction, Autopsies, Ballistics, Drugs and Explosives Detection, Latent Fingerprints, Product Tampering, and Questioned Document Examination

Along with Statistical Data, a Glossary of Forensics Terminology, and Listings of Sources for Further Help and Information

Edited by Annemarie S. Muth. 574 pages. 1999. 978-0-7808-0232-2.

"Given the expected widespread interest in its content and its easy to read style, this book is recommended for most public and all college and university libraries."

—E-Streams, Feb '01

"A wealth of information, useful statistics, references are up-to-date and extremely complete. This wonderful collection of data will help students who are interested in a career in any type of forensic field. It is a great resource for attorneys who need information about types of expert witnesses needed in a particular case. It also offers useful information for fiction and nonfiction writers whose work involves a crime. A fascinating compilation. All levels."

—CHOICE, Jan '00

"There are several items that make this book attractive to consumers who are seeking certain forensic data... This is a useful current source for those seeking general forensic medical answers."

—American Reference Books Annual, 2000

Gastrointestinal Diseases and Disorders Sourcebook, 2nd Edition

Basic Consumer Health Information about the Upper and Lower Gastrointestinal (GI) Tract, Including the Esophagus, Stomach, Intestines, Rectum, Liver, and Pancreas, with Facts about Gastroesophageal Reflux Disease, Gastritis, Hernias, Ulcers, Celiac Disease, Diverticulitis, Irritable Bowel Syndrome, Hemorrhoids, Gastrointestinal Cancers, and Other Diseases and Disorders Related to the Digestive Process

Along with Information about Commonly Used Diagnostic and Surgical Procedures, Statistics, Reports on Current Research Initiatives and Clinical Trials, a Glossary, and Resources for Additional Help and Information

Edited by Sandra J. Judd. 654 pages. 2006. 978-0-7808-0798-3.

"The text is designed for the general reader seeking information on prevention, disease warning signs, diagnostic and therapeutic questions... It is an excellent resource for the general reader to conveniently locate credible, coordinated and indexed information... The sourcebook will prove very helpful for patients, caregivers and should be available in every physician waiting room."

—Doody's Review Service, 2006

SEE ALSO *Diet and Nutrition Sourcebook, 3rd Edition, Digestive Diseases and Disorders Sourcebook*

Genetic Disorders Sourcebook, 4th Edition

Basic Consumer Health Information about Hereditary Diseases and Disorders, Including Facts about the Human Genome, Genetic Inheritance Patterns, Disorders Associated with Specific Genes, Such as Sickle Cell Disease, Hemophilia, and Cystic Fibrosis, Chromosome Disorders, Such as Down Syndrome, Fragile X Syndrome, and Turner Syndrome, and Complex Diseases and Disorders Resulting from the Interaction of Environmental and Genetic Factors, Such as Allergies, Cancer, and Obesity

Along with Facts about Genetic Testing, Suggestions for Parents of Children with Special Needs, Reports on Current Research Initiatives, a Glossary of Genetic Terminology, and Resources for Additional Help and Information

Edited by Sandra J. Judd. 600 pages. 2010. 978-0-7808-1076-1.

Head Trauma Sourcebook

Basic Information for the Layperson about Open-Head and Closed-Head Injuries, Treatment Advances, Recovery, and Rehabilitation

Along with Reports on Current Research Initiatives

Edited by Karen Bellenir. 414 pages. 1997. 978-0-7808-0208-7.

Headache Sourcebook

Basic Consumer Health Information about Migraine, Tension, Cluster, Rebound and Other Types of Headaches, with Facts about the Cause and Prevention of Headaches, the Effects of Stress and the Environment, Headaches during Pregnancy and Menopause, and Childhood Headaches

Along with a Glossary and Other Resources for Additional Help and Information

Edited by Dawn D. Matthews. 342 pages. 2002. 978-0-7808-0337-4.

"Highly recommended for academic and medical reference collections."

—Library Bookwatch, Sep '02

SEE ALSO *Pain Sourcebook, 3rd Edition*

Healthy Aging Sourcebook

Basic Consumer Health Information about Maintaining Health through the Aging Process, Including Advice on Nutrition, Exercise, and Sleep, Help in Making Decisions about Midlife Issues and Retirement, and Guidance Concerning Practical and Informed Choices in Health Consumerism

Along with Data Concerning the Theories of Aging, Different Experiences in Aging by Minority Groups, and Facts about Aging Now and Aging in the Future; and Featuring a Glossary, a Guide to Consumer Help, Additional Suggested Reading, and Practical Resource Directory

Edited by Jenifer Swanson. 537 pages. 1999. 978-0-7808-0390-9.

"Recommended reference source."

—Booklist, Feb '00

SEE ALSO *Adult Health Sourcebook, Physical and Mental Issues in Aging Sourcebook*

Healthy Children Sourcebook

Basic Consumer Health Information about the Physical and Mental Development of Children between the Ages of 3 and 12, Including Routine Health Care, Preventative Health Services, Safety and First Aid, Healthy Sleep, Dental Care, Nutrition, and Fitness, and Featuring Parenting Tips on Such Topics as Bedwetting, Choosing Day Care, Monitoring TV and Other Media, and Establishing a Foundation for Substance Abuse Prevention

Along with a Glossary of Commonly Used Pediatric Terms and Resources for Additional Help and Information.

Edited by Chad T. Kimball. 624 pages. 2003. 978-0-7808-0247-6.

"Should be required reading for parents and teachers."

—*E-Streams, Jun '04*

"It is hard to imagine that any other single resource exists that would provide such a comprehensive guide of timely information on health promotion and disease prevention for children aged 3 to 12."

—*American Reference Books Annual, 2004*

"This easy-to-read volume is a tremendous resource."

—*AORN Journal, May '05*

SEE ALSO *Childhood Diseases and Disorders Sourcebook, 2nd Edition*

Healthy Heart Sourcebook for Women

Basic Consumer Health Information about Cardiac Issues Specific to Women, Including Facts about Major Risk Factors and Prevention, Treatment and Control Strategies, and Important Dietary Issues

Along with a Special Section Regarding the Pros and Cons of Hormone Replacement Therapy and Its Impact on Heart Health, and Additional Help, Including Recipes, a Glossary, and a Directory of Resources

Edited by Dawn D. Matthews. 321 pages. 2000. 978-0-7808-0329-9.

"A good reference source and recommended for all public, academic, medical, and hospital libraries."

—*Medical Reference Services Quarterly, Summer '01*

"Contains very important information about coronary artery disease that all women should know. The information is current and presented in an easy-to-read format. The book will make a good addition to any library."

—*American Medical Writers Association Journal, Summer '00*

SEE ALSO *Cardiovascular Diseases and Disorders Sourcebook, 4th Edition, Women's Health Concerns Sourcebook, 3rd Edition*

Hepatitis Sourcebook

Basic Consumer Health Information about Hepatitis A, Hepatitis B, Hepatitis C, and Other Forms of Hepatitis, Including Autoimmune Hepatitis, Alcoholic Hepatitis, Nonalcoholic Steatohepatitis, and Toxic Hepatitis, with Facts about Risk Factors, Screening Methods, Diagnostic Tests, and Treatment Options

Along with Information on Liver Health, Tips for People Living with Chronic Hepatitis, Reports on Current Research Initiatives, a Glossary of Terms Related to Hepatitis, and a Directory of Sources for Further Help and Information

Edited by Sandra J. Judd. 570 pages. 2006. 978-0-7808-0749-5.

"The breadth of information found in this one book would not be readily found in another source. Highly recommended."

—*American Reference Books Annual, 2006*

SEE ALSO *Contagious Diseases Sourcebook, 2nd Edition*

Household Safety Sourcebook

Basic Consumer Health Information about Household Safety, Including Information about Poisons, Chemicals, Fire, and Water Hazards in the Home

Along with Advice about the Safe Use of Home Maintenance Equipment, Choosing Toys and Nursery Furniture, Holiday and Recreation Safety, a Glossary, and Resources for Further Help and Information

Edited by Dawn D. Matthews. 587 pages. 2002. 978-0-7808-0338-1.

"As a sourcebook on household safety this book meets its mark. It is encyclopedic in scope and covers a wide range of safety issues that are commonly seen in the home."

—*E-Streams, Jul '02*

Hypertension Sourcebook

Basic Consumer Health Information about the Causes, Diagnosis, and Treatment of High Blood Pressure, with Facts about Consequences, Complications, and Co-Occurring Disorders, Such as Coronary Heart Disease, Diabetes, Stroke, Kidney Disease, and Hypertensive Retinopathy, and Issues in Blood Pressure

Control, Including Dietary Choices, Stress Management, and Medications

Along with Reports on Current Research Initiatives and Clinical Trials, a Glossary, and Resources for Additional Help and Information

Edited by Dawn D. Matthews and Karen Bellenir. 588 pages. 2004. 978-0-7808-0674-0.

"Academic, public, and medical libraries will want to add the Hypertension Sourcebook to their collections."

—*E-Streams, Aug '05*

"The strength of this source is the wide range of information given about hypertension."

—*American Reference Books Annual, 2005*

SEE ALSO *Stroke Sourcebook, 2nd Edition*

Immune System Disorders Sourcebook, 2nd Edition

Basic Consumer Health Information about Disorders of the Immune System, Including Immune System Function and Response, Diagnosis of Immune Disorders, Information about Inherited Immune Disease, Acquired Immune Disease, and Autoimmune Diseases, Including Primary Immune Deficiency, Acquired Immunodeficiency Syndrome (AIDS), Lupus, Multiple Sclerosis, Type 1 Diabetes, Rheumatoid Arthritis, and Graves' Disease

Along with Treatments, Tips for Coping with Immune Disorders, a Glossary, and a Directory of Additional Resources

Edited by Joyce Brennfleck Shannon. 643 pages. 2005. 978-0-7808-0748-8.

"Highly recommended for academic and public libraries."

—*American Reference Books Annual, 2006*

"The updated second edition is a 'must' for any consumer health library seeking a solid resource covering the treatments, symptoms, and options for immune disorder sufferers... An excellent guide."

—*MBR Bookwatch, Jan '06*

SEE ALSO *AIDS Sourcebook, 4th Edition, Arthritis Sourcebook, 3rd Edition*

Infant and Toddler Health Sourcebook

Basic Consumer Health Information about the Physical and Mental Development of Newborns, Infants, and Toddlers, Including Neonatal Concerns, Nutrition Recommendations, Immunization Schedules, Common Pediatric Disorders, Assessments and Milestones, Safety Tips, and Advice for Parents and Other Caregivers

Along with a Glossary of Terms and Resource Listings for Additional Help

Edited by Jenifer Swanson. 570 pages. 2000. 978-0-7808-0246-9.

"As a reference for the general public, this would be useful in any library."

—*E-Streams, May '01*

"Recommended reference source."

—*Booklist, Feb '01*

Infectious Diseases Sourcebook

Basic Consumer Health Information about Non-Contagious Bacterial, Viral, Prion, Fungal, and Parasitic Diseases Spread by Food and Water, Insects and Animals, or Environmental Contact, Including Botulism, E. Coli, Encephalitis, Legionnaires' Disease, Lyme Disease, Malaria, Plague, Rabies, Salmonella, Tetanus, and Others, and Facts about Newly Emerging Diseases, Such as Hantavirus, Mad Cow Disease, Monkeypox, and West Nile Virus

Along with Information about Preventing Disease Transmission, the Threat of Bioterrorism, and Current Research Initiatives, with a Glossary and Directory of Resources for More Information

Edited by Karen Bellenir. 610 pages. 2004. 978-0-7808-0675-7.

"This reference continues the excellent tradition of the Health Reference Series in consolidating a wealth of information on a selected topic into a format that is easy to use and accessible to the general public."

—*American Reference Books Annual, 2005*

"Recommended for public and academic libraries."

—*E-Streams, Jan '05*

SEE ALSO Environmental Health Sourcebook, 3rd Edition

Injury and Trauma Sourcebook

Basic Consumer Health Information about the Impact of Injury, the Diagnosis and Treatment of Common and Traumatic Injuries, Emergency Care, and Specific Injuries Related to Home, Community, Workplace, Transportation, and Recreation

Along with Guidelines for Injury Prevention, a Glossary, and a Directory of Additional Resources

Edited by Joyce Brennfleck Shannon. 675 pages. 2002. 978-0-7808-0421-0.

"Practitioners should be aware of guides such as this in order to facilitate their use by patients and their families."

—*Doody's Health Sciences Book Review Journal, Sep-Oct '02*

"Recommended reference source."

—*Booklist, Sep '02*

"Highly recommended for academic and medical reference collections."

—*Library Bookwatch, Sep '02*

SEE ALSO *Emergency Medical Services Sourcebook, Sports Injuries Sourcebook, 3rd Edition*

Learning Disabilities Sourcebook, 3rd Edition

Basic Consumer Health Information about Dyslexia, Auditory and Visual Processing Disorders, Communication Disorders, Dyscalculia, Dysgraphia, and Other Conditions That Impede Learning, Including Attention Deficit/Hyperactivity Disorder, Autism Spectrum Disorders, Hearing and Visual Impairments, Chromosome-Based Disorders, and Brain Injury

Along with Facts about Brain Function, Assessment, Therapy and Remediation, Accommodations, Assistive Technology, Legal Protections, and Tips about Family Life, School Transitions, and Employment Strategies, a Glossary of Related Terms, and Directories of Additional Resources

Edited by Joyce Brennfleck Shannon. 613 pages. 2009. 978-0-7808-1039-6.

"Intended to be a starting point for people who need to know about learning disabilities. Each chapter on a specific disability includes readable, well-organized descriptions... The book is well indexed and a glossary is included. Chapters on organizations and helpful websites will aid the reader who needs more information."

—*American Reference Books Annual, 2009*

"This book provides the necessary information to better understand learning disabilities and work with children who have them... It would be difficult to find another book that so comprehensively explains learning disabilities without becoming incomprehensible to the average parent who needs this information."

—*Doody's Review Service, 2009*

SEE ALSO *Attention Deficit Disorder Sourcebook, Autism and Pervasive Developmental Disorders Sourcebook*

Leukemia Sourcebook

Basic Consumer Health Information about Adult and Childhood Leukemias, Including Acute Lymphocytic Leukemia (ALL), Chronic Lymphocytic Leukemia (CLL), Acute Myelogenous Leukemia (AML), Chronic Myelogenous Leukemia (CML), and Hairy Cell Leukemia, and Treatments Such as Chemotherapy, Radiation Therapy, Peripheral Blood Stem Cell and Marrow Transplantation, and Immunotherapy

Along with Tips for Life During and After Treatment, a Glossary, and Directories of Additional Resources

Edited by Joyce Brennfleck Shannon. 564 pages. 2003. 978-0-7808-0627-6.

"Unlike other medical books for the layperson... the language does not talk down to the reader... This volume is highly recommended for all libraries."

—*American Reference Books Annual, 2004*

"A fine title which ranges from diagnosis to alternative treatments, staging, and tips for life during and after diagnosis."

—*The Bookwatch, Dec '03*

SEE ALSO *Blood & Circulatory Disorders Sourcebook, 3rd Edition, Cancer Sourcebook, 5th Edition*

Liver Disorders Sourcebook

Basic Consumer Health Information about the Liver and How It Works; Liver Diseases, Including Cancer, Cirrhosis, Hepatitis, and

Toxic and Drug Related Diseases; Tips for Maintaining a Healthy Liver; Laboratory Tests, Radiology Tests, and Facts about Liver Transplantation

Along with a Section on Support Groups, a Glossary, and Resource Listings

Edited by Joyce Brennfleck Shannon. 580 pages. 2000. 978-0-7808-0383-1.

"This title is recommended for health sciences and public libraries with consumer health collections."

—*E-Streams, Oct '00*

"Recommended reference source."

—*Booklist, Jun '00*

SEE ALSO *Gastrointestinal Diseases and Disorders Sourcebook, 2nd Edition, Hepatitis Sourcebook*

Lung Disorders Sourcebook

Basic Consumer Health Information about Emphysema, Pneumonia, Tuberculosis, Asthma, Cystic Fibrosis, and Other Lung Disorders, Including Facts about Diagnostic Procedures, Treatment Strategies, Disease Prevention Efforts, and Such Risk Factors as Smoking, Air Pollution, and Exposure to Asbestos, Radon, and Other Agents

Along with a Glossary and Resources for Additional Help and Information

Edited by Dawn D. Matthews. 657 pages. 2002. 978-0-7808-0339-8.

"Highly recommended for academic and medical reference collections."

—*Library Bookwatch, Sep '02*

SEE ALSO *Asthma Sourcebook, 2nd Edition, Respiratory Disorders Sourcebook, 2nd Edition*

Medical Tests Sourcebook, 3rd Edition

Basic Consumer Health Information about X-Rays, Blood Tests, Stool and Urine Tests, Biopsies, Mammography, Endoscopic Procedures, Ultrasound Exams, Computed Tomography, Magnetic Resonance Imaging (MRI), Nuclear Medicine, Genetic Testing, Home-Use Tests, and More

Along with Facts about Preventive Care and Screening Test Guidelines, Screening and Assessment Tests Associated with Such Specific Concerns as Cancer, Heart Disease, Allergies, Diabetes, Thyroid Disfunction, and Infertility, a Glossary of Related Terms, and a Directory of Resources for Additional Help and Information

Edited by Karen Bellenir. 627 pages. 2008. 978-0-7808-1040-2

"This volume has a wide scope that makes it useful... Can be a valuable reference guide."

—*American Reference Books Annual, 2009*

"Would be a valuable contribution to any consumer health or public library."

—*Doody's Book Review Service, 2009*

Men's Health Concerns Sourcebook, 3rd Edition

Basic Consumer Health Information about Wellness in Men and Gender-Related Differences in Health, With Facts about Heart Disease, Cancer, Traumatic Injury, and Other Leading Causes of Death in Men, Reproductive Concerns, Sexual Dysfunction, Disorders of the Prostate, Penis, and Testes, Sex-Linked Genetic Disorders, and Other Medical and Mental Concerns of Men

Along with Statistical Data, a Glossary of Related Terms, and a Directory of Resources for Additional Information

Edited by Sandra J. Judd. 632 pages. 2009. 978-0-7808-1033-4.

"A good addition to any reference shelf in academic, consumer health, or hospital libraries."

—*ARBAOnline, Oct '09*

SEE ALSO *Prostate and Urological Disorders Sourcebook*

Mental Health Disorders Sourcebook, 4th Edition

Basic Consumer Health Information about the Causes and Symptoms of Mental Health Problems, Including Depression, Bipolar Disorder, Anxiety Disorders, Posttraumatic Stress Disorder, Obsessive-Compulsive Disorder, Eating Disorders, Addictions, and Personality and Psychotic Disorders

Along with Information about Medications and Treatments, Mental Health Concerns in

Children, Adolescents, and Adults, Tips on Living with Mental Health Disorders, a Glossary of Related Terms, and a Directory of Resources for Additional Help and Information

Edited by Amy L. Sutton. 680 pages. 2009. 978-0-7808-1041-9.

"Mental health concerns are presented in everyday language and intended for patients and their families as well as the general public... This resource is comprehensive and up to date... The easy-to-understand writing style helps to facilitate assimilation of needed facts and specifics on often challenging topics."

—*ARBAOnline, Oct '09*

"No health collection should be without this resource, which will reach into many a general lending library as well."

—*Internet Bookwatch, Oct '09*

SEE ALSO *Depression Sourcebook, 2nd Edition, Stress-Related Disorders Sourcebook, 2nd Edition*

Mental Retardation Sourcebook

Basic Consumer Health Information about Mental Retardation and Its Causes, Including Down Syndrome, Fetal Alcohol Syndrome, Fragile X Syndrome, Genetic Conditions, Injury, and Environmental Sources

Along with Preventive Strategies, Parenting Issues, Educational Implications, Health Care Needs, Employment and Economic Matters, Legal Issues, a Glossary, and a Resource Listing for Additional Help and Information

Edited by Joyce Brennfleck Shannon. 627 pages. 2000. 978-0-7808-0377-0.

"Public libraries will find the book useful for reference and as a beginning research point for students, parents, and caregivers."

—*American Reference Books Annual, 2001*

"The strength of this work is that it compiles many basic fact sheets and addresses for further information in one volume. It is intended and suitable for the general public."

—*E-Streams, Nov '00*

"An invaluable overview."

—*Reviewer's Bookwatch, Jul '00*

Movement Disorders Sourcebook, 2nd Edition

Basic Consumer Health Information about the Symptoms and Causes of Movement Disorders, Including Parkinson Disease, Amyotrophic Lateral Sclerosis, Cerebral Palsy, Muscular Dystrophy, Multiple Sclerosis, Myasthenia, Myoclonus, Spina Bifida, Dystonia, Essential Tremor, Choreatic Disorders, Huntington Disease, Tourette Syndrome, and Other Disorders That Cause Slowed, Absent, or Excessive Movements

Along with Information about Surgical and Nonsurgical Interventions, Physical Therapies, Strategies for Independent Living, a Glossary of Related Terms, and a Directory of Resources for Additional Help and Information

Edited by Amy L. Sutton. 618 pages. 2009. 978-0-7808-1034-1.

"The second updated edition of Movement Disorders Sourcebook is a winner, providing the latest research and health findings on all kinds of movement disorders in children and adults... a top pick for any health or general lending library's health reference collection."

—*California Bookwatch, Aug '09*

SEE ALSO *Muscular Dystrophy Sourcebook*

Multiple Sclerosis Sourcebook

Basic Consumer Health Information about Multiple Sclerosis (MS) and Its Effects on Mobility, Vision, Bladder Function, Speech, Swallowing, and Cognition, Including Facts about Risk Factors, Causes, Diagnostic Procedures, Pain Management, Drug Treatments, and Physical and Occupational Therapies

Along with Guidelines for Nutrition and Exercise, Tips on Choosing Assistive Equipment, Information about Disability, Work, Financial, and Legal Issues, a Glossary of Related Terms, and a Directory of Additional Resources

Edited by Joyce Brennfleck Shannon. 553 pages. 2007. 978-0-7808-0998-7.

Muscular Dystrophy Sourcebook

Basic Consumer Health Information about Congenital, Childhood-Onset, and Adult-Onset

Forms of Muscular Dystrophy, Such as Duchenne, Becker, Emery-Dreifuss, Distal, Limb-Girdle, Facioscapulohumeral (FSHD), Myotonic, and Ophthalmoplegic Muscular Dystrophies, Including Facts about Diagnostic Tests, Medical and Physical Therapies, Management of Co-Occurring Conditions, and Parenting Guidelines

Along with Practical Tips for Home Care, a Glossary, and Directories of Additional Resources

Edited by Joyce Brennfleck Shannon. 552 pages. 2004. 978-0-7808-0676-4.

"This book is highly recommended for public and academic libraries as well as health care offices that support the information needs of patients and their families."

—*E-Streams, Apr '05*

"Excellent reference."

—*The Bookwatch, Jan '05*

SEE ALSO *Movement Disorders Sourcebook, 2nd Edition*

Obesity Sourcebook

Basic Consumer Health Information about Diseases and Other Problems Associated with Obesity, and Including Facts about Risk Factors, Prevention Issues, and Management Approaches

Along with Statistical and Demographic Data, Information about Special Populations, Research Updates, a Glossary, and Source Listings for Further Help and Information

Edited by Wilma Caldwell and Chad T. Kimball. 360 pages. 2001. 978-0-7808-0333-6.

"The book synthesizes the reliable medical literature on obesity into one easy-to-read and useful resource for the general public."

—*American Reference Books Annual, 2002*

"Well suited for the health reference collection of a public library or an academic health science library that serves the general population."

—*E-Streams, Sep '01*

Osteoporosis Sourcebook

Basic Consumer Health Information about Primary and Secondary Osteoporosis and Juvenile Osteoporosis and Related Conditions, Including Fibrous Dysplasia, Gaucher Disease, Hyperthyroidism, Hypophosphatasia, Myeloma, Osteopetrosis, Osteogenesis Imperfecta, and Paget's Disease

Along with Information about Risk Factors, Treatments, Traditional and Non-Traditional Pain Management, a Glossary of Related Terms, and a Directory of Resources

Edited by Allan R. Cook. 568 pages. 2001. 978-0-7808-0239-1.

"This resource is recommended as a great reference source for public, health, and academic libraries, and is another triumph for the editors of Omnigraphics."

—*American Reference Books Annual, 2002*

"Will prove valuable to any library seeking to maintain a current, comprehensive reference collection of health resources... From prevention to treatment and associated conditions, this provides an excellent survey."

—*The Bookwatch, Aug '01*

SEE ALSO *Healthy Aging Sourcebook, Women's Health Concerns Sourcebook, 3rd Edition*

Pain Sourcebook, 3rd Edition

Basic Consumer Health Information about Acute and Chronic Pain, Including Nerve Pain, Bone Pain, Muscle Pain, Cancer Pain, and Disorders Characterized by Pain, Such as Arthritis, Temporomandibular Muscle and Joint (TMJ) Disorder, Carpal Tunnel Syndrome, Headaches, Heartburn, Sciatica, and Shingles, and Facts about Diagnostic Tests and Treatment Options for Pain, Including Over-the-Counter and Prescription Drugs, Physical Rehabilitation, Injection and Infusion Therapies, Implantable Technologies, and Complementary Medicine

Along with Tips for Living with Pain, a Glossary of Related Terms, and a Directory of Additional Resources

Edited by Joyce Brennfleck Shannon. 644 pages. 2008. 978-0-7808-1006-8.

"Excellent for ready-reference users and can be used for beginning students in health fields... appropriate for the consumer health collection in both public and academic libraries."

—*American Reference Books Annual, 2009*

SEE ALSO Arthritis Sourcebook, 3rd Edition; Back and Neck Sourcebook, 2nd Edition;

Headache Sourcebook; Sports Injuries Sourcebook, 3rd Edition

Pediatric Cancer Sourcebook

Basic Consumer Health Information about Leukemias, Brain Tumors, Sarcomas, Lymphomas, and Other Cancers in Infants, Children, and Adolescents, Including Descriptions of Cancers, Treatments, and Coping Strategies

Along with Suggestions for Parents, Caregivers, and Concerned Relatives, a Glossary of Cancer Terms, and Resource Listings

Edited by Edward J. Prucha. 575 pages. 1999. 978-0-7808-0245-2.

"An excellent source of information. Recommended for public, hospital, and health science libraries with consumer health collections."
—*E-Streams, Jun '00*

"A valuable addition to all libraries specializing in health services and many public libraries."
—*American Reference Books Annual, 2000*

SEE ALSO *Childhood Diseases and Disorders Sourcebook, 2nd Edition, Healthy Children Sourcebook*

Physical and Mental Issues in Aging Sourcebook

Basic Consumer Health Information on Physical and Mental Disorders Associated with the Aging Process, Including Concerns about Cardiovascular Disease, Pulmonary Disease, Oral Health, Digestive Disorders, Musculoskeletal and Skin Disorders, Metabolic Changes, Sexual and Reproductive Issues, and Changes in Vision, Hearing, and Other Senses

Along with Data about Longevity and Causes of Death, Information on Acute and Chronic Pain, Descriptions of Mental Concerns, a Glossary of Terms, and Resource Listings for Additional Help

Edited by Jenifer Swanson. 660 pages. 1999. 978-0-7808-0233-9.

"This is a treasure of health information for the layperson."
—*CHOICE Health Sciences Supplement, May '00*

"Recommended for public libraries."
—*American Reference Books Annual, 2000*

SEE ALSO *Healthy Aging Sourcebook*

Podiatry Sourcebook, 2nd Edition

Basic Consumer Health Information about Disorders, Diseases, and Deformities that Affect the Foot and Ankle, Including Sprains, Corns, Calluses, Bunions, Plantar Warts, Plantar Fasciitis, Neuromas, Clubfoot, Flat Feet, Achilles Tendonitis, and Much More

Along with Information about Selecting a Foot Care Specialist, Foot Fitness, Shoes and Socks, Diagnostic Tests and Corrective Procedures, Financial Assistance for Corrective Devices, a Glossary of Related Terms, and a Directory of Resources for Additional Help and Information

Edited by Ivy L. Alexander. 516 pages. 2007. 978-0-7808-0944-4.

"An excellent resource... Although there have been various types of 'foot books' published in the past, none are as comprehensive as this one. 5 Stars (out of 5)!"
—*Doody's Review Service, 2007*

"Perfect for both health libraries and general-interest lending collections."
—*Internet Bookwatch, Jul '07*

Pregnancy and Birth Sourcebook, 3rd Edition

Basic Consumer Health Information about Pregnancy and Fetal Development, Including Facts about Fertility and Conception, Physical and Emotional Changes during Pregnancy, Prenatal Care and Diagnostic Tests, High-Risk Pregnancies and Complications, Labor, Delivery, and the Postpartum Period

Along with Tips on Maintaining Health and Wellness during Pregnancy and Caring for Newborn Infants, a Glossary of Related Terms, and Directories of Resources for Additional Help and Information

Edited by Amy L. Sutton. 645 pages. 2009. 978-0-7808-1074-7.

SEE ALSO *Breastfeeding Sourcebook, Congenital Disorders Sourcebook, 2nd Edition, Family Planning Sourcebook, Women's Health Concerns Sourcebook, 3rd Edition*

Prostate and Urological Disorders Sourcebook

Basic Consumer Health Information about Urogenital and Sexual Disorders in Men, Including Prostate and Other Andrological Cancers, Prostatitis, Benign Prostatic Hyperplasia, Testicular and Penile Trauma, Cryptorchidism, Peyronie Disease, Erectile Dysfunction, and Male Factor Infertility, and Facts about Commonly Used Tests and Procedures, Such as Prostatectomy, Vasectomy, Vasectomy Reversal, Penile Implants, and Semen Analysis

Along with a Glossary of Andrological Terms and a Directory of Resources for Additional Information

Edited by Karen Bellenir. 604 pages. 2006. 978-0-7808-0797-6.

"Certain to be a popular pick among library reference holdings... No prior knowledge is assumed for any of the conditions or terms herein, making it a most accessible general-interest reference."

—*California Bookwatch, Apr '06*

SEE ALSO *Men's Health Concerns Sourcebook, 3rd Edition, Urinary Tract and Kidney Diseases and Disorders Sourcebook, 2nd Edition*

Prostate Cancer Sourcebook

Basic Consumer Health Information about Prostate Cancer, Including Information about the Associated Risk Factors, Detection, Diagnosis, and Treatment of Prostate Cancer

Along with Information on Non-Malignant Prostate Conditions, and Featuring a Section Listing Support and Treatment Centers and a Glossary of Related Terms

Edited by Dawn D. Matthews. 340 pages. 2001. 978-0-7808-0324-4.

"Recommended reference source."

—*Booklist, Jan '02*

"A valuable resource for health care consumers seeking information on the subject... All text is written in a clear, easy-to-understand language that avoids technical jargon. Any library that collects consumer health resources would strengthen their collection with the addition of the Prostate Cancer Sourcebook."

—*American Reference Books Annual, 2002*

SEE ALSO *Cancer Sourcebook, 5th Edition, Men's Health Concerns Sourcebook, 3rd Edition*

Rehabilitation Sourcebook

Basic Consumer Health Information about Rehabilitation for People Recovering from Heart Surgery, Spinal Cord Injury, Stroke, Orthopedic Impairments, Amputation, Pulmonary Impairments, Traumatic Injury, and More, Including Physical Therapy, Occupational Therapy, Speech/Language Therapy, Massage Therapy, Dance Therapy, Art Therapy, and Recreational Therapy

Along with Information on Assistive and Adaptive Devices, a Glossary, and Resources for Additional Help and Information

Edited by Dawn D. Matthews. 519 pages. 2000. 978-0-7808-0236-0.

"This is an excellent resource for public library reference and health collections."

—*American Reference Books Annual, 2001*

"Recommended reference source."

—*Booklist, May '00*

Respiratory Disorders Sourcebook, 2nd Edition

Basic Consumer Health Information about Infectious, Inflammatory, and Chronic Conditions Affecting the Lungs and Respiratory System, Including Pneumonia, Bronchitis, Influenza, Tuberculosis, Sarcoidosis, Asthma, Cystic Fibrosis, Chronic Obstructive Pulmonary Disease, Lung Abscesses, Pulmonary Embolism, Occupational Lung Diseases, and Other Bacterial, Viral, and Fungal Infections

Along with Facts about the Structure and Function of the Lungs and Airways, Methods of Diagnosing Respiratory Disorders, and Treatment and Rehabilitation Options, a Glossary of Related Terms, and a Directory of Resources for Additional Help and Information

Edited by Sandra L. Judd. 638 pages. 2008. 978-0-7808-1007-5.

"An excellent book for patients, their families, or for those who are just curious about respiratory disease. Public libraries and physician offices would find this a valuable resource as well. 4 Stars! (out of 5)"

—*Doody's Review Service, 2009*

"A great addition for public and school libraries because it provides concise health information... readers can start with this reference source and get satisfactory answers before proceeding to other medical reference tools for

more in depth information... A good guide for health education on lung disorders."

—*American Reference Books Annual, 2009*

SEE ALSO *Asthma Sourcebook, 2nd Edition, Lung Disorders Sourcebook*

Sexually Transmitted Diseases Sourcebook, 4th Edition

Basic Consumer Health Information about Chlamydial Infections, Gonorrhea, Hepatitis, Herpes, HIV/AIDS, Human Papillomavirus, Pubic Lice, Scabies, Syphilis, Trichomoniasis, Vaginal Infections, and Other Sexually Transmitted Diseases, Including Facts about Risk Factors, Symptoms, Diagnosis, Treatment, and the Prevention of Sexually Transmitted Infections

Along with Updates on Current Research Initiatives, a Glossary of Related Terms, and Resources for Additional Help and Information

Edited by Laura Larsen. 623 pages. 2009. 978-0-7808-1073-0.

"Extremely beneficial... The question-and-answer format along with the index and table of contents make this well-organized resource extremely easy to reference, read, and comprehend... an invaluable medical reference source for lay readers, and a highly appropriate addition for public library collections, health clinics, and any library with a consumer health collection"

—*ARBAOnline, Oct '09*

SEE ALSO *AIDS Sourcebook, 4th Edition, Contagious Diseases Sourcebook, 2nd Edition, Men's Health Concerns Sourcebook, 3rd Edition, Women's Health Concerns Sourcebook, 3rd Edition*

Sleep Disorders Sourcebook, 3rd Edition

Basic Consumer Health Information about Sleep Disorders, Including Insomnia, Sleep Apnea and Snoring, Jet Lag and Other Circadian Rhythm Disorders, Narcolepsy, and Parasomnias, Such as Sleep Walking and Sleep Talking, and Featuring Facts about Other Health Problems that Affect Sleep, Why Sleep Is Necessary, How Much Sleep Is Needed, the Physical and Mental Effects of Sleep Deprivation, and Pediatric Sleep Issues

Along with Tips for Diagnosing and Treating Sleep Disorders, a Glossary of Related Terms, and a List of Resources for Additional Help and Information

Edited by Sandra J. Judd. 600 pages. 2010. 978-0-7808-1084-6.

Smoking Concerns Sourcebook

Basic Consumer Health Information about Nicotine Addiction and Smoking Cessation, Featuring Facts about the Health Effects of Tobacco Use, Including Lung and Other Cancers, Heart Disease, Stroke, and Respiratory Disorders, Such as Emphysema and Chronic Bronchitis

Along with Information about Smoking Prevention Programs, Suggestions for Achieving and Maintaining a Smoke-Free Lifestyle, Statistics about Tobacco Use, Reports on Current Research Initiatives, a Glossary of Related Terms, and Directories of Resources for Additional Help and Information

Edited by Karen Bellenir. 595 pages. 2004. 978-0-7808-0323-7.

"Provides everything needed for the student or general reader seeking practical details on the effects of tobacco use."

—*The Bookwatch, Mar '05*

"Public libraries and consumer health care libraries will find this work useful."

—*American Reference Books Annual, 2005*

SEE ALSO *Respiratory Disorders Sourcebook, 2nd Edition*

Sports Injuries Sourcebook, 3rd Edition

Basic Consumer Health Information about Sprains and Strains, Fractures, Growth Plate Injuries, Overtraining Injuries, and Injuries to the Head, Face, Shoulders, Elbows, Hands, Spinal Column, Knees, Ankles, and Feet, and with Facts about Heat-Related Illness, Steroids and Sport Supplements, Protective Equipment, Diagnostic Procedures, Treatment Options, and Rehabilitation

Along with a Glossary of Related Terms and a Directory of Resources for Additional Help and Information

Edited by Sandra J. Judd. 623 pages. 2007. 978-0-7808-0949-9.

SEE ALSO *Fitness and Exercise Sourcebook, 3rd Edition, Podiatry Sourcebook, 2nd Edition*

Stress-Related Disorders Sourcebook, 2nd Edition

Basic Consumer Health Information about Stress and Stress-Related Disorders, Including Types of Stress, Sources of Acute and Chronic Stress, the Impact of Stress on the Body's Systems, and Mental and Emotional Health Problems Associated with Stress, Such as Depression, Anxiety Disorders, Substance Abuse, Posttraumatic Stress Disorder, and Suicide

Along with Advice about Getting Help for Stress-Related Disorders, Information about Stress Management Techniques, a Glossary of Stress-Related Terms, and a Directory of Resources for Additional Help and Information

Edited by Amy L. Sutton. 608 pages. 2007. 978-0-7808-0996-3.

"Accessible to the lay reader. Highly recommended for medical and psychiatric collections."

—*Library Journal, Mar '08*

"Well-written for a general readership, the 2nd Edition of Stress-Related Disorders Sourcebook is a useful addition to the health reference literature."

—*American Reference Books Annual, 2008*

SEE ALSO *Mental Health Disorders Sourcebook, 4th Edition*

Stroke Sourcebook, 2nd Edition

Basic Consumer Health Information about Stroke, Including Ischemic, Hemorrhagic, and Mini Strokes, as Well as Risk Factors, Prevention Guidelines, Diagnostic Tests, Medications and Surgical Treatments, and Complications of Stroke

Along with Rehabilitation Techniques and Innovations, Tips on Staying Healthy and Maintaining Independence after Stroke, a Glossary of Related Terms, and a Directory of Resources for Stroke Survivors and Their Families

Edited by Amy L. Sutton. 626 pages. 2008. 978-0-7808-1035-8.

"An encyclopedic handbook on stroke that is written in a language the layperson can understand... This is one of the most helpful, readable books on stroke. This volume is highly recommended and should be in every medical, hospital and public library; in addition, every family practitioner should have a copy in his or her office."

—*American Reference Books Annual, 2009*

SEE ALSO *Brain Disorders Sourcebook, 3rd Edition, Hypertension Sourcebook*

Surgery Sourcebook, 2nd Edition

Basic Consumer Health Information about Common Inpatient and Outpatient Surgeries, Including Critical Care and Trauma, Gastrointestinal, Gynecologic and Obstetric, Cardiac and Vascular, Neurologic, Ophthalmologic, Orthopedic, Reconstructive and Cosmetic, and Other Major and Minor Surgeries

Along with Information about Anesthesia and Pain Relief Options, Risks and Complications, Postoperative Recovery Concerns, and Innovative Surgical Techniques and Tools, a Glossary of Related Terms, and a Directory of Additional Resources

Edited by Amy L. Sutton. 645 pages. 2008. 978-0-7808-1004-4.

"Large public libraries and medical libraries would benefit from this material in their reference collections."

—*American Reference Books Annual, 2009*

SEE ALSO *Cosmetic and Reconstructive Surgery Sourcebook, 2nd Edition*

Thyroid Disorders Sourcebook

Basic Consumer Health Information about Disorders of the Thyroid and Parathyroid Glands, Including Hypothyroidism, Hyperthyroidism, Graves Disease, Hashimoto Thyroiditis, Thyroid Cancer, and Parathyroid Disorders, Featuring Facts about Symptoms, Risk Factors, Tests, and Treatments

Along with Information about the Effects of Thyroid Imbalance on Other Body Systems, Environmental Factors That Affect the Thyroid Gland, a Glossary, and a Directory of Additional Resources

Edited by Joyce Brennfleck Shannon. 573 pages. 2005. 978-0-7808-0745-7.

"Recommended for consumer health collections."

—*American Reference Books Annual, 2006*

"Highly recommended pick for Basic Consumer health reference holdings at all levels."

—*The Bookwatch, Aug '05*

SEE ALSO *Endocrine and Metabolic Disorders Sourcebook, 2nd Edition*

Transplantation Sourcebook

Basic Consumer Health Information about Organ and Tissue Transplantation, Including Physical and Financial Preparations, Procedures and Issues Relating to Specific Solid Organ and Tissue Transplants, Rehabilitation, Pediatric Transplant Information, the Future of Transplantation, and Organ and Tissue Donation

Along with a Glossary and Listings of Additional Resources

Edited by Joyce Brennfleck Shannon. 610 pages. 2002. 978-0-7808-0322-0.

"Recommended for libraries with an interest in offering consumer health information."

—*E-Streams, Jul '02*

"This is a unique and valuable resource for patients facing transplantation and their families."

—*Doody's Review Service, Jun '02*

Traveler's Health Sourcebook

Basic Consumer Health Information for Travelers, Including Physical and Medical Preparations, Transportation Health and Safety, Essential Information about Food and Water, Sun Exposure, Insect and Snake Bites, Camping and Wilderness Medicine, and Travel with Physical or Medical Disabilities

Along with International Travel Tips, Vaccination Recommendations, Geographical Health Issues, Disease Risks, a Glossary, and a Listing of Additional Resources

Edited by Joyce Brennfleck Shannon. 619 pages. 2000. 978-0-7808-0384-8.

"Recommended reference source."

—*Booklist, Feb '01*

"This book is recommended for any public library, any travel collection, and especially any collection for the physically disabled."

—*American Reference Books Annual, 2001*

SEE ALSO *Worldwide Health Sourcebook*

Urinary Tract and Kidney Diseases and Disorders Sourcebook, 2nd Edition

Basic Consumer Health Information about the Urinary System, Including the Bladder, Urethra, Ureters, and Kidneys, with Facts about Urinary Tract Infections, Incontinence, Congenital Disorders, Kidney Stones, Cancers of the Urinary Tract and Kidneys, Kidney Failure, Dialysis, and Kidney Transplantation

Along with Statistical and Demographic Information, Reports on Current Research in Kidney and Urologic Health, a Summary of Commonly Used Diagnostic Tests, a Glossary of Related Terms, and a Directory of Resources for Additional Help and Information

Edited by Ivy L. Alexander. 621 pages. 2005. 978-0-7808-0750-1.

"A good choice for a consumer health information library or for a medical library needing information to refer to their patients."

—*American Reference Books Annual, 2006*

SEE ALSO *Prostate and Urological Disorders Sourcebook*

Vegetarian Sourcebook

Basic Consumer Health Information about Vegetarian Diets, Lifestyle, and Philosophy, Including Definitions of Vegetarianism and Veganism, Tips about Adopting Vegetarianism, Creating a Vegetarian Pantry, and Meeting Nutritional Needs of Vegetarians, with Facts Regarding Vegetarianism's Effect on Pregnant and Lactating Women, Children, Athletes, and Senior Citizens

Along with a Glossary of Commonly Used Vegetarian Terms and Resources for Additional Help and Information

Edited by Chad T. Kimball. 337 pages. 2002. 978-0-7808-0439-5.

"Organizes into one concise volume the answers to the most common questions concerning vegetarian diets and lifestyles. This title is recommended for public and secondary school libraries."

—*E-Streams, Apr '03*

"Invaluable reference for public and school library collections alike."

—*Library Bookwatch, Apr '03*

"The articles in this volume are easy to read and come from authoritative sources. The book does not necessarily support the vegetarian diet but instead provides the pros and cons of this important decision... Recommended for public libraries and consumer health libraries."

—*American Reference Books Annual, 2003*

SEE ALSO *Diet and Nutrition Sourcebook, 3rd Edition*

Women's Health Concerns Sourcebook, 3rd Edition

Basic Consumer Health Information about Issues and Trends in Women's Health and Health Conditions of Special Concern to Women, Including Endometriosis, Uterine Fibroids, Menstrual Irregularities, Menopause, Sexual Dysfunction, Infertility, Cancer in Women, and Other Such Chronic Disorders as Lupus, Fibromyalgia, and Thyroid Disease

Along with Statistical Data, Tips for Maintaining Wellness, a Glossary, and a Directory of Resources for Further Help and Information

Edited by Sandra J. Judd. 679 pages. 2009. 978-0-7808-1036-5.

"This useful resource provides information about a wide range of topics that will help women understand their bodies, prevent or treat disease, and maintain health... A detailed index helps readers locate information. This is a useful addition to public and consumer health library collections"

—*ARBAOnline, Jun '09*

SEE ALSO *Breast Cancer Sourcebook, 3rd Edition, Cancer Sourcebook for Women, 4th Edition, Healthy Heart Sourcebook for Women*

Workplace Health and Safety Sourcebook

Basic Consumer Health Information about Workplace Health and Safety, Including the Effect of Workplace Hazards on the Lungs, Skin, Heart, Ears, Eyes, Brain, Reproductive Organs, Musculoskeletal System, and Other Organs and Body Parts

Along with Information about Occupational Cancer, Personal Protective Equipment, Toxic and Hazardous Chemicals, Child Labor, Stress, and Workplace Violence

Edited by Chad T. Kimball. 610 pages. 2000. 978-0-7808-0231-5.

"As a reference for the general public, this would be useful in any library."

—*E-Streams, Jun '01*

"Provides helpful information for primary care physicians and other caregivers interested in occupational medicine... General readers; professionals."

—*CHOICE, May '01*

Worldwide Health Sourcebook

Basic Information about Global Health Issues, Including Malnutrition, Reproductive Health, Disease Dispersion and Prevention, Emerging Diseases, Risky Health Behaviors, and the Leading Causes of Death

Along with Global Health Concerns for Children, Women, and the Elderly, Mental Health Issues, Research and Technology Advancements, and Economic, Environmental, and Political Health Implications, a Glossary, and a Resource Listing for Additional Help and Information

Edited by Joyce Brennfleck Shannon. 597 pages. 2001. 978-0-7808-0330-5.

"Named an Outstanding Academic Title."

—*CHOICE, Jan '02*

"Yet another handy but also unique compilation in the extensive Health Reference Series, this is a useful work because many of the international publications reprinted or excerpted are not readily available. Highly recommended."

—*CHOICE, Nov '01*

SEE ALSO *Traveler's Health Sourcebook*

Teen Health Series

Complete Catalog

List price $69 per volume. School and library price $62 per volume.

Abuse and Violence Information for Teens

Health Tips about the Causes and Consequences of Abusive and Violent Behavior

Including Facts about the Types of Abuse and Violence, the Warning Signs of Abusive and Violent Behavior, Health Concerns of Victims, and Getting Help and Staying Safe

Edited by Sandra Augustyn Lawton. 411 pages. 2008. 978-0-7808-1008-2.

"A useful resource for schools and organizations providing services to teens and may also be a starting point in research projects."

—*Reference and Research Book News, Aug '08*

"Violence is a serious problem for teens... This resource gives teens the information they need to face potential threats and get help—either for themselves or for their friends."

—*American Reference Books Annual, 2009*

Accident and Safety Information for Teens

Health Tips about Medical Emergencies, Traumatic Injuries, and Disaster Preparedness

Including Facts about Motor Vehicle Accidents, Burns, Poisoning, Firearms, Natural Disasters, National Security Threats, and More

Edited by Karen Bellenir. 420 pages. 2008. 978-0-7808-1046-4.

"Aimed at teenage audiences, this guide provides practical information for handling a comprehensive list of emergencies, from sport injuries and auto accidents to alcohol poisoning and natural disasters."

—*Library Journal, Apr 1, '09*

"Useful in the young adult collections of public libraries as well as high school libraries."

—*American Reference Books Annual, 2009*

SEE ALSO *Sports Injuries Information for Teens, 2nd Edition*

Alcohol Information for Teens, 2nd Edition

Health Tips about Alcohol and Alcoholism

Including Facts about Alcohol's Effects on the Body, Brain, and Behavior, the Consequences of Underage Drinking, Alcohol Abuse Prevention and Treatment, and Coping with Alcoholic Parents

Edited by Lisa Bakewell. 410 pages. 2009. 978-0-7808-1043-3.

"This handbook, written for a teenage audience, provides information on the causes, effects, and preventive measures related to alcohol abuse among teens... The chapters are quick to make a connection to their teenage reading audience. The prose is straightforward and the book lends itself to spot reading. It should be useful both for practical information and for research, and it is suitable for public and school libraries."

—*ARBAOnline, Jun '09*

SEE ALSO *Drug Information for Teens, 2nd Edition*

Allergy Information for Teens

Health Tips about Allergic Reactions Such as Anaphylaxis, Respiratory Problems, and Rashes

Including Facts about Identifying and Managing Allergies to Food, Pollen, Mold, Animals, Chemicals, Drugs, and Other Substances

Edited by Karen Bellenir. 410 pages. 2006. 978-0-7808-0799-0.

"This is a comprehensive, readable text on the subject of allergic diseases in teenagers. 5 Stars (out of 5)!"

—*Doody's Review Service, Jun '06*

"This authoritative and useful self-help title is a solid addition to YA collections, whether for personal interest or reports."

—*School Library Journal, Jul '06*

Asthma Information for Teens, 2nd Ed.

Health Tips about Managing Asthma and Related Concerns

Including Facts about Asthma Causes, Triggers and Symptoms, Diagnosis, and Treatment

Edited by Kim Wohlenhaus. 400 pages. 2010. 978-0-7808-1086-0.

Body Information for Teens

Health Tips about Maintaining Well-Being for a Lifetime

Including Facts about the Development and Functioning of the Body's Systems, Organs, and Structures and the Health Impact of Lifestyle Choices

Edited by Sandra Augustyn Lawton. 458 pages. 2007. 978-0-7808-0443-2.

Cancer Information for Teens, 2nd Edition

Health Tips about Cancer Awareness, Symptoms, Prevention, Diagnosis, and Treatment

Including Facts about Common Cancers Affecting Teens, Causes, Detection, Coping Strategies, Clinical Trials, Nutrition and Exercise, Cancer in Friends or Family, and More

Edited by Karen Bellenir and Lisa Bakewell. 445 pages. 2010. 978-0-7808-1085-3.

Complementary and Alternative Medicine Information for Teens

Health Tips about Non-Traditional and Non-Western Medical Practices

Including Information about Acupuncture, Chiropractic Medicine, Dietary and Herbal Supplements, Hypnosis, Massage Therapy, Prayer and Spirituality, Reflexology, Yoga, and More

Edited by Sandra Augustyn Lawton. 407 pages. 2007. 978-0-7808-0966-6.

"This volume covers CAM specifically for teenagers but of general use also. It should be a welcome addition to both public and academic libraries."

—American Reference Books Annual, 2008

"This volume provides a solid foundation for further investigation of the subject, making it useful for both public and high school libraries."

—VOYA: Voice of Youth Advocates, Jun '07

Diabetes Information for Teens

Health Tips about Managing Diabetes and Preventing Related Complications

Including Information about Insulin, Glucose Control, Healthy Eating, Physical Activity, and Learning to Live with Diabetes

Edited by Sandra Augustyn Lawton. 410 pages. 2006. 978-0-7808-0811-9.

"A comprehensive instructional guide for teens... some of the material may also be directed towards parents or teachers. 5 stars (out of 5)!"

—Doody's Review Service, 2006

"Students dealing with their own diabetes or that of a friend or family member or those writing reports on the topic will find this a valuable resource."

—School Library Journal, Aug '06

"This text is directed to the teen population and would be an excellent library resource for a health class or for the teacher as a reference for class preparation. It can, however, serve a much wider audience. The clinical educator on diabetes may find it valuable to educate the newly diagnosed client regardless of age. It also would be an excellent reference and education tool for a preventive medicine seminar on diabetes."

—Physical Therapy, Mar '07

Diet Information for Teens, 2nd Edition

Health Tips about Diet and Nutrition

Including Facts about Dietary Guidelines, Food Groups, Nutrients, Healthy Meals, Snacks, Weight Control, Medical Concerns Related to Diet, and More

Edited by Karen Bellenir. 432 pages. 2006. 978-0-7808-0820-1.

"A very quick and pleasant read in spite of the fact that it is very detailed in the information it gives... A book for anyone concerned about diet and nutrition."

—American Reference Books Annual, 2007

SEE ALSO *Eating Disorders Information for Teens, 2nd Edition*

Drug Information for Teens, 2nd Edition

Health Tips about the Physical and Mental Effects of Substance Abuse

Including Information about Marijuana, Inhalants, Club Drugs, Stimulants, Hallucinogens, Opiates, Prescription and Over-the-Counter Drugs, Herbal Products, Tobacco, Alcohol, and More

Edited by Sandra Augustyn Lawton. 468 pages. 2006. 978-0-7808-0862-1.

"As with earlier installments in Omnigraphics' Teen Health Series, Drug Information for Teens is designed specifically to meet the needs and interests of middle and high school students... Strongly recommended for both academic and public libraries."

—*American Reference Books Annual, 2007*

"Solid thoughtful advice is given about how to handle peer pressure, drug-related health concerns, and treatment strategies."

—*School Library Journal, Dec '06*

SEE ALSO *Alcohol Information for Teens, 2nd Edition, Tobacco Information for Teens, 2nd Edition*

■

Eating Disorders Information for Teens, 2nd Edition

Health Tips about Anorexia, Bulimia, Binge Eating, And Other Eating Disorders

Including Information about Risk Factors, Diagnosis and Treatment, Prevention, Related Health Concerns, and Other Issues

Edited by Sandra Augustyn Lawton. 377 pages. 2009. 978-0-7808-1044-0.

"This handy reference offers basic information and addresses specific disorders, consequences, prevention, diagnosis and treatment, healthy eating, and more. It is written in a conversational style that is easy to understand... Will provide plenty of facts for reports as well as browsing potential for students with an interest in the topic.

—*School Library Journal, Jun '09*

"Written in a straightforward style that will appeal to its teenage audience. The author does not play down the danger of living with an eating disorder and urges those struggling with this problem to seek professional help. This work, as well as others in this series, will be a welcome addition to high school and undergraduate libraries."

—*American Reference Books Annual, 2009*

SEE ALSO *Diet Information for Teens, 2nd Edition*

■

Fitness Information for Teens, 2nd Edition

Health Tips about Exercise, Physical Well-Being, and Health Maintenance

Including Facts about Conditioning, Stretching, Strength Training, Body Shape and Body Image, Sports Nutrition, and Specific Activities for Athletes and Non-Athletes

Edited by Lisa Bakewell. 432 pages. 2009. 978-0-7808-1045-7.

"This no-nonsense guide packs a great deal into its pages... This is a helpful reference for basic diet and exercise information for health reports or personal use."

—*School Library Journal, April 2009*

"An excellent source for general information on why teens should be active, making time to exercise, the equipment people might need, various types of activities to try, how to maintain health and wellness, and how to avoid barriers to becoming healthier... This would still be an excellent addition to a public library ready-reference collection or a high school health library collection."

—*American Reference Books Annual, 2009*

"This easy to read, well-written, up-to-date overview of fitness for teenagers provides excellent wellness and exercise tips, information, and directions... It is a useful tool for them to obtain a base knowledge in fitness topics and different sports."

—*Doody's Review Service, 2009*

SEE ALSO *Diet Information for Teens, 2nd Edition, Sports Injuries Information for Teens, 2nd Edition*

■

Learning Disabilities Information for Teens

Health Tips about Academic Skills Disorders and Other Disabilities That Affect Learning

Including Information about Common Signs of Learning Disabilities, School Issues, Learning to Live with a Learning Disability, and Other Related Issues

Edited by Sandra Augustyn Lawton. 400 pages. 2006. 978-0-7808-0796-9.

"This book provides a wealth of information for any reader interested in the signs, causes, and consequences of learning disabilities, as well as related legal rights and educational interventions... Public and academic libraries should want this title for both students and general readers."

—*American Reference Books Annual, 2006*

Mental Health Information for Teens, 3rd Edition

Health Tips about Mental Wellness and Mental Illness

Including Facts about Mental and Emotional Health, Depression and Other Mood Disorders, Anxiety Disorders, Behavior Disorders, Self-Injury, Psychosis, Schizophrenia, and More

Edited by Karen Bellenir. 400 pages. 2010. 978-0-7808-1087-7.

SEE ALSO *Stress Information for Teens, Suicide Information for Teens, 2nd Edition*

Pregnancy Information for Teens

Health Tips about Teen Pregnancy and Teen Parenting

Including Facts about Prenatal Care, Pregnancy Complications, Labor and Delivery, Postpartum Care, Pregnancy-Related Lifestyle Concerns, and More

Edited by Sandra Augustyn Lawton. 434 pages. 2007. 978-0-7808-0984-0.

Sexual Health Information for Teens, 2nd Edition

Health Tips about Sexual Development, Reproduction, Contraception, and Sexually Transmitted Infections

Including Facts about Puberty, Sexuality, Birth Control, Chlamydia, Gonorrhea, Herpes, Human Papillomavirus, Syphilis, and More

Edited by Sandra Augustyn Lawton. 430 pages. 2008. 978-0-7808-1010-5.

"This offering represents the most up-to-date information available on an array of topics including abstinence-only sexual education and pregnancy-prevention methods... The range of coverage—from puberty and anatomy to sexually transmitted diseases—is thorough and extensive. Each chapter includes a bibliographic citation, and the three back sections containing additional resources, further reading, and the index are all first-rate... This volume will be well used by students in need of the facts, whether for educational or personal reasons."

—*School Library Journal, Nov '08*

"Presents information related to the emotional, physical, and biological development of both males and females that occurs during puberty. It also strives to address some of the issues and questions that may arise... The text is easy to read and understand for young readers, with satisfactory definitions within the text to explain new terms."

—*American Reference Books Annual, 2009*

Skin Health Information for Teens, 2nd Edition

Health Tips about Dermatological Concerns and Skin Cancer Risks

Including Facts about Acne, Warts, Hives, and Other Conditions and Lifestyle Choices, Such as Tanning, Tattooing, and Piercing, That Affect the Skin, Nails, Scalp, and Hair

Edited by Edited by Kim Wohlenhaus. 418 pages. 2009. 978-0-7808-1042-6.

"The material in this work will be easily understood by teenagers and young adults. The publisher has liberally used bulleted lists and sidebars to keep the reader's attention... A useful addition to school and public library collections."

—*ARBAOnline, Oct '09*

Sleep Information for Teens

Health Tips about Adolescent Sleep Requirements, Sleep Disorders, and the Effects of Sleep Deprivation

Including Facts about Why People Need Sleep, Sleep Patterns, Circadian Rhythms, Dreaming, Insomnia, Sleep Apnea, Narcolepsy, and More

Edited by Karen Bellenir. 355 pages. 2008. 978-0-7808-1009-9.

"Clear, concise, and very readable and would be a good source of sleep information for anyone—not just teenagers. This work is highly recommended for medical libraries, public school libraries, and public libraries."
—American Reference Books Annual, 2009

SEE ALSO *Body Information for Teens*

Sports Injuries Information for Teens, 2nd Edition

Health Tips about Acute, Traumatic, and Chronic Injuries in Adolescent Athletes

Including Facts about Sprains, Fractures, and Overuse Injuries, Treatment, Rehabilitation, Sport-Specific Safety Guidelines, Fitness Suggestions, and More

Edited by Karen Bellenir. 429 pages. 2008. 978-0-7808-1011-2.

"An engaging selection of informative articles about the prevention and treatment of sports injuries... The value of this book is that the articles have been vetted and are often augmented with inserts of useful facts, definitions of technical terms, and quick tips. Sensitive topics like injuries to genitalia are discussed openly and responsibly. This revised edition contains updated articles and defines sport more broadly than the first edition."
—School Library Journal, Nov '08

"This work will be useful in the young adult collections of public libraries as well as high school libraries... A useful resource for student research."
—American Reference Books Annual, 2009

SEE ALSO *Accident and Safety Information for Teens*

Stress Information for Teens

Health Tips about the Mental and Physical Consequences of Stress

Including Information about the Different Kinds of Stress, Symptoms of Stress, Frequent Causes of Stress, Stress Management Techniques, and More

Edited by Sandra Augustyn Lawton. 392 pages. 2008. 978-0-7808-1012-9.

"Understanding what stress is, what causes it, how the body and the mind are impacted by it, and what teens can do are the general categories addressed here... The chapters are brief but informative, and the list of community-help organizations is exhaustive. Report writers will find information quickly and easily, as will those who have personal concerns. The print is clear and the format is readable, making this an accessible resource for struggling readers and researchers."
—School Library Journal, Dec '08

"The articles selected will specifically appeal to young adults and are designed to answer their most common questions."
— American Reference Books Annual, 2009

SEE ALSO *Mental Health Information for Teens, 3rd Edition*

Suicide Information for Teens, 2nd Edition

Health Tips about Suicide Causes and Prevention

Including Facts about Depression, Risk Factors, Getting Help, Survivor Support, and More

Edited by Kim Wohlenhaus. 400 pages. 2010. 978-0-7808-1088-4.

SEE ALSO *Mental Health Information for Teens, 3rd Edition*

Tobacco Information for Teens, 2nd Edition

Health Tips about the Hazards of Using Cigarettes, Smokeless Tobacco, and Other Nicotine Products

Including Facts about Nicotine Addiction, Nicotine Delivery Systems, Secondhand Smoke, Health Consequences of Tobacco Use, Related Cancers, Smoking Cessation, and Tobacco Use Statistics

Edited by Karen Bellenir. 400 pages. 2010. 978-0-7808-1153-9.

SEE ALSO *Drug Information for Teens, 2nd Edition*